Expert praise for *The PDR® Family Guide Encyclopedia of Medical Care™*

"Should be a great asset to any family with concerns over various health problems."
—EDWARD E. WALLACH, M.D.
  J. Donald Woodruff Professor of Gynecology
  The Johns Hopkins University School of Medicine

"For everyone confused by medical jargon, this book provides simple, easy-to-understand explanations of specific illnesses, their symptoms, and their treatment. . . . Puts *you* in control of your health and medical care."
—MACE L. ROTHENBERG, M.D.
  Associate Professor
  The University of Texas Health Science
  Center at San Antonio

*Please turn the page
for more acclaim. . . .*

"Provides a solid foundation of basic information on commonly encountered conditions, from the benign to the life-threatening."
—MITCHELL R. LESTER, M.D.
Director, Pediatric Asthma Center
Children's Hospital
Boston, MA

"This indispensable family guide arms consumers with crucial information on hundreds of common medical problems and procedures. With its step-by-step instructions for follow-up care and its vital warnings about complications and emergencies, it is a ready reference that no household can afford to be without."
—GREGG J. BERDY, M.D.
Clinical Instructor in Ophthalmology
Washington University School of Medicine
St. Louis, MO

"This family medical book covers a wide array of subjects common to us all. In easily understood language, it gives straightforward recommendations and valuable information that health-care practitioners may forget—or not have time—to pass on to the patient."
—RICHARD G. FISCELLA, R. Ph., MPH
Clinical Associate Professor
College of Pharmacy
University of Illinois at Chicago

"A comprehensive, well-organized, and clearly written guide to hundreds of symptoms, diseases, medical procedures, and surgical operations. An ideal user-friendly reference to enhance your understanding of your medical condition and its proper care."
—PAUL MISKOVITZ, M.D.
Clinical Associate Professor of Medicine
Cornell University Medical College

Also published by Ballantine Books:

THE PDR® FAMILY GUIDE TO
  OVER-THE-COUNTER DRUGS ™

The PDR® Family Guide Encyclopedia of Medical Care™

BALLANTINE BOOKS • NEW YORK

A Ballantine Book
Published by The Ballantine Publishing Group
Copyright © 1997 by Medical Economics Company, Inc.

http://www.randomhouse.com/BB/

Library of Congress Catalog Card Number: 98-93464

ISBN 0-345-42009-8

This edition published by arrangement with Three Rivers Press, a division of Crown Publishers, Inc.

Manufactured in the United States of America

First Ballantine Books Edition: January 1999

10 9 8 7 6 5 4 3 2 1

Officers of Medical Economics Company: *President and Chief Executive Officer:* Curtis B. Allen; *Vice President, New Media:* L. Suzanne BeDell; *Vice President, Corporate Human Resources:* Pamela M. Bilash; *Vice President and Chief Information Officer:* Steven M. Bressler; *Senior Vice President, Finance, and Chief Financial Officer:* Thomas W. Ehardt; *Vice President, Directory Services:* Stephen B. Greenberg; *Vice President, New Business Planning:* Linda G. Hope; *Executive Vice President, Healthcare Publishing and Communications:* Thomas J. Kelly; *Executive Vice President, Magazine Publishing:* Lee A. Maniscalco; *Vice President, Group Publisher:* Terrence W. Meacock; *Vice President, Production:* David A. Pitler; *Vice President, Group Publisher:* Thomas C. Pizor; *Vice President, Magazine Business Management:* Eric Schlett; *Senior Vice President, Operations:* John R. Ware

Bulk copy inquiries are invited. Contact the Commercial Sales Department at 1-800-442-6657.

Contents

The PDR® Family Guide
Encyclopedia of Medical Care™

Contributors and Consultants

Editor-in-Chief: David W. Sifton
Director of Professional Services: Mukesh Mehta, R Ph
Art Director: Robert Hartman

Associate Editor: Jayne Jacobson
Assistant Editors: Ann Ben Larbi; Paula Benus; Gwynned L. Kelly
Editorial Production: Vice President of Production: David Pitler;
Contracts and Support Services Director: Marjorie A. Duffy; Director
of Production, Annuals: Carrie Williams; Manager of Production, Annuals: Kimberly Hiller-Vivas; Electronic Publishing Coordinator:
Joanne M. Pearson; Electronic Publishing Designer: Kevin J. Leckner

Medical Economics Company Directory Services

Vice President of Directory Services: Stephen B. Greenberg;
Director of Product Management: David P. Reiss; Senior Product
Manager: Mark A. Friedman; Associate Product Manager: Bill
Shaughnessy: National Sales Manager, Trade Group: Bill Gaffney;
Promotion Manager: Donna R. Lynn

Publisher's Note

Foreword

There are plenty of first-aid books that will help you handle an emergency *before* you get to a doctor; but *after* you've been treated, you're pretty much on your own. This is the first book designed specifically to fill that gap.

Why would you need a medical book after the doctor has already made a diagnosis? Think about it. If you're like most people, half of the most important questions about your condition don't occur to you until hours—or even days—after your doctor visit. Worse yet, you may feel a nagging suspicion that you've already been given the answers, and therefore be reluctant to call the doctor again. (You could well be right, too. Doctors tend to cover a lot of information in a very short time; and under the stress and pressure of a medical exam, you're more than likely to miss much of what you're being told.)

For whatever reason, people frequently leave the doctor's office with more questions than when they arrived. That's where this new and different kind of medical encyclopedia fits in. It focuses on all the questions that pop up once you really start giving some thought to your condition. It summarizes the care that's needed after your initial treatment, tells what additional tests and treatments may be required, and gives you a forecast for recovery. If you're going to need a stay in the hospital, it gives you a preview of the equipment and procedures you're likely to encounter, tells what special preparations are usually required before you go, and leaves you with a reminder of the measures you need to take once you're back home.

Most importantly, it spells out—for each individual condition—the symptoms that should send you back to the doctor as soon as possible, plus the signs of trouble that signal a major emergency. This crucial information alone is something every household should have.

Medicine has a language all its own—a shorthand that can make even the simplest statement impossible to understand. In this book, we've attempted to eliminate or clarify all medical terminology. Only the key medical terms that you're likely to hear most frequently have been left unchanged; and whenever one of these terms does appear, you'll find it accompanied by a clear "translation." The goal has been to provide you with information that you can use immediately, without guesswork and without a dictionary.

For your additional convenience, we've also included detailed instructions for some of the most commonly encountered home-care problems, such as cast care, crutches, and bathing your baby. And to help you avoid needless injury and illness, there are also tips on important safety measures, including the best ways to make your home poison-proof, prevent burns, and use car safety seats correctly.

This book won't answer all of your questions— no book can—and it certainly is no substitute for a talk with your doctor. But in between visits, when a worrisome new symptom appears or you've forgotten some detail about the right care, we think you'll be glad you have the book handy. This is one home reference that you'll find indispensable whenever illness or injury strikes.

How to Use This Book

For just about everyone, even a minor medical problem immediately raises a host of troubling questions: What's gone wrong? How serious is it? What treatment is needed? How long will it take to recover? What can be done in the meantime? Under ideal circumstances, a visit to your doctor should provide you with the answers to all these questions and more. But in the real world, it rarely works out that way. The doctor is probably overloaded with patients and you're under stress. When the doctor explains the condition, you miss half of what's said. You forget the questions you most wanted to ask. Then, before you know it, the visit is over, the doctor is out the door, and you're on your way home.

It's for such moments that this book was created. If you can't remember how often to clean a wound, here's a book that will tell you. If you develop a new symptom, you'll now have a way to find out whether it's harmless or serious—and whether you should do nothing or call the doctor immediately. And if you're scheduled for a hospital procedure, here's where you'll find a reassuring preview of what to expect and how to prepare.

To make your search as easy as possible, the book includes brief profiles of over 350 of the most common medical problems and procedures, arranged alphabetically by their everyday names and cross-referenced by their formal medical titles. The profiles cover everything from wart removal to stroke. They summarize selected key facts under a series of standard headings designed to help you quickly locate the precise information you need.

Most profiles have two major sections, "What You Should Know" and "What You Should Do." When the problem is likely to require a stay in the hospital, a third section, "If You're Heading for the Hospital" also appears. Here's a closer look at what you'll typically find in each section.

What You Should Know

Each profile begins with a brief overview of the problem, including, if appropriate, information on whom the disease is most likely to strike, the way it's spread, and how long it will take to clear up. The profile then turns to several of people's greatest concerns.

Causes

Under this heading, you'll find a quick summary of the usual reasons for the problem, plus a list of other diseases and conditions that could also prove to be the culprit.

Signs/Symptoms

A medical ailment rarely causes only one symptom. Each illness typically provokes a characteristic set of problems that may or may not all show up in the same patient. Under this heading, you'll first find a list of the symptoms that are most likely to appear, followed by other symptoms that could develop, but don't occur in every case. Because totally different diseases sometimes produce the same set of symptoms, this list won't provide you with a definite diagnosis. For that, there's no substitute for a medical exam and testing. However, the list can give you a fairly reliable idea of what you may be facing.

Care

Under this heading, you'll get a brief summary of the treatment that's usually required. You'll find out whether the problem can be treated at home, whether the doctor will need to give tests, what kinds of drugs might be prescribed, and whether you might need a stay in the hospital.

This information is designed to give you a general idea of what to expect. It does not include every available treatment option or describe special measures that vary from case to case. Every patient is unique; and so is every treatment plan. So, although your doctor's recommendations may be similar to what you see here, you'll often find that they're a little different because they've been tailored to fit your specific needs.

What You Should Do

In this section you'll find a series of tips for home care during the recovery period. These are the measures that doctors and nurses generally recommend for an illness of your type. You'll find them useful if your doctor hasn't gone into enough detail or you've forgotten what was said. If your doctor's instructions are different from those you find here, don't be alarmed. There are innumerable reasons why an individual care plan will be different from the norm. If you have serious doubts, however, don't hesitate to check with your doctor. You may have misunderstood—or there may actually have been a mistake!

Also found in this section are tips for preventing the problem from recurring. And at the end of the section, you'll find two important sets of guidelines for dealing with a change in your condition:

Call Your Doctor If . . .

If you develop any of the symptoms listed under this heading, it's a signal to contact your doctor. Chances are that you will need additional treatment or care. The problems shown here are not dangerous...but they can't be ignored, either.

Seek Care Immediately If . . .

The symptoms listed here are emergencies that should send you to the ER or Urgent Care Center **as soon as possible**. They are **not** problems that can wait for a doctor's appointment. If you experience such symptoms, don't hesitate to call 911 or the operator for help.

If You're Heading for the Hospital . . .

This section gives you a preview of what you'll encounter if your condition requires a stay in the hospital. Any hospitalization—even for a minor operation—is bound to be an upsetting experience filled with odd equipment and strange demands. The information presented here will help to prepare you for what lies ahead. The more you know in advance, the more comfortable you'll be when you actually arrive.

Before You Go

If any special preparations are needed prior to departure for the hospital, you'll find them briefly summarized here.

What to Expect While You're There

Under this heading you'll find an overview of some of the routine measures you'll face, as well as brief thumbnail descriptions of the procedures, equipment, and medications typically employed for your particular problem. The list is not all-inclusive, and some of the tests and procedures that are described here may not be necessary in your case. Still, what you undergo may seem a little more familiar after you've reviewed this list. You may also find that the information makes a useful checklist for discussion with your doctor.

After You Leave

Shown here are the guidelines you'll probably have to follow once you've returned home. These are the restrictions and measures that doctors typically recommend after the type of treatment you're likely to undergo. Your doctor will probably have additional tips and warnings, particularly if you've received special treatment. However, you can regard the recommendations shown here as a basic foundation for your recovery.

Signs and Symptoms Index

This handy index can help you pinpoint some of the most likely reasons for an unexplained set of symptoms. Arranged alphabetically by symptom, it lists all the ailments in the book that are known to cause each problem, along with the page number of the related disease profile.

Although this index may give you some clues about the nature of your illness, it won't give you a firm diagnosis. When you check the index, you'll quickly find that an isolated symptom such as "headache" can be the result of any number of totally unrelated conditions. To narrow down the possibilities, you'll therefore need to look up each of your symptoms and see which ailments have all of them in common. And when you're finished, you'll probably find that several totally different illnesses could still be the cause.

This is one of the things that make medicine so difficult. It's also the reason that this index can be used only as a general guide. To be certain of almost any diagnosis, you need the testing and judgment that only a doctor can provide.

The Doctor-Patient Partnership

In the end, no book can ever be a substitute for a visit to the doctor. Only a doctor can weigh all the diverse aspects of your condition and choose the treatment most likely to meet your needs. What we hope this book can do, however, is serve as a reminder of your doctor's advice and a springboard for further discussion. Your doctor, after all, can respond only to the problems and concerns you mention. And a seemingly unimportant question could turn out to be a crucial aspect of your particular case.

This book is offered as an aid in this cooperative effort with your doctor. We hope it suggests the right questions to ask, while allaying any needless fears you might have. Most of all, we hope it helps in some small way to make all of your treatments as effective as possible—and your recovery speedy and complete.

Encyclopedia of Medical Care

Abdominal Pain in Adults

WHAT YOU SHOULD KNOW

Pain felt in the abdomen can come from inside or outside the belly. The pain may be a sign of a serious problem or be the result of something as harmless as gas. Doctors often cannot find the source.

Causes

Abdominal pain can be caused by a blockage or swelling of your appendix, chemicals and swelling that irritate nerves and body tissues, stretching of nerve fibers, infection with bacteria, or an irritation from stomach acids.

Signs/Symptoms

The pain may take the form of cramps that come and go or it may be constant. It may feel like stabbing, aching, or burning in your abdomen. Pain may also spread to your back or chest. Sometimes the pain may be accompanied by nausea, vomiting, diarrhea, or fever.

Care

Depends on the cause. Your doctor will need to ask a number of questions and examine your abdomen. X-rays and tests on your blood, urine, and stool may be necessary. You may have to stay in the hospital, and you may even need surgery.

WHAT YOU SHOULD DO

• If the doctor is not sure of what's causing the pain, you may need to return later or make an appointment with another doctor for more tests.
• If the doctor prescribes antibiotics, continue to take them until they are all gone—even if you feel well. Always take medicines exactly as directed.
• Take your temperature every 4 hours.
• As long as you still have pain, do not eat any solid foods or drink large amounts of liquids. If you get thirsty, you may take small sips of fluids or suck on ice.

Seek Care Immediately If . . .

• Your pain gets worse or becomes focused in one area.
• You throw up blood or find blood in your stool.
• You feel dizzy or faint.
• Your abdomen becomes swollen.

- You have a high temperature.
- You have trouble urinating.
- You have trouble breathing.

Abdominal Pain in Children

WHAT YOU SHOULD KNOW

Abdominal pain can occur anywhere between the bottom of your child's ribcage and his or her groin. Often there is no apparent cause, but the pain could signal a serious problem.

Causes
The pain may merely be the result of overeating, gas, or constipation. On the other hand, it could be a sign of food poisoning, a stomach infection, or appendicitis.

Signs/Symptoms
The pain can be "sharp as a knife" or dull. It can stay in the same place or move around. The pain can be constant or it can go away and then come back. It may be accompanied by nausea, vomiting, fever, diarrhea, and fainting.

WHAT YOU SHOULD DO

- Watch the child closely. If the pain is worse after 1 hour, call the doctor.
- Have the child rest in bed until he or she feels better.
- Take the child's temperature every 4 hours.
- Do not give any medication without first asking your doctor.
- Give clear fluids if the child can take them. Avoid giving solid food for 24 hours.

Call Your Doctor If . . .
- The pain has lasted more than 1 hour.
- Your child has a high temperature.

Seek Care Immediately If . . .
- The pain increases or is only in one specific area.
- The child begins to vomit blood or you find blood in the stool.
- The child is walking bent-over or holding the abdomen, or refuses to walk.
- The pain is in the testicle or scrotum.
- The abdomen becomes swollen or tender to the touch.

• The child has difficulty passing urine.
• The child is short of breath.

Abnormal Uterine Bleeding

See Dysfunctional Uterine Bleeding

Abortion, Spontaneous

See Miscarriage

Abortion, Threatened

See Threatened Miscarriage

Abrasions

See Scrapes

Abrasions, Corneal

See Corneal Abrasion

Abscess

WHAT YOU SHOULD KNOW

An abscess (AB-ses) is an infected pocket of pus. You can develop an abscess anywhere on your body. Common sites include the armpit, rectum, vaginal lips, face, and area around the tonsils in the throat. Nursing mothers sometimes develop an abscess on the breast.

Causes
A bacterial infection.

Signs/Symptoms
You're likely to experience pain, soreness, redness, swelling, or fever. The abscess may feel like a soft, moveable lump under your skin.

Care
The usual treatment is to cut open the abscess and allow the pus to drain. You will need to take an antibiotic to treat the infection.

Risks
Following treatment, the area around the abscess could become infected. You also might have more bleeding than normal.

IF YOU'RE HEADING FOR THE DOCTOR . . .

What to Expect While You're There
You may encounter the following procedures and equipment while you're there.

• **Taking Your Vital Signs:** These include your temperature, blood pressure, pulse (counting your heartbeats), and respirations (counting your breaths). A stethoscope is used to listen to your heart and lungs. Your blood pressure is taken by wrapping a cuff around your arm.

• **Incision and Drainage of Abscess:**
  —You may be asked to lie on a table, depending on where the abscess is located. You will be given numbing medicine to prevent pain, and, perhaps, medication to relax you during the procedure.
  —After cleaning the area, the doctor will cut a small hole in or around the abscess to let the pus drain out.
  —Sometimes it is necessary to cut the abscess open and to remove unhealthy skin. To keep the pus and other liquid draining out of the abscess, the doctor may insert a gauze wick or a tube. The drain may be left in for 1 or more days.
  —To determine the type of bacteria causing the infection, the doctor may send a sample of the pus to a laboratory.
  —It is important for the abscess to heal from the inside out. If the skin covering the abscess heals first, a pocket may be left under the skin, inviting development of another infection. Carefully follow your doctor's treatment plan.

• **Medicine:**
  —**Antibiotics** may be given by IV, in a shot, or by mouth to fight infection.
  —**Fever medicine** such as acetaminophen or ibuprofen may be given by mouth or in your rectum to lower your temperature.
  —**Pain medicine** may be given as a shot or by mouth. If the pain does not subside or comes back, call your doctor.

After You Leave
• If you are drowsy from your medicine, do not drive.
• Apply heat to help relieve the pain. Use warm, wet compresses or a warm heating pad 3 or 4 times a day for 20 minutes.
• When you bathe, cover the dressing with plastic. After the drain is removed, you may wash the wound gently with mild unscented soap.

Call Your Doctor If . . .
• You develop increased swelling, redness, drainage, or bleeding.
• You have severe pain in the area of the abscess that lasts for 24 hours.

Seek Care Immediately If . . .
• You have a high temperature.
• You have signs of infection such as muscle aches, dizziness, or a generally ill feeling.

Abscess, Dental

See Dental Abscess

Abscess, Perirectal

See Perirectal Abscess

Abscess, Peritonsillar

See Peritonsillar Abscess

Achilles Tendon Rupture

WHAT YOU SHOULD KNOW

The Achilles tendon is the cord that attaches the heel to the calf muscles. It runs up the back side of the ankle, and can be torn (ruptured) by a sudden strain. If the tear is small, it will usually take about 8 to 12 weeks to heal.

Causes

The ruptures usually occur during athletics or in an accident. Running, jumping, and tripping can all cause a tear.

Signs/Symptoms

You can expect pain, tenderness, swelling, or bruising behind the ankle. You may find it difficult to move your foot, and it's usually painful to walk.

Care

Your doctor will probably order an x-ray. If you have a small tear, treatment may consist of a cast or splint followed by exercise therapy to bring the tendon back up to strength. If the injury is large, surgery may be needed to fix the tear, again followed by exercise therapy.

You'll need to use crutches for a while. If you tore some skin when you were injured, you may need a tetanus shot.

WHAT YOU SHOULD DO

- Use your crutches as long as directed. Do not stop using them on your own.
- To reduce the swelling, keep the injured foot on pillows while lying down and on a stool when sitting.
- Apply ice to the injury for 15 to 20 minutes each hour for the first 1 to 2 days. Put the ice in a plastic bag and place a towel between the bag of ice and your skin.
- If you are given a plaster or fiberglass cast:
  —Do not try to scratch the skin under the cast by pushing a sharp or pointed object down the cast.
  —Check the skin around the cast every day. You may put lotion on any red or sore areas.
  —If your fiberglass cast gets a little wet, it can be dried off with a hair dryer.
- If you are given a plaster splint:
  —Wear the splint until your doctor says you may take it off or until your follow-up examination.
  —You may loosen the elastic around the splint if your toes become numb or begin tingling.
- If you put pressure on any part of the cast or splint, it may break.
- Keep the cast or splint dry. Cover it with a plastic bag when you bathe. Do not lower it into water.
- If the doctor prescribes pain medicine that makes you drowsy, don't drive. You also may take over-the-counter medicines for pain. Take all medications exactly as directed.
- If you are given a tetanus shot, your arm may get swollen, red, and warm to the touch at the site of the shot. This is a normal reaction to the medicine.

Call Your Doctor If . . .
- Your cast or splint gets damaged or breaks.
- You have severe pain that won't go away.
- You have more swelling than you did before treatment.
- The skin or toenails of the injured foot turn blue or gray, or become cold or numb.
- There is a bad smell coming from your cast or splint.
- There are new stains coming from under the cast or splint.

Acromioclavicular Separation

See Separated Shoulder

Activated Charcoal

WHAT YOU SHOULD KNOW

Activated charcoal, available in black powder or liquid form, keeps your body from absorbing certain drugs or poisons swallowed by accident. The drugs or poisons stick to the charcoal and pass out of your body with it during regular bowel movements. Stools and anything thrown up will be black until all the charcoal has cleared the body.

WHAT YOU SHOULD DO

• To prevent constipation, your first dose of charcoal may be mixed with a laxative.
• You may also be able to avoid constipation by drinking plenty of liquids.

Call Your Doctor If . . .
• You have stomach pain that lasts several days.
• You have not had a bowel movement in several days.
• Your vomiting does not stop for several days.
• You have a fever and stomach pain accompanied by constipation.
• You notice blood in your stools.

Seek Care Immediately If . . .
• You have trouble breathing or have severe stomach pain.
• You feel as if you are going to pass out.
• You develop a high temperature.

Acute Bronchitis

WHAT YOU SHOULD KNOW

Acute Bronchitis (bron-KITE-is) is swelling and irritation of the windpipe (trachea) or the airways to the lungs. It occurs most often in the winter and usually starts as a cold. The cold then spreads from the nose and throat to the windpipe and airways.

Causes
This disease is usually caused by germs (virus or bacteria) spread through the air or by contact with someone who is infected. Other causes are allergies or breathing air that contains chemical fumes,

dust, or smoke. Your chances of getting bronchitis increase if you have lung disease, smoke, go out in cold, humid weather, do not eat healthy foods, or have become run down from another illness.

Signs/Symptoms

The most common symptom is a dry cough. Later in the illness the cough may bring up sputum. Other complaints may include a low fever (less than 101 degrees F—38.3 degrees C), burning chest pain or pressure behind the breastbone, noisy breathing (wheezing), and trouble breathing.

Care

Most people can be treated at home. Care may include cough medicine to control the cough (suppressants) and cough expectorants to thin the sputum. Antibiotics may also be needed to fight an infection caused by bacteria. You may need to be put into the hospital if you get pneumonia or chronic bronchitis, or if you fail to get better.

Risks

If you don't follow your doctor's directions, your illness can get worse or turn into pneumonia. Remember, acute bronchitis can be cured with medicine.

WHAT YOU SHOULD DO

- Always take your medicine as directed. If you feel it is not helping, call your doctor. Do not quit taking it on your own.
- If you are taking antibiotics, continue to take them until they are all gone even if you feel well.
- If you are taking medicine that makes you drowsy, do not drive or use heavy equipment.
- If you use medicine that you inhale, follow the steps below:
  —First, shake the inhaler.
  —Breathe out slowly, all the way.
  —Put the mouthpiece of the inhaler in your mouth or 2 inches away (about half a finger's length), or use the spacer (a piece of plastic-like tubing that attaches to the inhaler).
  —Breathe in and push down on the inhaler at the same time (to create the mist).
  —Hold your breath for about 10 seconds.
  —Breathe out slowly through puckered lips or through your nose.
  —If you need to take 2 puffs, wait 2 to 5 seconds before taking the second one.

—Gargling after using your inhaler may reduce burning in your throat.

• Quit smoking. It increases your chances of getting lung diseases such as bronchitis, and harms the heart and lungs. If you are having trouble quitting, ask your doctor for help.

• If you are coughing up sputum and milk seems to make your sputum thicker, avoid dairy foods.

• If you do not have to limit the amount of liquids you drink, drink 8 to 10 (soda-can size) glasses of water each day. This helps thin the sputum so it can be coughed up more easily.

• To help keep your lungs free of infection, take 2 or 3 deep breaths and then cough. Do this often during the day.

• Use a humidifier to help keep the air moist and your sputum thin. This makes it easier to cough up the sputum. You must keep the humidifier free of fungus. Clean it every day.

• Stay inside during very cold or hot weather, or on days when the air pollution is high. This will help you breathe easier and help control your cough.

• Rest until you feel better. You may return to work or school when your temperature is around 98.6 degrees F (37 degrees C).

Call Your Doctor If . . .

• Your cough does not go away in a few days.

• You have a rash, itching, swelling, or stomach pain or any other problems that might be caused by your medicine.

• You cough up gray, green, or bloody sputum.

Seek Care Immediately If . . .

• You have chills, increasing chest pain, trouble breathing while resting, or vomiting.

• Your lips or nailbeds turn blue or pale.

• You are coughing and cannot stop, or your constant coughing makes you feel light-headed.

IF YOU'RE HEADING FOR THE HOSPITAL . . .

What to Expect While You're There

You may encounter the following procedures and equipment during your stay.

• **Activity:** At first you will need to rest in bed, with a few pillows to keep you sitting up a little. This will help your breathing. Do not lie flat. Once you are breathing more easily, you will be allowed to increase your exercise.

• **Oxygen:** You may need extra oxygen at this time. It is given either by a mask or nasal prongs. Tell your doctor if the oxygen is drying out your nose or if the nasal prongs bother you.

- **Pulse Oximeter:** While you are getting oxygen, you may be hooked up to a pulse oximeter (ox-IM-uh-ter). It is placed on your ear, finger, or toe and is connected to a machine. It measures the oxygen in your blood.
- **IV:** A tube placed in your vein for giving medicine or liquids. It will be capped or have tubing connected to it.
- **Medicines:** The drugs below will help you breathe easier. They can be taken by mouth or given in your IV.
  - **—Antibiotics:** If you have an infection in the lungs, you'll be given antibiotics to clear it up.
  - **—Bronchodilators** (bronk-o-DIE-lay-tors)**:** The medicines may be needed to help open your lung's airways.
  - **—Steroids** (STAIR-oids)**:** You may be given one of these drugs to decrease the swelling and inflammation of the tissue in your lungs.
- **Breathing Treatments:** A machine will be used to help you inhale medicine. A therapist will help with these treatments. They will help open your airways so you can breathe easier. At first you may need them frequently. As you get better, you may only need them when you are having trouble breathing.
- **Postural Drainage:** A nurse may tap your back briskly with his or her hands. This helps loosen the sputum in your lungs so you can cough it up more easily.
- **Taking Vital Signs:** These include your temperature, blood pressure, pulse (counting your heartbeats), and respirations (counting your breaths). A stethoscope is used to listen to your heart and lungs. Your blood pressure is taken by wrapping a cuff around your arm.
- **ECG:** Also called a heart monitor, an electrocardiograph (e-lec-tro-CAR-dee-o-graf), or EKG. The patches on your chest are hooked up to a TV-type screen or a small portable box (telemetry unit). This screen shows a tracing of each heartbeat. Your heart will be watched for signs of injury or damage.
- **12 Lead ECG:** This test makes tracings from different parts of your heart. It can help your doctor decide whether there is a heart abnormality.
- **Chest X-ray:** This picture of your lungs and heart will be used to monitor your condition.
- **Blood Gases:** Blood taken from an artery in your wrist, elbow, or groin is tested for oxygen.
- **Blood:** Usually taken for testing from a vein in your hand or from the bend in your elbow.

After You Leave
Follow the directions listed under "What You Should Do."

Acute Kidney Failure

See Kidney Failure, Acute

Alcohol Abuse

WHAT YOU SHOULD KNOW

Many people can stop drinking after one or two beers or glasses of wine, vodka, whiskey, or other alcoholic beverages. Some people, however, can't stop, and are at great risk of alcoholism.

Alcoholism affects both your body and your life. Excessive drinking over a long period can lead to dependency—so great a need for alcohol that you will become physically ill if you abruptly stop drinking. Constant drunkenness can lead to loss of job and family, serious accidents, and arrest. Large amounts of alcohol consumed year after year also result in severe damage to the liver, brain, and heart. Without treatment, an alcoholic faces increasing illness and a needlessly early death.

Causes
The cause of alcoholism is unknown. It may be present from birth. If women drink while they are pregnant, their infants can be born with fetal alcohol syndrome, a serious condition that affects the development of their brains and may cause serious illness.

Signs/Symptoms
Tip-offs of an alcohol problem include the need to drink more and more to get the same feeling or "buzz," drinking daily until you get drunk, drinking in the morning and whenever you feel stress, and hiding the amount you drink. Alcoholics often react with guilt and anger when other people say something about their drinking. Drinking starts to control their lives; they may skip work or drive drunk. Another typical symptom: insomnia and bad dreams.

As the problem gets worse, alcoholics begin to have blackouts, forgetting where they were and what they were doing. Other possible symptoms include liver, stomach, pancreas, and heart problems. Deprived of a drink, they may develop the condition called delirium tremens (DTs). Typical symptoms include shaking hands; sweating; nervousness, confusion, or depression; hallucinations, and seizures.

Care

Your doctor may give you a checkup to see if you have any other illnesses or injuries. Therapy may include a drug that makes you sick when you drink. You also may need treatment for withdrawal symptoms; and your doctor will probably ask you to see a counselor or join a support group.

WHAT YOU SHOULD DO

• If you have been abusing alcohol, the first step to quitting is to admit you have a problem. Be honest and open with family and close friends. Ask for their help.

• Stay away from people who use and abuse alcohol and who encourage others to drink.

• The Alcoholics Anonymous (AA) program can provide you with essential support. Take advantage of it.

• Get the help of a counselor and keep seeing him or her.

• Don't give up. It can take many months or years of treatment for some people to stop drinking.

• Eat a healthy diet, drink 6 to 8 glasses of water a day, and get plenty of rest.

• Find new things to do. Get out of the house every day. Go for walks outside.

Call Your Doctor If . . .

• You cannot fight the need to drink alcohol. Call your doctor, a counselor, friend, or family member you trust RIGHT AWAY.

• You feel your problems are getting the best of you and you can't deal with them on your own.

• You get an upset stomach and start vomiting.

Seek Care Immediately If . . .

• You have severe chest pain, sweating, or trouble breathing.

• You get a severe pain in your head or stomach or develop pain, a numb or prickly feeling, or burning in your arms or legs.

• You have hallucinations, pass out, or have a seizure.

Allergic Rhinitis

See Hay Fever

Allergic Shock

See Anaphylaxis

Allergy, Drug

See Drug Allergy

Allergy, Food

See Food Allergy

Anal Fissure

WHAT YOU SHOULD KNOW

An anal fissure is a tear in the lining of the anus. The problem can happen to anyone, at any age, including infancy. Most fissures heal within 4 to 6 weeks on their own.

Causes

The fissures are usually caused by very large or hard bowel movements.

Signs/Symptoms

The chief symptoms are pain and bleeding during bowel movements. The pain may last for hours afterward, then go away until the next bowel movement. Because of this pain, children may try to "hold it in," rather than go to the bathroom. You may see bloody streaks on toilet paper, underwear, or diapers. There may be itching around the anus.

Care

There are a number of steps you take at home to help the fissure heal. You may need surgery if it fails to heal.

Risks

Without treatment, you could end up with permanent scarring that may cause pain and bleeding whenever you move your bowels.

WHAT YOU SHOULD DO

- Various over-the-counter medications can help. Take only as directed by your doctor.
  - 0.50 percent hydrocortisone cream to help relieve irritation. Apply to the anal area.
  - A numbing ointment to help relieve pain. Apply to the anal area.
  - Oral pain-killers such as acetaminophen for additional relief.
  - A stool softener to prevent constipation until the fissure heals,
- Soaking in a warm bath can also lessen the pain.

- To hasten healing and avoid a recurrence:
  —Try to keep your stool soft by eating high-fiber foods (fruits, vegetables, bran, whole-wheat grains).
  —Drink 6 to 8 glasses (soda-can sized) of water to keep the stool from drying out.
  —Do not strain too hard during bowel movements.
  —Avoid anal sex.

Call Your Doctor If . . .

- Bleeding from the rectal area increases in amount or occurs more than 3 times, or blood is mixed throughout the stool.
- A high temperature develops.
- The fissure becomes more painful or shows no improvement after 3 days of treatment.

IF YOU'RE HEADING FOR THE HOSPITAL . . .

What to Expect While You're There

You may encounter the following procedures and equipment during your stay.

- **Taking Vital Signs:** These include your temperature, blood pressure, pulse (counting your heartbeats), and respirations (counting your breaths). A stethoscope is used to listen to your heart and lungs. Your blood pressure is taken by wrapping a cuff around your arm.
- **Blood:** Usually taken from a vein in your hand or from the bend in your elbow. Tests will be done on the blood.
- **IV:** A tube placed in your vein for giving medicine or liquids. It will be capped or have tubing connected to it.
- **Pulse Oximeter:** While you are getting oxygen, you may be hooked up to a pulse oximeter (ox-IM-uh-ter). It is placed on your ear, finger, or toe and is connected to a machine that measures the oxygen in your blood.
- **ECG:** Also called a heart monitor, an electrocardiograph (e-lec-tro-CAR-dee-o-graf), or EKG. The patches on your chest are hooked up to a TV-type screen or a small portable box (telemetry unit). This screen shows a tracing of each heartbeat. Your heart will be watched for signs of injury or damage that could be related to your illness.
- **Foley Catheter** (CATH-uh-ter): This tube will drain urine from your bladder if you are unable to urinate. The catheter will be taken out when you can get to the bathroom and urinate on your own.
- **Activity:** You may need to rest in bed. Once you are feeling better, you will be allowed to get up.

• **Medicines**
  —**Antibiotics** may be prescribed to fight infection. They can be given through an IV, in a shot, or by mouth.
  —**Pain medicine** may also be given in your IV, as a shot, or by mouth. If the pain does not go away or comes back, tell a doctor right away.

Anal Itching

WHAT YOU SHOULD KNOW

Although itching around the anus can be a problem in itself, it is often a sign of some other disease or condition.

Causes
Although the reason cannot always be pinned down, anal itching is often caused by stool, moisture, soaps, or clothing that irritates the skin. It also can result from a tear in the skin, swollen anal veins (in adults), or parasites such as pinworms. Anal itching makes the skin red and swollen.

Signs/Symptoms
Itching around the anus may become worse at night. Skin in the area may be red and swollen.

Care
Depends on the cause of the itching. If it is not a symptom of some other problem, the basic goal is to keep the area clean and dry.

WHAT YOU SHOULD DO

• Don't rub or scratch the area. This makes the itching worse.
• After every bowel movement and at bedtime, gently clean the anal area. Use a moistened tissue, cotton ball, or soft wash cloth. You also may use premoistened anal cleansing pads or tissues made for cleaning up babies. Don't use soap. Gently pat the area dry.
• Put a thin strip of cotton directly on the anus. This helps absorb moisture and stool. The cotton should be thin enough so that you can't feel it. Don't use a cotton ball or sanitary pad. You may dust the cotton with corn starch or baby powder. Change the cotton several times a day.
• Wear underwear made of cotton or with a cotton crotch. Don't wear tight-fitting clothes and underwear.
• Some foods and beverages may make the problem worse. Examples are beer, tea, coffee, milk, cola, tomatoes, citrus fruits, nuts, chocolate, and spicy foods. Avoid any that seem to increase the itching.

• Don't use products that may irritate the anal skin. These include perfumed or colored toilet paper, deodorant sprays, and perfumed soaps.
• Don't use any medicine, cream, or lotion on the anal area without checking with your doctor. Many products used to treat the itching can sometimes make it worse.

Call Your Doctor If . . .
• The itching is not better in a few days or if it gets worse.
• You have a high temperature.
• The skin around the anus becomes red, swollen, or tender. This may be a sign of infection.
• Other members of your family also start itching.

Anaphylaxis

WHAT YOU SHOULD KNOW

Anaphylaxis (AN-uh-fuh-LAX-is), also called allergic shock, is a severe reaction to stings and bites, medicines, foods, and other substances to which you are allergic. It usually comes on suddenly. **Anaphylaxis can kill you. It is an emergency.**

Causes
Anaphylaxis may be caused by foods such as nuts, shell fish, fruits, eggs, fruit, or milk; medicines, such as penicillin, aspirin, or dyes used to take x-rays; and stings or bites from bees, wasps, hornets, some spiders, or biting ants. Even exercise can sometimes trigger this reaction.

Signs/Symptoms
Typically, you'll begin to have trouble breathing, suffer chest pain, or feel swelling or tingling around your mouth. Other signs include itchy or red skin, a throbbing heartbeat, sweating, faintness, or a blackout. Your tongue may swell and cause you to choke. A few people also develop stomach cramps, nausea, vomiting, or diarrhea.

These signs may appear seconds or minutes after the offending substance has gotten into your body. The attack may last from a few seconds to a few hours.

Care
Call 911 or 0 (operator) for help. Anaphylaxis is an **emergency.** You will need CPR if your heart or breathing stops; and emergency care givers will need to give you epinephrine (EP-ih-NEF-rin) by in-

jection or intravenously to slow down the movement of the allergen through your blood stream and to help you breathe more easily.

If you have been stung by an insect, scrape the stinger out with a knife or your fingernail. Don't squeeze the stinger. It may still have some venom in it and squeezing can spread the venom into your skin.

After emergency treatment, you may need to stay in the hospital for 12 to 24 hours. If you are sent home from the emergency room, you should have someone stay with you for at least 24 hours. Symptoms of anaphylaxis can sometimes return within a few hours of the attack.

Risks
If not treated immediately, anaphylaxis may end in shock, heart failure, and death.

IF YOU'RE HEADING FOR THE HOSPITAL . . .

What to Expect While You're There
You may encounter the following procedures and equipment during your stay:
- **Taking Vital Signs:** These include your temperature, blood pressure, pulse (counting your heartbeats), and respirations (counting your breaths). A stethoscope is used to listen to your heart and lungs. Your blood pressure is taken by wrapping a cuff around your arm.
- **Pulse Oximeter:** A pulse oximeter (ox-IM-uh-ter) may be placed on your ear, finger, or toe and connected to a machine that measures the oxygen in your blood.
- **Oxygen:** You may need extra oxygen at this time. It is given either by a mask or nasal prongs. Tell your doctor if the oxygen is drying out your nose or if the nasal prongs bother you.
- **Ventilator:** A special machine used to help with breathing.
- **IV:** A tube placed in your vein for giving medicine or liquids. It will be capped or have tubing connected to it.
- **Blood:** Usually taken from a vein in your hand or from the bend in your elbow and sent to a laboratory for testing.
- **Breathing Treatments:** A special machine will be used to help you inhale medicine. A doctor will help with these treatments. You will need the medicine to help open your airways and restore your breathing. At first you may need the treatments frequently. As you get better, you may only need them when you are having trouble breathing.
- **ECG:** Also called a heart monitor, an electrocardiograph (e-LEC-tro-CAR-dee-o-graf), or EKG. The patches on your chest are hooked up to a TV-type screen or a small portable box (telemetry

unit) that shows a tracing of each heartbeat. Your heart will be monitored until danger from the reaction has passed.
- **Medications**
  - **Heart Medicines** may be needed to restore normal heartbeat and function.
  - **Steroids** may be given to decrease the swelling and redness (inflammation) of the tissue.
  - **Anti-Nausea Medicine** may be needed to control vomiting and prevent loss of too much body fluid.
  - **Bronchodilators** may be needed to help open your lung's airways.

After You Leave
- If the cause of the attack isn't apparent, you'll need to undergo tests to identify the triggering substance (or insect) and avoid it in the future.
- You may be given a kit for emergency treatment of anaphylaxis. The kit contains epinephrine that you can inject yourself if you have another serious reaction. Ask your doctor to show you how to use the kit, and teach your friends or family how to use it in case they have to give you the shot. Keep your kit with you at all times.
- You should wear a medic-alert bracelet or necklace indicating that you have had anaphylaxis. Emergency care givers will be able to treat you quickly in case you cannot talk during an attack.
- Be sure to tell all medical personnel that you have a serious allergy. Stay in your doctor's office for at least 15 minutes after getting an injection containing medicine you have never had before. Always know the names of the medicines you are taking.
- Read labels on food and medicine carefully to see if they contain the substance to which you are sensitive. Be very careful about what you eat. Allergens such as nuts or fruit may be hidden in prepared food like meat dishes or cookies.
- Always wait at least 2 hours after eating before starting to exercise.
- If you are allergic to bee or wasp stings, avoid gardening, tree-trimming, or lawn-mowing. Do not wear perfume, hair spray, or brightly colored clothes when you are outside; bees and wasps like sweet smells and bright colors. Also, always wear shoes.

Call Your Doctor If . . .
- You think you have a food or drug allergy. Your signs may show up in seconds or minutes after eating a food or taking a medicine. Even mild symptoms can rapidly develop into a life-threatening reaction.

• An allergic rash, hives, or itching does not go away in a few days, or you develop new symptoms.
• The area around an insect sting gets red, warm, sore, and swollen. These are signs of infection.

Seek Care Immediately If . . .
• You begin to have any of the symptoms of an anaphylactic reaction.

Angina

WHAT YOU SHOULD KNOW

Angina pectoris is chest pain that occurs when your heart does not get enough oxygen. The pain is usually caused by a spasm or blockage of the arteries in the heart.

There are different kinds of angina, including stable and unstable angina. If they are not treated, you could have a heart attack.

• **Stable Angina**
This is the most common form. The chest pain may feel crushing, tight, or heavy. It may spread to the neck, jaw, shoulders, back, or left arm. The pain may also feel like indigestion (burning), occurring under the breastbone.

The pain commonly starts below the breastbone and on the left side of the body. It may spread down into your arm or up into your jaw or shoulder blade. It often starts slowly, lasting only a few minutes. It may be caused by cold or hot air or cold wind. Chest pain may also occur after you get upset.

• **Unstable Angina**
This is pain that comes back often or hurts more every time it returns. It may start while you are resting or exercising, and may continue even after resting.

Care
If you have "stable angina," you can be treated with medicine that opens up the arteries to the heart and lowers the amount of oxygen it needs. Your medicines should help lessen your pain and how often you have it.

If you still have pain after taking your medicine, call your doctor. It is important that your treatment helps you lead a normal life.

If you have "unstable angina," you will be put in the hospital. During your stay, your heartbeat will be monitored and you will be given pain medicine.

You also may need a stress test (to watch your heart during exercise) or a cardiac catheterization (a look at the arteries in your heart).

Depending on the results of the tests, your doctor may recommend an angioplasty (opening up a blocked artery in your heart) or surgery on your heart if the arteries are severely blocked.

Risks

Without treatment, your angina may get worse, and you could have a heart attack.

WHAT YOU SHOULD DO

- Always take your medicine as directed. If you feel it is not helping, call your doctor. Do not quit taking it.
- You may be directed to take aspirin regularly. Aspirin helps thin the blood so blood clots don't form. Do not take acetaminophen or ibuprofen instead.
- Your doctor also may prescribe nitroglycerin (ny-tro-GLIS-er-in). It may give you a headache or make you feel a little dizzy. Take it while sitting or lying down.
- A diet low in fat, salt, and cholesterol is very important. It keeps your heart healthy and strong. Ask your doctor what you should and should not eat.
- It may take time getting used to a new diet. Special cookbooks may help you and the cook in your family find new recipes.
- Quit smoking. It harms the heart and lungs. If you are having trouble quitting, call your doctor to talk about other ways to quit.
- Exercise daily. It helps make the heart stronger, lowers blood pressure, and keeps you healthy. If your exercise plan is too hard or easy, talk to your doctor.
- Weighing too much can make the heart work harder. Talk to your doctor about a plan to lose weight.
- Since it is hard to avoid stress, learn to control it. Ways to relax are: deep breathing, relaxing the muscles, imagery (dreaming), and talking to someone about things that upset you.
- If you have other illnesses like diabetes or high blood pressure, you need to control them. Take medicines as directed. Because of these illnesses, you have a higher chance of getting a heart attack.
- For more information about the heart, call the **American Heart Association at 1-800-AHA-USA1 (1-800-242-8721)** or call your local **Red Cross**.

Call Your Doctor If . . .

- You have any questions or concerns about your illness or medicine.
- Your chest pain:
  —Is more painful each time you have it or occurs more often.

—Lasts longer than 10 to 15 minutes even after you rest.
—Does not go away after taking your nitroglycerin or other medicine as directed.
—Wakes you from your sleep.
—Occurs during exercise and doesn't go away with rest.
• Your medicine is making you light-headed or dizzy, sweaty, or nauseated.

Seek Care Immediately If . . .
• You have chest pain that spreads to your arms, jaw, or back, and you are sweating, sick to your stomach (nauseated), and have trouble breathing. These are signs of a heart attack. **THIS IS AN EMERGENCY. Call 911 or 0 (operator)** to get to the nearest hospital or clinic. **Do not drive yourself!**
• You have any of the problems listed under "Call If" and you live in an area that does not have an ambulance or is far away from a hospital.
• You feel dizzy or you faint.

IF YOU'RE HEADING FOR THE HOSPITAL . . .

What to Expect While You're There
You may encounter the following procedures and equipment during your stay.
• **Taking Vital Signs:** These include your temperature, blood pressure, pulse (counting your heartbeats), and respirations (counting your breaths). A stethoscope is used to listen to your heart and lungs. Your blood pressure is taken by wrapping a cuff around your arm.
• **Pulse Oximeter:** While you are getting oxygen, you may be hooked up to a pulse oximeter (ox-IM-uh-ter). It is placed on your ear, finger, or toe and is connected to a machine. It measures the oxygen in your blood.
• **ECG:** Also called a heart monitor, an electrocardiograph (e-LEK-tro-CAR-dee-o-graf), or EKG. The patches on your chest are hooked up to a TV-type screen or a small portable box (telemetry unit). The TV-type screen shows a tracing of each heartbeat. Your heart will be watched for signs of injury or damage.
• **12 Lead ECG:** This test makes tracings from different parts of your heart. It can help your doctor gauge the seriousness of the problem.
• **Oxygen:** Your body may need extra oxygen at this time. It is given either by a mask or nasal prongs. Tell your care giver if the oxygen is drying out your nose or if the nasal prongs bother you.
• **IV:** A tube placed in your vein for giving medicine or liquids. It will be capped or have tubing connected to it.

- **Blood:** Usually taken from a vein in your hand or from the bend in your elbow. Tests will be done on the blood.
- **Blood Gases:** Blood is taken from an artery in your wrist, elbow, or groin. It is tested for the amount of oxygen in your blood.
- **Chest X-ray:** This is a picture of your lungs and heart. The care givers use it to see how your heart and lungs are handling the illness.
- **Medicine:**
  —**Nitroglycerin:** Lessens the amount of oxygen your heart needs. Also opens the arteries to your heart so it gets more oxygen. As a result, the pain usually lessens or goes away. But, the "nitro" may also give you a headache or make you dizzy.
  It may be taken by placing it under your tongue or attaching a medicine-filled patch to your chest, arm, or back.
  —**Heart Medicines:** May also be given depending on what is causing your angina.
- **Other Tests:** May be needed to find out what is causing your chest pain.
  —**Stress Test:** Used to watch your heart during exercise.
  —**ECHO:** Also called an echocardiogram (ek-oh-CAR-dee-o-gram). This uses sound waves to view your heart while it is beating. It can help care givers decide what is causing your heart failure.
  —**Cardiac Catheterization** (cath-uh-ter-i-ZAY-shun): A test used to study the arteries sending blood to your heart.
- **Angioplasty:** May be needed to open up a blocked artery to your heart.
- **Surgery:** May be needed if the arteries to your heart are severely blocked.

Animal Bite

WHAT YOU SHOULD KNOW

After an animal bite, the greatest fear is infection with rabies. However, other infections, including tetanus (lockjaw), also are possible. It's important to have your doctor check the bite.

Signs/Symptoms

You are likely to have bleeding, pain, swelling, redness, and bruising at the site of the bite.

Care

Your doctor may need to have the animal checked for disease. To prevent tetanus, you may need a shot. The doctor also may prescribe antibiotics for other infections.

WHAT YOU SHOULD DO

- Keep the area around the bite clean. Wash it with soap and water 3 or 4 times a day.
- To decrease pain and swelling, you can put ice on the bite during the first 1 or 2 days. Sit or lie so the area of the bite is raised above your heart (You can put pillows under an injured leg when lying in bed).
- You may take over-the-counter medications such as acetaminophen or ibuprofen to relieve the pain.
- If you have been given a tetanus shot, your arm may get swollen, red, and warm to the touch at the shot site. This is a normal response to the medicine in the shot.

Call Your Doctor If . . .

- There is numbness or tingling in the area of the bite.
- There are signs of infection (redness, red streaking or pus coming from the wound, or warmth or swelling in the area of the bite).
- You develop a high temperature.
- You have pain or difficulty moving the injured part.
- You get tender lumps in the groin or under the arm.

Seek Care Immediately If . . .

- You are having trouble talking, walking, or breathing.
- You are having trouble swallowing and your jaw and neck are stiff.

Ankle Arthroscopy

WHAT YOU SHOULD KNOW

Arthroscopy (arth-ROS-co-PEE) is an examination of the inside of a joint, such as an ankle, using a surgical tool called an arthroscope (ARTH-row-scope) that is inserted into the joint through a small incision. An arthroscope is a small, soft tube with a light and lenses on the tip. Your doctor will perform this procedure if there's a possibility that your ankle joint is injured or diseased, or if you need to have bone or cartilage removed or tendons or ligaments repaired. After the arthroscopy, you may have some pain and swelling for a few days.

Risks

There is a chance that the procedure will cause bleeding, infection, or injury to another part of your ankle. A problem in a leg vein could cause a blood clot to form.

IF YOU'RE HEADING FOR THE HOSPITAL . . .

Before You Go

- You will need to stop eating and drinking in preparation for this procedure. The doctor will tell you exactly when to begin fasting.

What to Expect While You're There

You may encounter the following procedures and equipment during your stay:

- **Taking Your Vital Signs:** These include your temperature, blood pressure, pulse (counting your heartbeats), and respirations (counting your breaths). A stethoscope is used to listen to your heart and lungs. Your blood pressure is taken by wrapping a cuff around your arm.
- **IV:** A tube placed in your vein for giving medicine or liquids. It will be capped or have tubing connected to it.
- **During Your Arthroscopy . . .**
  —You will be taken to the operating room. The hair around your ankle will be shaved and the area will be scrubbed with soap and water.
  —You will need to lie still and move as little as possible during the procedure. Your doctor will give you numbing medicine, so you will feel little pain. You may be put to sleep with anesthetic medication.
  —An elastic bandage will be wrapped tightly around your leg and foot to help drain blood from your leg. A rubber cuff may be put around your leg to slow the flow of blood into your ankle. Doctors sometimes pump liquid into the ankle joint to further decrease blood flow to the ankle.
  —Your doctor will then make a small hole in the skin at your ankle and put the arthroscope through it. In some cases the arthroscope may have to be inserted into a second area of your ankle. During this part of the procedure, you may feel pressure or a thumping sensation.
  —Your doctor may repair or remove some of the tissue in your ankle joint.
  —When the arthroscope is taken out, your doctor will close the hole with sutures (a type of thread) and put a bandage on the wound.

—Your arthroscopy will take about 30 to 45 minutes. You may be given medicine to help relieve your pain.

After You Leave

• When you leave the hospital, you may still be drowsy from the medicine. Do not drive during this period.

• Stay off your feet as much as possible for 24 to 48 hours. Keep your leg raised on 2 pillows whenever possible for the next 2 days.

• For the first 24 hours, apply an ice pack to the area to reduce pain and swelling. Put ice in a plastic bag and place a towel between the bag of ice and your skin or the bandage. Keep the ice pack on your ankle for up to 2 hours at a time.

• You'll need to walk with crutches for one week; put as much weight on your ankle as comfort permits.

• Keep your dressing dry and clean. After 4 days, remove the wrap and dressing.

• After your bandage is off, you may bathe or shower as usual. Wash the incision gently with soap and water.

• To prevent development of blood clots, move your legs often while resting in bed.

• You may begin drinking or eating as soon as you are up to it.

• Resume work and normal activity as soon as possible.

• Avoid vigorous exercise such as jogging or bicycling for 6 weeks after the procedure.

Call Your Doctor If . . .

• Swelling, drainage, or bleeding gets worse in the area of the incision.

• You develop signs of infection such as a headache, muscle aches, dizziness, or a generally ill feeling.

• You suffer really bad pain that is not helped by medicine.

• You develop a high temperature.

Ankle Fracture

See Broken Ankle

Ankle Sprain

See Sprained Ankle

Anxiety Attack

See Panic Attack

Apgar Score

WHAT YOU SHOULD KNOW

An Apgar (AP-gar) score is a quick reading of your baby's condition at birth. At 1 and 5 minutes after birth, the baby is checked for skin color, heart rate, movement, breathing, and reflexes. Each is rated from 0 to 2. The Apgar score is the total of the ratings.

The score at 5 minutes gives a better picture of how well your baby did during labor and delivery. Babies born before the due date or at a high altitude may have a lower score. The Apgar cannot predict how well your child will grow and develop.

Aphthous Ulcers

See Canker Sores

Appendicitis

WHAT YOU SHOULD KNOW

Appendicitis (uh-pen-dih-SIGH-tis) is an inflammation of the appendix that affects about 1 in 500 people each year. It is most common in young adults 15 to 25 years old.

Causes
If the appendix is blocked, an infection occurs. An infected appendix becomes swollen, reddened, and filled with pus.

Signs/Symptoms
Abdominal pain (usually in the right lower side of the belly), fever, nausea, and vomiting.

Care
It may be hard for the doctor to decide whether you have appendicitis. You will probably need some blood tests, plus an examination called abdominal ultrasound. You may have surgery to remove your appendix right away, or the operation may occur later. If your signs and symptoms get worse, you will need to see your doctor immediately.

Risks
You can die from untreated appendicitis. But the risks of serious illness or death are small if you follow your doctor's advice.

WHAT YOU SHOULD DO

Call Your Doctor If . . .
• You have a high temperature.
• Your stomach pain gets worse or you are vomiting.
• You faint, are dizzy, or have a headache.
• You have blood in your stool or in your vomit.

Seek Care Immediately If . . .
• You feel dizzy or confused, are urinating less, or have a dry mouth
  and tongue. These are signs of dehydration.

IF YOU'RE HEADING FOR THE HOSPITAL . . .

What to Expect While You're There
You may encounter the following procedures and equipment during
your stay.
• **Abdominal Ultrasound:** This painless test is done while you are
  lying down. A dab of a jelly-like lotion is placed on your stomach.
  The person doing the test will gently move a small handle through
  the lotion and across the skin. A TV-like screen is attached to the
  handle.
• **Medicines:**
  —**Antibiotic medicine** may be given to fight infection.
  —**Pain medicine** will also be prescribed. If the pain does not go
    away or comes back, tell a doctor right away.
  —These medicines may be given in your IV, as a shot, or by mouth.
• **Taking Vital Signs:** These include your temperature, blood pres-
  sure, pulse (counting your heartbeats), and respirations (counting your breaths). A stethoscope is used to listen to your heart and
  lungs. Your blood pressure is taken by wrapping a cuff around
  your arm.
• **Pulse Oximeter:** You may be hooked up to a pulse oximeter (ox-
  IM-uh-ter). It is placed on your ear, finger, or toe and is connected to
  a machine that measures the oxygen in your blood.
• **Activity:** You will be asked to stay in bed before surgery except to
  go to the bathroom. After surgery, you will be encouraged to get out
  of bed with help. As you feel better, you can walk more.
• **IV:** A tube placed in your vein for giving medicine or liquids. It will
  be capped or have tubing connected to it.
• **Blood:** Usually taken from a vein in your hand or from the bend in
  your elbow. Tests will be done on the blood.
• **Chest X-ray:** As a precaution, a picture of your lungs and heart will
  be taken before surgery.

- **After Surgery:**
  —You will be returned to your hospital room when you awake. Ask for medicine if you are having pain. You may want to have someone stay with you to give comfort and support.
  —You will go home as soon as you are able to eat, drink, and care for yourself.

After You Leave
- Always take your medicine as directed by your doctor. If you feel it is not helping, call your doctor. Do not quit taking it on your own.
- If you are taking antibiotics, continue to take them until they are all gone—even if you feel well.
- You will need to take your temperature frequently.
- Do not take a laxative (medicine to help you move your bowels) or an enema.
- Do not take pain or fever medicine, such as aspirin, acetaminophen, or ibuprofen.
- Follow your doctor's advice about resting, eating, or drinking liquids.

Arm Fracture

See Broken Arm

Arthritis

See Osteoarthritis

Arthroscopy of the Ankle

See Ankle Arthroscopy

Arthroscopy of the Knee

See Knee Arthroscopy

Asthma

WHAT YOU SHOULD KNOW

Asthma causes the airways of the lungs to swell and become narrower. This can make it hard to breathe and cause wheezing as you breathe in and out. Asthma cannot be cured, but it can be relieved with medicine. Repeat attacks are common.

Causes
Triggers may include pollen, dust, animals, molds, some foods, lung infections, smoke, exercise, high amounts of air pollution, or stress.

Signs/Symptoms
Common symptoms include trouble breathing, a tight feeling in the chest, and wheezing.

During a bad asthma attack, you may sweat and have real diffi-culty breathing. Your lips and nailbeds may turn a pale or blue color, your heart may beat faster and you may become very anxious. If this happens, call **911 or 0 (operator)** to get help immediately.

Care
Most of the time you can care for yourself at home. But if medicine fails to improve your breathing, you must be treated in the emergency department or in the hospital. While there, you may need oxygen, medicine, and breathing treatments.

Risks
Asthma is rarely fatal if you take your medicine and follow your doctor's orders.

WHAT YOU SHOULD DO

• If you use a medicine that you inhale, here are some tips:
  —First, shake the inhaler.
  —Breathe out slowly, all the way.
  —Put the mouthpiece of the inhaler in your mouth or 2 inches away (about half a finger's length), or use the spacer (a piece of plastic-like tubing that attaches to the inhaler).
  —Breathe in and push down on the inhaler at the same time (to create the mist).
  —Hold your breath for about 10 seconds.
  —Breathe out slowly through puckered lips or through your nose.
  —If you need to take 2 puffs, wait 2 to 5 seconds before taking the second one.
  —Gargling after using your inhaler may reduce the amount of burning in your throat.
• When you have an attack:
  —Use your inhaler. If this does not help, repeat the inhaler one more time after waiting the number of minutes recommended by your doctor. If the second try doesn't work, check to see whether the inhaler is empty. It's empty if it floats in a bowl of water.

—It may help your breathing if you straddle a chair backwards, placing your elbows up on the back of the chair.
- If you do not know what causes your attacks:
  —Keep writing down the time of your attack. Also notice what is around you when it occurs.
  —Consider allergy testing if you have not had it done already.
- Always take your medicine as directed by your doctor. If you feel it is not helping, call your doctor. Do not quit taking it on your own.
- Try to avoid pollen, dust, animals, molds, smoke, and anything else that could cause an attack.
- Keep the amount of dust in your home at a minimum. One way is to hire a company to clean out the air ducts and vents in your house.
- Replace your pillows or mattress with materials that don't cause allergies. Look for bedding that is made of "urethane" or foam rubber and is labeled "nonallergenic."
- If you do not have to limit the amount of liquids you drink, drink 8 to 10 (soda-can size) glasses of water each day. This helps thin the sputum so it can be coughed up more easily.
- If animals are the cause of your asthma, you may need to find another home for your pets.
- Quit smoking. It harms the lungs. If you are having trouble quitting, ask your doctor for help.
- Exercise daily. It helps make the heart stronger, lowers blood pressure, and keeps you healthy. If your exercise plan seems too hard or easy, check with your doctor.
- Excess weight can make the heart and lungs work harder. If you need to lose weight, ask your doctor for the plan that's best for you.

Call Your Doctor If . . .
- You have wheezing and trouble breathing even when taking your medicine regularly.
- You develop a high temperature.
- You have muscle aches or chest pain.
- Your sputum turns yellow, green, gray, or bloody, or becomes too thick to cough up.
- You have any problems that may be caused by your medicine (such as a rash, itching, swelling, or trouble breathing).
- Wheezing, trouble breathing, or coughing gets worse, even though you are taking your medicine.
- You have followed directions above and still cannot breathe, **Call 911 or 0 (operator)** to get to the nearest hospital or clinic. **Do not drive yourself!**

What to Expect While You're There

You may encounter the following procedures and equipment during your stay.

- **Taking Vital Signs:** These include your temperature, blood pressure, pulse (counting your heartbeats), and respirations (counting your breaths). A stethoscope is used to listen to your heart and lungs. Your blood pressure is taken by wrapping a cuff around your arm.

- **Oxygen:** Your body may need extra oxygen at this time. It is given either by a mask or nasal prongs. Tell your doctor if the oxygen is drying out your nose or if the nasal prongs bother you.

- **Pulse Oximeter:** While you are getting oxygen, you may be hooked up to a pulse oximeter (ox-IM-uh-ter). It is placed on your ear, finger, or toe and is connected to a machine that measures the oxygen in your blood.

- **Breathing Treatments:** A machine will be used to help you inhale medicine. A therapist will help with these treatments. They will help open your airways so you can breathe easier. At first you may need them frequently. As you get better, you may only need them when you are having trouble breathing.

- **IV:** A tube placed in your vein for giving medicine or liquids. It will be capped or have tubing connected to it.

- **Blood:** Usually taken from a vein in your hand or from the bend in your elbow. Tests will be done on the blood.

- **Blood Gases:** Blood is taken from an artery in your wrist, elbow, or groin. It is tested for the amount of oxygen it contains.

- **ECG:** Also called a heart monitor, an electrocardiograph (e-LEK-tro-CAR-dee-o-graf), or EKG. The patches on your chest are hooked up to a TV-type screen or a small portable box (telemetry unit). This screen shows a tracing of each heartbeat. Your heart will be watched for signs of injury or damage that could be related to your illness.

- **12 Lead ECG:** This test makes tracings from different parts of your heart. It can help your doctor decide whether there is a heart problem.

- **Chest X-ray:** This picture of your lungs and heart shows how they are handling the illness.

- **Medicine:** Many different kinds of medicines may be needed.
  - **Inhalants:** These medicines are breathed in to help open your airways.
  - **Antibiotics:** If an infection is causing breathing problems, you'll be given antibiotics to clear it up.

—**Breathing Medicine:** This medicine may be given in your IV first, and then in pill form. Like an inhalant, it will open your airways.

• **Activity:** It is best to stay in bed until you are breathing easier. Then you can slowly increase your exercise.

Atherosclerosis, Coronary

See Coronary Artery Disease

Athlete's Foot

WHAT YOU SHOULD KNOW

Athlete's foot is also known as tinea (TIN-ee-uh) pedis (PEED-us) ringworm. This skin infection usually disappears after 3 weeks of treatment, but often returns repeatedly.

Causes
The infection is caused by a fungus, and may be spread to others by sharing towels or shower stalls.

Signs/Symptoms
Typically, you'll notice an itchy, gray-white or red rash on the bottom of the feet and between the toes. You may find dead skin between the toes.

Care
Athlete's foot medications will kill the infection. To prevent additional attacks, keep your feet clean and dry.

WHAT YOU SHOULD DO

• Apply medicine exactly as directed.
• Keep your feet clean, cool, and dry. Wash them daily and dry well, especially between your toes.
• Change your shoes and socks every day. Use cotton or wool socks. It is helpful to go barefoot or wear sandals during treatment; wearing canvas tennis shoes also can help.
• Soaking your feet in Burow's solution (available in drug and grocery stores) for 20 to 30 minutes 2 times a day will dry out the blisters.
• To keep the infection from returning, continue to wear cotton or wool socks and dry your feet well after washing.

Call Your Doctor If . . .
• You develop a high temperature.
• You think the infection is spreading.
• The athlete's foot is not better in 7 days or completely cured in 30 days.

Atopic Dermatitis

See Eczema

Atrial Fibrillation

WHAT YOU SHOULD KNOW

The heart has 4 chambers in it. The upper chambers are called atria (A-tree-uh) and the lower chambers are called ventricles (VEN-trick-uls). When the heart "beats," the atria push blood into the ventricles and the ventricles push blood out of the heart.

During atrial fibrillation, the atria quiver uselessly instead of maintaining their normal beat. (The ventricles still beat, but not as regularly.) Because the atria are no longer pushing all their blood into the ventricles, the ventricles may not fill up properly. If this happens, the rest of the body may not get enough of the oxygen-rich blood it needs.

Causes
Atrial fibrillation can be a result of valve disease, hardening of the arteries, thyroid disease, or heart failure. Another cause is swelling and irritation of the outside of the heart. If the cause is treated, your heart rate may return to normal. However, there is a chance that no cause will be found.

Signs/Symptoms
Many people have no symptoms at all, but some may feel weak, dizzy, or faint. Others may feel pain or fluttering in the chest, trouble breathing, or nausea.

Care
Treatment may begin in the office, emergency department, or hospital. If your heart rate is around 100 beats per minute, you may be treated in your doctor's office. But if your heart rate is faster or causing other problems, you will be admitted to the hospital.

Hospital Care

Your heart rate will be watched on a TV-type screen and you will be given oxygen, an IV (a small tube placed in your vein), and medicine to slow down your heart rate. If the medicine fails to slow your heart rate enough, you may need to have cardioversion (car-dee-o-VER-shun)—an electrical shock to your heart. Your doctor will also try to find out the cause of the problem.

Risks

When the atria fail to beat normally, blood can pool in them, causing clots to form. These clots could make their way to your brain and cause a stroke—a serious risk of atrial fibrillation. They could also cause a heart attack or lodge in a lung, and the danger of heart failure increases as well. The sooner you are treated the better your chance of avoiding these problems.

WHAT YOU SHOULD DO

- Ask your doctor how to count your pulse, and make sure it is strong and regular.
- If you take aspirin regularly, continue to take it. Aspirin helps thin the blood so blood clots won't form. Do not take acetaminophen or ibuprofen instead.
- A diet low in fat, salt, and cholesterol is very important. It keeps your heart healthy and strong. Ask your doctor for guidelines on what to eat. It may take time getting used to a new diet. Special cookbooks may help you and the cook in your family find new recipes.
- Quit smoking. It harms the heart and lungs. If you are having trouble stopping, ask your doctor for help.
- Exercise daily. It helps make the heart stronger, lowers blood pressure, and keeps you healthy. If your exercise plan seems too hard or too easy, talk to your doctor.
- Do not have sex if you are tired, or if you have just eaten a big meal. Avoid sex if you have been drinking, if you are angry with your mate, or if the room temperature is too cold or too hot. If you get chest pain during sex, stop.
- Weighing too much can make the heart work harder. If you need to lose weight, ask your doctor for a weight-reduction plan.
- Since it is hard to avoid stress, learn to control it. Learn new ways to relax (deep breathing, relaxing muscles, meditation, or biofeedback). Don't hesitate to talk to someone about things that upset you.
- If you have other illnesses like diabetes or high blood pressure, you

need to control them. Take medicines as directed. Because of these illnesses, you have a higher chance of getting a heart attack.
• For more information about the heart, call the **American Heart Association at 1-800-AHA-USA1 (1-800-242-8721)** or call your local **Red Cross**.

Call Your Doctor If . . .
• You have chest pain during exercise that doesn't go away with rest.
• You are dizzy or nauseated after taking your medicine, or you have other problems that you think may be caused by your medicine.
• You have trouble breathing while resting, you have swelling in your feet or ankles, or you are more tired than usual.
• You are bleeding from your gums or nose, or have blood in your urine or stools. This may be due to your medications.

Seek Care Immediately If . . .
• Your heart rate increases or becomes irregular and you faint or feel like fainting.
• Your pulse is much higher or lower than usual.
• You feel dizzy, have numbness or weakness of your face or limbs, or have trouble seeing or speaking.
• You have chest pain that spreads to your arms, jaw, or back, accompanied by sweating, nausea, and difficulty breathing. These are signs of a heart attack. **THIS IS AN EMERGENCY. Call 911 or 0 (operator)** to get to the nearest hospital or clinic. **Do not drive yourself!**

IF YOU'RE HEADING FOR THE HOSPITAL . . .

What to Expect While You're There
You may encounter the following procedures and equipment during your stay.
• **Taking Vital Signs:** These include your temperature, blood pressure, pulse (counting your heartbeats), and respirations (counting your breaths). A stethoscope is used to listen to your heart and lungs. Your blood pressure is taken by wrapping a cuff around your arm.
• **Oxygen:** Your body may need extra oxygen at this time. It is given either by a mask or nasal prongs. Tell your doctor if the oxygen is drying out your nose or if the nasal prongs bother you.
• **Pulse Oximeter:** While you are getting oxygen, you may be hooked up to a pulse oximeter (ox-IM-uh-ter). It is placed on your ear, finger, or toe and is connected to a machine that measures the oxygen in your blood.

- **Blood:** Usually taken from a vein in your hand or from the bend in your elbow. Tests will be done on the blood.
- **IV:** A tube placed in your vein for giving medicine or liquids. It will be capped or have tubing connected to it.
- **ECG:** Also called a heart monitor, an electrocardiograph (e-lec-tro-CAR-dee-o-graf), or EKG. Patches placed on your chest are hooked up to a TV-type screen or a small portable box (telemetry unit). This screen shows a tracing of each heartbeat. Your heart will be watched carefully until your heartbeat returns to normal.
- **12 Lead ECG:** This test makes tracings from different parts of your heart. It can help your doctor gauge the seriousness of the problem.
- **Chest X-ray:** This picture of your lungs and heart shows how they are handling the illness.
- **Medicines:**
  - **—Heart Medicine:** Drugs to slow your heart rate will be given in your IV. If you get dizzy, feel pain, or have other side effects after getting this medicine, call your doctor right away.
  - **—Heparin:** This drug keeps the blood thin so no clots can form. It is given in your IV. Later, the doctor my prescribe other blood thinners that may be taken by mouth.
- **Cardioversion** (car-dee-o-VER-shun): This procedure uses an electric shock to the heart to return it to a normal rate. It may be needed if medicine fails to slow your heart rate. Before cardioversion, you will be given medicine to make you sleepy. Then the shock is administered. If it works, your heart rate and rhythm will return to normal. However, you may still need medicine to keep your heart rate under control.

Atrial Flutter

WHAT YOU SHOULD KNOW

The heart has 4 chambers in it. The upper chambers are called atria (A-tree-uh) and the lower chambers are called ventricles (VEN-trick-uls). When the heart "beats," the atria push blood into the ventricles and the ventricles push blood out of the heart.

Usually, the atria and ventricles work at the same time. But in people with the condition called atrial flutter, the atria "beat" more often than the ventricles. This means that the atria have a shorter time to push all of their blood into the ventricles; and because of this, the ventricles may not fill up with enough blood. The body, then, may not get enough oxygen-rich blood.

This may or may not be a problem, depending on how fast the

atria are beating. The faster they beat the more problems your body will have getting enough oxygen.

Causes

Atrial flutter can be the result of valve disease, hardening of the arteries, thyroid disease, or heart failure. Another cause is swelling and irritation of the outside of the heart. If the cause is treated, your heart rate may return to normal. There is a chance that no cause will be found.

Signs/Symptoms

Many people have no symptoms at all, but others may feel weak, dizzy, or faint. Some people may feel pain or fluttering in the chest, have trouble breathing, or develop nausea.

Care

If your heart is beating too fast, treatment may begin in the office, emergency department, or hospital. Your heart rate will be watched on a TV-type screen and you will be given oxygen, an IV (a small tube placed in your vein), and medicine to slow down your heart rate.

If the medicine doesn't work well enough, you may need to have cardioversion (car-dee-o-VER-shun). This is an electrical shock to your heart. Your doctor will also try to find out the cause of your atrial flutter.

Risks

If a fast atrial flutter goes untreated, your body will not get the oxygen it needs to work well. As a result, you could end up with worse heart or lung problems (such as a heart attack or fluid in the lungs). The sooner you have treatment, the better chance you have of avoiding problems.

WHAT YOU SHOULD DO

- Ask your doctor how to count your pulse, and make sure it is strong and regular.
- If you take aspirin regularly, continue to take it. Aspirin helps thin the blood so blood clots don't form. Do not take acetaminophen or ibuprofen instead.
- A diet low in fat, salt, and cholesterol is very important. It keeps your heart healthy and strong. Ask your doctor for guidelines on what to eat. It may take time getting used to a new diet. Special cookbooks may help you and the cook in your family find new recipes.

- Quit smoking. It harms the heart and lungs. If you are having trouble stopping, call your doctor to talk about other ways to quit.
- Exercise daily. It helps make the heart stronger, lowers blood pressure, and keeps you healthy. If your exercise plan seems too hard or too easy, talk to your doctor.
- Do not have sex if you are tired or if you have just eaten a big meal. Avoid sex if you have been drinking, if you are angry with your mate, or if the room temperature is too cold or too hot. If you get chest pain during sex, stop.
- Weighing too much can make the heart work harder. If you need to lose weight, ask your doctor for a diet plan.
- Since it is hard to avoid stress, learn to control it. Learn new ways to relax (deep breathing, relaxing muscles, meditation, or biofeedback). Don't hesitate to talk to someone about things that upset you.
- If you have other illnesses, such as diabetes or high blood pressure, you need to control them. Take medicines as directed. Because of these illnesses, you have a higher chance of getting a heart attack.
- For more information about the heart, call the **American Heart Association at 1-800-AHA-USA1 (1-800-242-8721)** or call your local **Red Cross**.

Call Your Doctor If . . .
- You have chest pain during exercise that doesn't go away with rest.
- You are dizzy or nauseated after taking medicine, or you have other problems that you think may be caused by the medicine.
- You have trouble breathing while resting, you have swelling in your feet or ankles, or you are more tired than usual.

Seek Care Immediately If . . .
- Your heart rate increases or becomes irregular and you faint or feel like fainting.
- After counting for 1 minute, your pulse is higher or lower than usual.
- You have chest pain that spreads to your arms, jaw, or back, accompanied by sweating, nausea, and difficulty breathing. These are signs of a heart attack. **THIS IS AN EMERGENCY. Call 911 or 0 (operator)** to get to the nearest hospital or clinic. **Do not drive yourself!**

IF YOU'RE HEADING FOR THE HOSPITAL . . .

What to Expect While You're There
You may encounter the following procedures and equipment during your stay.

- **Taking Vital Signs:** These include your temperature, blood pressure, pulse (counting your heartbeats), and respirations (counting your breaths). A stethoscope is used to listen to your heart and lungs. Your blood pressure is taken by wrapping a cuff around your arm.
- **Oxygen:** Your body may need extra oxygen at this time. It is given either by a mask or nasal prongs. Tell your doctor if the oxygen is drying out your nose or if the nasal prongs bother you.
- **Pulse Oximeter:** While you are getting oxygen, you may be hooked up to a pulse oximeter (ox-IM-uh-ter). It is placed on your ear, finger, or toe and is connected to a machine that measures the oxygen in your blood.
- **Blood:** Usually taken from a vein in your hand or from the bend in your elbow. Tests will be done on the blood.
- **IV:** A tube placed in your vein for giving medicine or liquids. It will be capped or have tubing connected to it.
- **ECG:** Also called a heart monitor, an electrocardiograph (e-lec-tro-CAR-dee-o-graf), or EKG. Patches placed on your chest are hooked up to a TV-type screen or a small portable box (telemetry unit). This screen shows a tracing of each heartbeat. Your heart will be watched for signs of injury or damage that could be related to your illness.
- **12 Lead ECG:** This test makes tracings from different parts of your heart. It can help your doctor gauge the seriousness of the problem.
- **Chest X-ray:** This picture of your lungs and heart shows how they are handling the illness.
- **Medicines:** Heart medicine will be given in your IV to slow your heart rate. If you get dizzy, feel pain, or have other side effects after getting your medicine, call your doctor right away.
- **Cardioversion** (car-dee-o-VER-shun): This procedure uses an electric shock to the heart to return it to a normal rate. It may be needed if medicine fails to slow your heart rate. Before cardioversion, you will be given medicine to make you sleepy. Then the shock is administered. If it works, your heart rate and rhythm will return to normal. However, you may still need medicine to keep your heart rate under control.

Atrial Tachycardia

See Supraventricular Tachycardia

Back Pain

WHAT YOU SHOULD KNOW

Low back pain (also called low back *sprain*) is usually caused by muscle strain. The pain may come on suddenly at the moment of injury or develop gradually over time. With care, your back should return to normal. However, backaches tend to recur, and some last over a long period of time.

Causes

There are numerous causes. A strain may occur while you are lifting, or happen during a fall. An infection, a ruptured disk, or nerve damage may be at fault. Other causes include osteoporosis ("brittle bone" disease), tumors, hardening and stiffening of the spinal cord, and childbirth. Sometimes no cause can be found.

Signs/Symptoms

Pain and stiffness may be constant or intermittent. It may be more noticeable when you bend over or first get out of bed.

Care

Get plenty of rest and follow your doctor's treatment plan. You may need physical therapy to strengthen your back muscles and medication to ease the pain. For certain problems, such as a ruptured disk, surgery may be needed.

WHAT YOU SHOULD DO

- Apply ice to the injury for 10 to 20 minutes each hour for the first 1 to 2 days. Put the ice in a plastic bag and place a towel between the bag of ice and your skin.
- After the first 1 or 2 days, you may apply heat to the injury to help relieve pain. Use a warm heating pad, whirlpool bath, or warm, moist towels for 10 to 20 minutes every hour for 48 hours.
- Stay in bed until your doctor says it is safe to get up.
- Resume normal activities when you can do them without feeling pain.
- When picking things up, never bend from the waist; instead, bend at the hips and knees.
- When sleeping:
  —Sleep on a firm mattress or put a 1/2- to 1-inch piece of plywood between the mattress and box springs.
  —Do not use a waterbed; it will not support your back correctly.

—Sleep with a pillow under your knees or sleep on your side with your knees bent.
- Wear low-heeled shoes.
- Excess weight puts strain on the back. If you are overweight, try to bring your weight down to normal.
- The right kind of exercises will strengthen your back and reduce the chances of another strain. However, some types of exercise can cause further injury. Check with your doctor before undertaking any exercise program.

Call Your Doctor If . . .
- You have shooting pains into your buttocks, groin, or legs.

Seek Care Immediately If . . .
- You have trouble urinating or lose control of your bladder or bowels.
- You develop numbness or weakness in your legs or feet.

Bacteremia

See Sepsis

Bacterial Meningitis

WHAT YOU SHOULD KNOW

Bacterial (back-TEER-e-ul) meningitis (men-in-JIE-tis) is an infection that causes swelling and irritation of the tissue around the brain and spinal cord. Although it can be a very serious disease, with treatment, it will probably clear up in 2 to 3 weeks.

Causes
The bacteria that cause this disease spread to the brain from other parts of the body. The most common causes are the *Neisserria meningitidis*, pneumococcus, and *Haemophilus influenzae* bacteria. These bacteria can pass from one person to another.

Signs/Symptoms
Symptoms include fever, chills, sweating, headache, stiff neck, vomiting, red or purple skin rash, confusion, irritability, or tiredness. In addition, your eyes may be bothered by light.

Care
Antibiotic medicine will be prescribed to treat your infection. You may be put in the hospital for tests and care. After 2 to 3 weeks, you may return to normal activity.

Risks

Without treatment, this disease can be fatal—and if you don't get treatment soon enough, you may end up with brain damage (hearing loss, learning problems, difficulty talking, seizures, or paralysis).

WHAT YOU SHOULD DO

- Take antibiotics exactly as directed until they are all gone. Finish the prescription even if you feel well.
- If any of your medicines make you drowsy, do not drive.
- Stay away from others until your doctor says you can no longer spread your illness.
- Although no special diet is needed, you should drink about 6 to 8 glasses (soda-can sized) of water a day, even if you don't feel like it. Do not drink alcohol.
- Eat healthy foods and get lots of rest.
- To ease headaches, rest in a dark, quiet room.
- Wash your hands each time you go to the bathroom and before eating to keep from spreading germs.
- As soon as you feel better, you may resume your normal activities.
- Get shots to prevent the flu and pneumonia.

Call Your Doctor If . . .

- You have new symptoms (such as a rash, itching, swelling, or trouble breathing) that started when you began taking medicine. You may be allergic to the medicine.
- You have a high temperature while you are taking medicine.

Seek Care Immediately If . . .

- Someone in your family develops a severe headache, stiff neck, fever, and changes in vision. They may have picked up the disease from you.
- You or someone in your family becomes confused or difficult to wake up, or has a high temperature.
- You or someone in your family has seizures.

IF YOU'RE HEADING FOR THE HOSPITAL . . .

What to Expect While You're There

You may encounter the following procedures and equipment during your stay.

- **Activity:** You will be required to stay in bed in a darkened room. You may not be allowed to have certain visitors if the doctors think they could catch your infection.
- **Isolation:** To keep from spreading the infection, you will be kept

away from others. Nurses and others around you will wear face masks and gowns to keep from getting the disease.

- **Neuro Signs:** The doctor will check your eyes and memory, and see how easily you awaken. These are important signs that tell how well the brain is responding to the infection.
- **Lumbar Puncture:** Also called spinal tap. Fluid is taken from your spine and sent for tests.
- **Body Fluid Cultures:** Blood, urine, throat, and nose fluids may be tested. This will help the doctor decide which antibiotic will be the best treatment.
- **Taking Vital Signs:** These include your temperature, blood pressure, pulse (counting your heartbeats), and respirations (counting your breaths). A stethoscope is used to listen to your heart and lungs. Your blood pressure is taken by wrapping a cuff around your arm.
- **Pulse Oximeter:** While you are getting oxygen, you may be hooked up to a pulse oximeter (ox-IM-uh-ter). It is placed on your ear, finger, or toe and is connected to a machine that measures the oxygen in your blood.
- **Blood:** Usually taken from a vein in your hand or from the bend in your elbow. Tests will be done on the blood.
- **Blood Gases:** Blood is taken from an artery in your wrist, elbow, or groin. It is tested to see how much oxygen it contains.
- **Chest X-ray:** This picture of your lungs and heart shows how well they are handling the illness.
- **CT Scan:** Also called a "CAT" scan, this is an x-ray using a computer. It will be used to take pictures of your brain and check the progress of the infection.
- **IV:** A tube placed in your vein for giving medicine or liquids. It will be capped or have tubing connected to it.
- **ECG:** Also called a heart monitor, an electrocardiograph (e-LEK-tro-CAR-dee-o-graf), or EKG. The patches on your chest are hooked up to a TV-type screen or a small portable box (telemetry unit). This screen shows a tracing of each heartbeat.
- **Medicines:**
  - **Antibiotics** will be prescribed to fight the infection. They may be given by IV, in a shot, or by mouth.
  - **Pain medicine** may be given in your IV, as a shot, or by mouth. If the pain does not go away or comes back, tell a doctor right away.
  - **Fever medicine**, usually acetaminophen, will be given to bring down your fever. It may be given by mouth or in your rectum.
  - **Anti-nausea medicine** may be given to get rid of your nausea

and control your vomiting so you don't lose too much body fluid (become dehydrated).

After You Leave
Follow the guidelines listed under "What You Should Do."

Bacterial Meningitis in Children

WHAT YOU SHOULD KNOW

Bacterial meningitis (men-in-JIE-tis) is a serious infection of the tissues around the brain and spinal cord. It can begin and spread quickly. It is seen most often in children 6 to 12 months of age. This infection is not as common as it once was because most children now get shots (immunizations) to prevent it. If a child does get this disease, it will pass in 2 to 3 weeks when given proper treatment and care.

Causes
The bacteria that cause this disease often get a foothold in other parts of the body, such as the ear, nose, or throat, then move to the brain. A child may also get the disease after a head injury.

Signs/Symptoms
Typical symptoms include a high fever (usually 101 to 106 degrees F, 38.3 to 41.1 degrees C), vomiting, stiff neck, back pain, fussiness, headache, sleepiness, confusion, red or purple skin rash, no interest in eating, and, perhaps, eyes that hurt when exposed to light. A high-pitched cry is a sign of meningitis in babies.

Care
The child will need a stay in the hospital to be carefully watched and treated with antibiotics.

Risks
Bacterial meningitis can be fatal. However, the risks of serious illness or death are smaller with the right treatment and care.

IF YOU'RE HEADING FOR THE HOSPITAL . . .

What to Expect While You're There
You may encounter the following procedures and equipment during your stay.
• **Room:** A quiet room with dim lights may make your child more comfortable. To keep from spreading the disease, he or she will be kept away from others. Care givers will wear a face mask and gown

to keep from getting the disease. This may scare the child, but it is a necessary safety measure.

- **Emotional Support:** You may stay with your child to provide comfort and support. The child will feel safer in the hospital with you close by.
- **Hand Washing:** Wash your hands after each visit with your child to keep from spreading the infection.
- **Antibiotics:** These bacteria-killing medicines will be given by IV for at least 10 days to fight the infection.
- **Neuro Signs:** The doctor will watch your child's eye movements, check to see if the child is fully awake, and take note of how he or she moves around. These are important signs of how well the brain is handling the infection.
- **Lumbar Puncture:** Also called a spinal tap. In this procedure, fluid is taken from the child's spine and sent for tests.
- **CT Scan** (also called a "CAT" scan)**:** This computer-assisted x-ray will be used to examine the brain.
- **EEG** (also called an electroencephalogram (e-lek-tro-en-SEF-uh-lo-gram)**:** This is a brain wave study. It will be used to check for any possible damage to the brain.
- **Taking Vital Signs:** These include your child's temperature, blood pressure, pulse (counting the heartbeats), and respirations (counting the breaths). A stethoscope is used to listen to the child's heart and lungs. Blood pressure is taken by wrapping a cuff around the child's arm. None of these procedures cause any pain.
- **Pulse Oximeter:** Your child may be hooked up to a pulse oximeter (ox-IM-uh-ter). It is placed on the ear, finger, or toe and is connected to a machine that measures the oxygen in the child's blood.
- **Oxygen:** May be given using nasal prongs or a face mask.
- **IV:** A tube placed in your child's veins for giving medicine or liquids. It will be capped or have tubing connected to it.
- **Intake/Output:** Nurses will carefully watch how much liquid your child is getting and how much he or she is urinating.
- **ECG:** Also called a heart monitor, an electrocardiograph (e-LEK-tro-CAR-dee-o-graf), or EKG. The patches on your child's chest are hooked up to a TV-type screen. This screen shows a tracing of each heartbeat. The heart will be watched for signs of injury or damage related to the infection.
- **Blood:** Usually taken from a vein in your child's hand or from the bend in the elbow. Tests will be done on this blood.
- **Blood Gases:** Blood is taken from an artery in the wrist, elbow, or groin. It is tested to see how much oxygen is in it.

• **Chest X-rays:** These pictures of the heart and lungs will show how they are handling the illness.

After You Leave

• Be sure to give your child the medicine prescribed by your doctor exactly as directed. Finish all the medicine even if the child is feeling better.
• Encourage the child to rest, drink liquids, and eat healthy foods. He or she can slowly return to normal activity.
• Make an appointment to see the doctor. It is very important to keep this follow-up appointment. Your doctor will check for any lasting effects of the infection.
• Meningitis can cause hearing problems, so your child's hearing should be tested. Ask your doctor how often this should be done.
• Family members and others in close contact with your child may be asked to take antibiotics. This will keep the infection from spreading to others.

Call Your Doctor If . . .

• The child has a high temperature.
• New signs or symptoms appear, such as rash, swelling, or trouble breathing. These may be a side effect of the child's medicine.

Seek Care Immediately If . . .

• The child has a seizure.
• You feel the child is getting sicker.
• Anyone else in the family develops symptoms of meningitis such as fever, vomiting, stiff neck, back pain, fussiness, headache, sleepiness, or confusion.

Bacterial Pneumonia

WHAT YOU SHOULD KNOW

Bacterial pneumonia is an infection that causes irritation, swelling, and congestion in the lungs. It is also called bacterial pneumonitis (new-mo-NI-tis). It occurs most often in the winter.

Causes

This type of pneumonia results when bacteria are inhaled and settle in the lungs.

Signs/Symptoms

This illness usually follows a cold. It often starts suddenly with a high fever (over 102 degrees F or 38.9 degrees C) and chills. Difficult or painful breathing and a cough with bloody or yellow sputum are common symptoms. Other signs may include fast breathing, tiredness, abdominal pain, and blue or pale lips and nailbeds.

Care

If you have no other illnesses or problems, you can be treated at home. This care will include antibiotics, a humidifier to loosen your sputum (making it easier to cough up), and rest.

If your condition gets worse, or if you have other problems (such as diabetes or heart failure), you may need a stay in the hospital. There your care will be similar, but you can be carefully watched.

Risks

Without treatment, the infection could spread and become a threat to your life. Your lung problems could become worse—possibly even fatal.

WHAT YOU SHOULD DO

• Take your antibiotics as directed until they are all gone—even if you feel well. If you don't think they are helping, call your doctor. Do not quit taking them on your own.

• If you are taking medicine that makes you drowsy, do not drive or use heavy equipment.

• If you are coughing up sputum and milk seems to make the sputum thicker, do not eat or drink foods that contain milk.

• To help free your lungs of infection, take 2 or 3 deep breaths and then cough. Do this often during the day.

• If you do not have to limit the amount of liquids you drink, drink 8 to 10 (soda-can size) glasses of water each day. This helps thin the sputum so it can be coughed up more easily.

• Use a humidifier to help keep the air moist and your sputum thin. This makes it easier to cough up the sputum. You must keep the humidifier free of fungus. Clean it every day.

• Stay inside during very cold or hot weather, or on days when the air pollution is high. This will make it easier to breathe and will help control your cough.

• Rest at home until you feel better. You may return to work or school when your temperature is around 98.6 degrees F (37 degrees C). Slowly increase your activity. You may feel weak and tired for up to 6 weeks after your illness.

• If you have chest pain, apply a heating pad (set on low) or warm

cloths to the sore area for 10 to 20 minutes, 2 to 3 times a day. This may ease the pain, making it easier to breathe.
- Because you have had pneumonia, it may be easier for you to get other lung infections. Try to stay away from people who have colds or the flu. Get shots against flu and pneumonia.
- Quit smoking. It harms the lungs. If you are having trouble quitting, ask your doctor for help.
- Make an appointment for another chest x-ray, if your doctor thinks one is necessary.

Call Your Doctor If . . .
- You have a high temperature.
- Your medicine does not relieve your chest pain within a few days.
- You get nauseated, or have vomiting or diarrhea.
- You are coughing up bloody or pink, frothy sputum.
- You have problems, such as a rash, itching, swelling, or stomach pain, that may be caused by your medicine.
- Another family member shows signs of pneumonia.

Seek Care Immediately If . . .
- You have a lot of trouble breathing or have blue or pale skin, lips, or nailbeds.
- You have a severe headache, neck stiffness, or feel confused.
- You continue to have fever and chills and feel worse even when taking your medicine.

IF YOU'RE HEADING FOR THE HOSPITAL . . .

What to Expect While You're There
You may encounter the following procedures and equipment during your stay.
- **Activity:** At first you will need to rest in bed, with a few pillows to keep you sitting up a little. This will help your breathing. Do not lie flat. Once you are breathing more easily, you will be allowed to increase your exercise.
- **Taking Vital Signs:** These include your temperature, blood pressure, pulse (counting your heartbeats), and respirations (counting your breaths). A stethoscope is used to listen to your heart and lungs. Your blood pressure is taken by wrapping a cuff around your arm.
- **Oxygen:** Your body may need extra oxygen at this time. It is given either by a mask or nasal prongs. Tell your doctor if the oxygen is drying out your nose or if the nasal prongs bother you.
- **Pulse Oximeter:** While you are getting oxygen, you may be hooked up to a pulse oximeter (ox-IM-uh-ter). It is placed on your ear,

finger, or toe and is connected to a machine that measures the oxygen in your blood.

- **ECG:** Also called a heart monitor, an electrocardiograph (e-LEK-tro-CAR-dee-o-graf), or EKG. The patches on your chest are hooked up to a TV-type screen or a small portable box (telemetry unit). This screen shows a tracing of each heartbeat. Your heart will be watched for signs of injury or damage that could be related to your illness.
- **12 Lead ECG:** This test makes tracings from different parts of your heart. It can help your doctor decide whether there is a heart problem.
- **Chest X-ray:** This picture of your lungs and heart shows how well they are handling your illness.
- **Blood:** Usually taken from a vein in your hand or from the bend in your elbow. Tests will be done on the blood.
- **Blood Gases:** Blood is taken from an artery in your wrist, elbow, or groin and tested for the amount of oxygen it contains.
- **IV:** A tube placed in your vein for giving medicine or liquids. It will be capped or have tubing connected to it.
- **Medicines:**
    —**Antibiotics** are given to fight infection. They may be given in your IV, in a shot, or by mouth.
    —**Expectorants** (ex-PEK-ter-ants) may also be given to help thin your sputum so it is easier to cough up.
- **Coughing and Deep Breathing:** It is important to do this often because it helps clear your lungs of infection.
    —To ease your pain during coughing and deep breathing, you may need to loosely wrap your rib cage with a 6-inch elastic bandage.
    —Holding a pillow tightly against your chest when you cough can help reduce the pain. Lying on the side that is hurting may also help ease the pain.
- **Heat:** A warm towel or heating pad (set on low) may help ease your chest pain.
- **Sputum Sample:** If you are coughing up sputum, your doctor may need to send a sample to the lab. From this sample, the lab can determine which kind of bacteria is causing your illness. This helps the doctor choose the medicine you need.
- **Postural Drainage:** Periodically, a nurse may tap briskly on your back with his or her hands. This helps loosen the sputum in your lungs so you can cough it up more easily.

After You Leave
Follow the directions listed under "What You Should Do."

Bacterial Vaginosis

WHAT YOU SHOULD KNOW

Bacterial (back-TEER-e-ul) vaginosis (vag-in-O-sis) is an infection of the vagina. It is sometimes spread by having sex and may be spread in other ways as well. With treatment, you should be well in 5 to 7 days. You may get this infection again.

Causes
This infection is caused by germs that live naturally in your vagina. If the healthy balance of germs is upset, these germs have a chance to grow and cause infection. Many things can change the balance of a healthy vagina. Some causes may be douching, certain soaps or bubble baths, antibiotic medicines, or diabetes. Other causes range from having sex to using feminine hygiene sprays or powders.

Signs/Symptoms
The most common sign is a white, gray, or yellow vaginal discharge with a "fishy" smell that may seem the strongest after you have sex. Other signs may be itching, redness, or swelling of the vagina and vulva (area around the vagina).

Care
Antibiotic medicine is used to treat this infection. Your partner(s) may also need to be treated.

WHAT YOU SHOULD DO

- Take the medicine your doctor prescribes exactly as directed.
- Keep your genital area clean and dry. Take showers instead of tub baths. Use plain, unscented soap.
- Don't use feminine hygiene sprays or powders. Don't douche during treatment unless your doctor recommends it. After the infection is cleared up, don't douche more often than once a week.
- Don't have sex while you are being treated. Otherwise, the infection could be passed back and forth between you and your partner(s).
- Wear underpants and pantyhose that have a cotton lining in the crotch.
- After urination and bowel movements, wipe from front to back to prevent the spread of germs.
- Avoid activities that make you sweaty, especially during hot, humid weather.

Call Your Doctor If . . .
• Your symptoms become worse or last longer than a few days.
• You have vaginal bleeding that is not menstrual bleeding.
• Your symptoms come back after treatment.
• You have any problems that you suspect are related to the medicine you are taking.

Barbiturate Abuse

WHAT YOU SHOULD KNOW

Barbiturates, also called sedatives or "downers," are often prescribed to decrease nervousness or to help you sleep better. However, using them for a long time or taking more than the recommended amount can lead to addiction or dependency. You'll begin to feel that you must have more of the drug; and if you abruptly stop taking it, you'll become physically ill.

Long-term abuse of barbiturates can interfere with your ability to function. You'll find you have trouble thinking, talking, walking, and remembering things; and you'll run the risk of dying from an overdose.

To kick this habit, you need to gradually reduce your intake under medical supervision. Attempting to go "cold turkey" on your own could be difficult and even dangerous.

Causes
Taking a barbiturate for several months or years, or taking larger doses than prescribed, will lead to physical addiction. Pregnant women who take these drugs can pass the addiction to their babies.

Signs/Symptoms
If you abuse barbiturates, you may feel sleepy; have trouble thinking, talking and walking; and develop bruises on your arms and legs from falling. The longer you keep taking the drug, the more you will feel you need it. If you stop taking the drug, you'll have symptoms of withdrawal.

The first effects of withdrawal are restlessness, weakness, and shakiness. Later, you may feel nervous and develop insomnia, an upset stomach, vomiting, sweating, or sensitivity to bright lights or loud noises. Sudden withdrawal sometimes leads to hallucinations and seizures.

Care
Your doctor may slowly reduce the amount of barbiturates you take each day. During this period, you may need to stay in the hospital.

Counseling can help you kick this habit. Your doctor can prescribe medications to ease the withdrawal symptoms.

WHAT YOU SHOULD DO

• If prescribed a barbiturate, be careful to follow your doctor's instructions. Do not increase the dose or take the drug any longer than absolutely necessary.
• The first step to quitting is to admit you have a problem. Be honest and open with family and close friends. Ask for their help.
• Don't try to stop taking the drug all at once. You will need medical help to get you through a gradual withdrawal period.
• Tell your doctor exactly how much of the drug you have been taking. Also tell your doctor if you are taking any other medications. Don't hesitate to be honest. Doctors are familiar with the problem.
• Support-group meetings and counseling can help you quit. Take advantage of both.
• Eat a healthy diet, drink 6 to 8 glasses of water a day, and get plenty of rest.
• Don't smoke or drink coffee or alcohol. They can make you nervous and increase your withdrawal symptoms.
• Don't dwell on the problem. Find new things to do. Get out of the house every day. Go for walks outside.

Call Your Doctor If . . .
• You cannot fight the need to take more drugs. Call your doctor, a counselor, friend, or family member you trust RIGHT AWAY.
• You feel your problems are getting the best of you and you can't deal with them on your own.

Seek Care Immediately If . . .
• You have chest pain, sweating, or trouble breathing.
• You develop an urge to hurt yourself or someone else.
• You get a severe headache or develop pain, a numb or prickly feeling, or burning in your arms or legs.
• You have hallucinations, pass out, or have a seizure.

Barium Enema

WHAT YOU SHOULD KNOW

A barium enema is an x-ray test of the large bowel. Barium is used to help the intestine show-up better on x-ray film.

Risks
If the barium is not cleared from your bowel, your bowel could become blocked. However, if you follow the directions given to you after the barium enema, you should not have any problems.

IF YOU'RE HEADING FOR THE HOSPITAL . . .

Before You Go
Your doctor will put you on a limited diet and give you medicine to completely clean out your bowel.
• **Diet:** The day before the test, you should drink liquids only; the day of the test, don't eat anything.
• **Medicine:** The day before and the day of the test, you may need to take laxatives. Be sure to take them exactly as ordered by your doctor.

What to Expect While You're There
• Before the x-ray is taken, an x-ray technician will gently put a tube into your rectum. Barium (a white chalky liquid) will flow into the large bowel through this tube. The tube may cause a feeling of pressure or discomfort, or make you feel like you need to have a bowel movement.
• A technician will be taking the x-rays. You will be placed in many positions during the test (lying on your back, side, and stomach). This part of the session takes about 45 minutes.
• After the x-ray, you'll be asked to go to the bathroom to pass the barium that is left in your bowel. The technician will then take another x-ray to check for any remaining barium.

After You Leave
• It is important that all the barium be cleared from your bowel. To do this:
  —Drink 2 or 3 glasses of water after the test.
  —Take either a mild laxative or use a cleansing enema after the test, as recommended by your doctor.
• The barium will turn your stool a lighter color. After the barium is cleared from your body, your stools will return to normal.

Call Your Doctor If . . .
• You have pain or discomfort in your lower abdomen or stomach.
• You have pencil-thin stools.
• Your stools are not normal within a few days.

Seek Care Immediately If . . .
• You have severe abdominal pain, nonstop throwing up, or bloody vomit or stools.

Barium Swallow

WHAT YOU SHOULD KNOW

A barium swallow is an x-ray of the throat and esophagus (eh-SOF-uh-gus), the tube connecting the throat to the stomach. Barium blocks x-rays so that the outline of the throat and esophagus will show up on the film. The pictures are used to help pinpoint your problem.

Risks
If your body does not get rid of the barium, it can harden and block your bowel, causing pain and other problems. Barium can also cause the body to lose water, leading to dehydration. To avoid these problems, follow your doctor's instructions carefully.

IF YOU'RE HEADING FOR THE HOSPITAL . . .

Before You Go
• Your doctor will tell you when you must stop eating or drinking anything, including water. Follow these instructions exactly.
• If your doctor says you may take your medicine as usual, swallow it with only a sip of water.
• You may be asked to take a laxative before the test. This will help to clear the barium from your bowel.
• For 2 to 3 days before the test, eat high-fiber foods, such as fruits, grains, and vegetables, and drink at least 6 to 8 (soda-can size) glasses of water per day. This also helps your body get rid of the barium.

What to Expect While You're There
• **Taking Vital Signs:** Before the test, a nurse will take your temperature, blood pressure, pulse (counting your heartbeat), and respirations (counting your breaths). A stethoscope is used to listen to your heart and lungs. Your blood pressure may be taken by wrapping a cuff around your arm.
• **During the Barium Swallow:**
  —You will be given 1 or 2 large barium "milkshakes" to drink. Because barium tastes chalky, flavoring such as strawberry may be added to the milkshake.
  —You will be asked to lie on a table, and straps will be put around

you to hold you in place. The table will then be moved to many different positions.

—The x-rays will be taken as the barium flows down your esophagus and into your stomach.

—The test takes about 15 to 30 minutes. Follow-up pictures may need to be taken about 6 hours after you swallowed the barium.

After You Leave

• You may need to take a mild laxative after the test to help clear out the barium.

• Drink 2 to 3 glasses (soda-can size) of water after the test to help flush the barium from your body.

• Your stools will be chalky and light-colored for 24 to 72 hours after the test.

• If you have a colostomy, irrigate it after the last x-ray is taken and again in the morning. The last x-ray may be taken as late as 6 hours after you first swallowed barium.

Call Your Doctor If . . .

• You have not passed barium in your stool within 2 to 3 days after the exam.

• Your have pain in your lower belly or stomach.

• Your stool is pencil-thin, or there is a change in your bowel habits.

Barotitis Media

WHAT YOU SHOULD KNOW

Barotitis (BEAR-o-TI-tis) media (me-DEE-uh) is an injury to the middle ear (the area behind the eardrum) that results when a blockage develops in the tube that normally equalizes pressure within the ear (the eustachian tube that runs from the middle ear to the back of the nose). When normal air flow is blocked, pressure can build in the ear. The condition is not serious, and usually clears up in a few hours or days. In some cases, however, it may last a long time.

Causes

The problem can result from air pressure changes that occur during scuba or sky diving, airplane flights, or trips through the mountains. Barotitis media can also be caused by an injury to the ear.

Signs/Symptoms

You may experience hearing loss, plugged ears, ear pain, dizziness, or ringing in the ears.

Care

Usually no care is needed, but if the problem persists, you may need medicine for an infection, for pain, or to unplug the ears.

WHAT YOU SHOULD DO

• Don't take any medicine without your doctor's approval.
• Do not put anything into your ears to clean or unplug them.
• Do not swim or dive until your doctor says it is okay.
• Avoid flying or scuba-diving when you have a head cold.
• If you must fly:
  —Call your doctor for medicine to keep your ears unplugged.
  —Chew gum or suck on candy when the airplane is taking off and landing. This will force you to swallow often and will equalize the air pressure in your middle and outer ears.
  —Take a breath, hold your nose, close your mouth. This will force air into the eustachian tube.
  —To prevent the problem in an infant, breastfeed or give the baby a bottle of water or juice on takeoff and landing.

Call Your Doctor If . . .

• You get a painful headache or a really bad earache, you feel dizzy, or you have blood or pus-like drainage from the ear.
• You develop a high temperature.
• Your symptoms do not get better or they become worse.

Bartholin's Cyst

WHAT YOU SHOULD KNOW

Bartholin's (BAR-tul-ins) glands are two small glands in the folds of skin that cover the opening of the vagina. Occasionally a cyst, or fluid-filled sac, develops in one of the glands or the tube leading to it. The fluid inside this cyst may become infected.

Care

The doctor will open the cyst and drain it.

WHAT YOU SHOULD DO

• A small piece of gauze is left over the area so that it can continue to drain. Do not remove the gauze until the doctor says it's okay.
• Put warm, moist towels on the area or sit in a tub of warm water. This helps ease the pain and discomfort. Do this for 10 to 20 minutes several times a day.

• You may want to use a panty liner to keep from staining your underwear.

Call Your Doctor If . . .
• You have pain, redness, swelling, drainage, or bleeding in the area of the cyst and it is getting worse.
• You have tenderness or pain in the folds of skin around your vagina (the labia), you have pain with sex, or your labia are swollen.
• You get chills or a have a high temperature.

Bathing Babies

See Tub Bathing Your Baby

Bell's Palsy

WHAT YOU SHOULD KNOW

In Bell's palsy, one side of the face suddenly becomes paralyzed. The problem results from a swollen, irritated nerve that weakens facial muscles. Fortunately, it is not serious, and although complete healing may take many months, most people do get better.

Causes
Doctors are not sure why the nerve swells and becomes irritated, but they suspect the problem may be a disruption in the blood supply. Other possible causes include a virus, immune disease, or exposure to cold weather.

Signs/Symptoms
You'll feel a sudden weakness on one side of the face. You may begin drooling and feel pain behind the ear. You may not be able to move your mouth or the eye on the affected side of the head. Your face may look droopy; the affected eye may not close completely.

Care
To rule out other problems, the doctor may order an x-ray or CT scan (computer-assisted x-ray) of your head. You'll probably need medication to reduce swelling in the nerve and eyedrops to keep the affected eye from drying out.

WHAT YOU SHOULD DO

• Be sure to use the prescribed medications exactly as directed.
• If you cannot close your eyelid, wear wrap-around plastic goggles to

protect the eye from dirt, dust, and dryness. At night, wear an eye patch or tape the eyelid shut.

• Applying heat to the affected side helps relieve pain. Use an electric heating pad set on warm or a towel soaked in warm water, then wrung out. Apply the heat for 15 minutes, twice a day. Cover or close the eye during these treatments.

• Use facial massage and exercises when muscle strength returns. Gently rub the muscles of the forehead, cheek, lip, and eye. Open and close the eye, wink, and smile wide. Do these exercises for 15 or 20 minutes several times a day.

• You may perform your normal activities. Rest does not help Bell's palsy.

Seek Care Immediately If . . .

• Your eye stays red and irritated or becomes more painful.
• You cannot stop drooling.
• You develop a high temperature.

Benign Prostatic Hyperplasia

See Enlarged Prostate

Benzodiazepine Abuse

WHAT YOU SHOULD KNOW

Benzodiazepines (BEN-zo-die-AZ-a-peens) are a type of tranquilizing medication frequently prescribed for anxiety or trouble sleeping. If you use benzodiazepines for several months or take more pills than prescribed, you may become dependent on them. Benzodiazepine abuse can interfere with thinking and memory, and may lead to depression. You also face the danger of an accidental overdose.

If you stop taking benzodiazepines suddenly, you will become ill. It is better to taper off gradually.

Causes

Dependence on benzodiazepines takes hold in two ways. It can develop gradually if you take low doses for several months or years, or set in quickly if you take higher doses than you are supposed to.

Signs/Symptoms

If you become dependent on a benzodiazepine, you will feel an intense craving for it and get sick if you do not take it. You may also need to take more and more of the drug to get the same feeling that a smaller dosage used to provide.

If you stop taking the drug suddenly you may develop withdrawal symptoms such as shaking, nervousness, insomnia, upset stomach, vomiting, fast heartbeat, sweating, and (sometimes) sensitivity to bright lights or loud noises. Some people have seizures or hallucinations.

Care
Your doctor is likely to gradually reduce your daily dosage. You may need counseling to help you stop using the drug and other medicines to help ease the withdrawal symptoms.

WHAT YOU SHOULD DO

- Don't take more of any drug than your doctor directs; and never take a benzodiazepine for an extended period of time. Ask your doctor how long it's safe to continue taking the drug.
- Tell your doctor exactly how much of the drug you have been taking. Also tell your doctor if you are taking any other medications. Don't hesitate to be honest. Doctors are familiar with the problem.
- Don't try to stop taking the drug all at once.
- The first step to quitting is to admit you have a problem. Be honest and open with family and close friends. Ask for their help.
- Stay away from people who use drugs and who encourage others to use them.
- Support-group meetings and counseling can help you quit. Take advantage of both.
- Eat a healthy diet, drink 6 to 8 glasses of water a day, and get plenty of rest.
- Don't smoke or drink coffee or alcohol. They can make you nervous and increase your withdrawal symptoms.
- Don't dwell on the problem. Find new things to do. Get out of the house every day. Go for walks outside.

Call Your Doctor If . . .
- You cannot fight the need to take more drugs; call your doctor, a counselor, friend, or a family member you trust RIGHT AWAY.
- You feel your problems are getting the best of you and you can't deal with them on your own.

Seek Care Immediately If . . .
- You pass out or have a seizure.
- You start using the drugs again.

Bicycle Helmets

WHAT YOU SHOULD KNOW

One of every seven children has a head injury in a bike accident. The best protection is a well-fitting helmet that meets the safety rules of the American National Standards Institute or the Snell Memorial Foundation.

WHAT YOU SHOULD DO

• Get your child a helmet as soon as he or she starts learning to ride.
• The helmet may have a foam shell or a hard shell. Buy only a tested, approved helmet. It should have an approval sticker from either SNELL or ANSI Z90.4.
• Make sure the helmet is the right size. It should fit snugly so it will not move around on the head or come off in a fall.
• The helmet should be worn over the forehead, not tipped back. The front edge should be only 1 inch above the eyebrows.
• Have the child hang the helmet from the handlebars when not riding the bicycle. This helps the child remember to put it on before every ride.
• Over time, the foam fitting pads inside the helmet wear down and may need to be replaced to ensure a snug fit.
• It's a good idea to replace the entire helmet every 3 to 5 years, especially if it is worn in the sun a lot.

Bicycle Safety

WHAT YOU SHOULD KNOW

You can avoid a bicycle injury easily by learning a few safety rules and using proper clothing and gear. A few of the basics:

Don't wear loose clothing or a long coat; they can get caught in the bicycle chain. Put clips or rubber bands around the bottom of pants legs. When riding at night, wear light-colored clothing. Wearing armbands, legbands, or vests that glow in the dark helps assure that drivers will see you. **Always** wear a helmet when riding your bike.

Learn and obey all traffic rules, signals, and signs if you ride in the street. Teach bicycle safety to your children by setting a good example. Don't let children under age 8 ride in the street. They should ride on bike paths and sidewalks instead.

WHAT YOU SHOULD DO

- Follow these **SAFETY RULES**:
  —Obey all street signs. Use the correct hand signals before you turn or stop.
  —Ride single-file on the right side of the street with traffic. Always keep at least one hand on the handlebars.
  —Always stay a car door's width away from parked cars. Watch out for opening doors.
  —Be alert for vehicles turning right or oncoming vehicles turning left in front of you.
  —Watch for vehicles exiting a driveway.
  —Never assume that you have the right of way.
  —Always cross train tracks straight on. Don't ride over sewer grates.
  —Don't ride in puddles, potholes, sand, gravel on the pavement, or glass and debris that might cause loss of control.
  —Don't carry anyone on the handlebars or back fender.
  —If you are transporting a young child, use a child seat attached to the back of the bike or a trailer.
  —Don't hold onto any other moving vehicle while riding.
- Always use the following **EQUIPMENT**:
  —Make sure the bicycle fits the rider.
  —Wear eye protection to guard against bugs, flying gravel, and the sun's rays.
  —Carry your things in a backpack or on a bicycle rack to keep your hands free for steering and to keep packages out of the way of moving bicycle parts.
  —Wear riding gloves to protect your hands in case of a fall.
  —Equip your bicycle with back and side red reflectors, a white front headlight, and a rear-view mirror.
  —Make sure the brakes and tires are in good working order.
  —Take a water bottle with you, especially on long rides.

Biliary Colic

See Gallstones

Biopsy, Skin

See Skin Biopsy

Birthmark Removal

See Mole Removal

Bite, Animal

See Animal Bite

Bite, Brown Recluse Spider

See Brown Recluse Spider Bite

Bite, Cat

See Cat Scratch or Bite

Bite, Human

See Human Bite

Bite, Insect

See Insect Stings

Bite, Marine Life

See Marine-Life Stings and Bites

Bite, Snake

See Snake Bite

Bite, Tick

See Tick Bite

Black Eye

WHAT YOU SHOULD KNOW

A black eye—known medically as a periorbital hematoma (HE-muh-TOW-muh)—is the result of bleeding underneath the skin around the eye following a hard blow to the eye or the area near the eye. The blood under the skin, also known as a contusion, looks black or blue at the surface. The eyelid, eyeball, bones around the eye, or eye muscle may be involved. It may take 2 to 3 weeks for the bruising around the eye to go away.

Signs/Symptoms

The bruise may be accompanied by red, painful swelling of the eye or area near the eye. You may have bleeding or bruising in the eye, and may notice vision changes.

Care

Generally, no specific medical treatment is needed. Simply follow the guidelines listed below.

WHAT YOU SHOULD DO

• Apply ice to the injury for 10 to 20 minutes each hour for the first 1 to 2 days. Put the ice in a plastic bag and place a towel between the bag of ice and your skin.
• After the first 1 to 2 days, you may apply heat to the injury to help relieve pain. Use a warm heating pad or warm, moist towels for 10 to 20 minutes every hour for 48 hours.
• Sleeping with your head raised on 2 pillows may help ease the discomfort.
• You may use nonprescription medicines such as aspirin, acetaminophen and ibuprofen to ease the swelling and discomfort.
• Wear dark glasses temporarily to protect your eyes from bright light and sunlight.
• You may continue your normal daily activities.

Seek Care Immediately If . . .

• You develop nausea and vomiting.
• You develop dizziness, faintness, confusion, or stumbling.
• You have any changes in your vision (such as double vision or loss of vision).

Blepharitis

WHAT YOU SHOULD KNOW

Blepharitis (BLEF-uh-RYE-tis) is an irritation of the edges of your eyelids. It may affect your eyelids, eyelashes, the glands that oil your lids, and the whites of your eyes. Blepharitis is a hard disease to treat. It may take 8 to 12 months to clear up, and could last indefinitely.

Causes

Infection and allergies are the most likely causes. Other diseases, such as diabetes, may also trigger the problem.

Signs/Symptoms

You're likely to have burning, itching, and soreness of the eyelids, plus the feeling that there's a foreign body in your eye. The eyelids may be red, warm, swollen and have greasy scales on them. Overnight, your lids may be glued shut by matter that has drained from the eyelids and dried. You may have flaking around your lashes or lose lashes. Bright light may hurt your eyes.

Care
If an infection is the cause, you may need antibiotics.

WHAT YOU SHOULD DO

- Wash your eyelids with warm salt water or a warm soapless shampoo in the morning and at night.
  - Carefully remove the scales from the eyelids daily. To do this, use a cotton tipped swab. There may be bleeding after you remove the scales.
  - Use a clean towel each time you dry your eyelids.
- To ease discomfort and speed healing, apply a warm washcloth to the eyelid several times a day for 10 to 20 minutes.
- Do not wear eye makeup until the eyelid has healed.
- To relieve discomfort, you may use nonprescription medicines such as acetaminophen or ibuprofen.

Call Your Doctor If . . .
- You have pain in your eye.
- Your eyesight changes.
- You have any new symptoms.
- Your symptoms continue for longer than 2 weeks.

Blood in the Urine

WHAT YOU SHOULD KNOW

Hematuria (HE-muh-TUR-e-uh), or blood in the urine, is a sign of a problem. In most cases, medical treatment can clear up the condition.

Causes
A urinary infection, kidney stones, some medicines, or an injury to your back or lower abdomen can bring blood to the urine. Hematuria can also result from an enlarged prostate gland or a disorder or injury of the kidneys or bladder.

Signs/Symptoms
The urine may be pink, red, or tea-colored.

Care
To pinpoint the cause of the bleeding, the doctor will order tests of the urine and may take x-rays of your kidneys.

WHAT YOU SHOULD DO

- If your doctor prescribes any medicines, take them exactly as directed. Some medications may change the color of urine; others may make you sleepy. If you feel tired or cannot concentrate, do not drive or operate heavy machinery.
- Call your doctor in a few days to find out the results of the tests that were performed on your urine. If a cause for the bleeding cannot be found, it is important that you get follow-up care.

Call Your Doctor If . . .
- You develop a high temperature.
- You have any new problems that may be related to the medication you are taking.
- The bleeding gets worse or becomes bright red.
- The bleeding does not go away in a few hours.
- You develop abdominal pain or swelling, nausea, or vomiting.

Seek Care Immediately If . . .
- You are dizzy, feel weak, or faint.
- You haven't passed urine for a long time.

Boils

WHAT YOU SHOULD KNOW

A boil, known medically as a furuncle (FUR-un-cul), is an infected hair follicle (the place in the skin where a hair is formed). Boils are common and grow deep into the skin's layers. They are usually found on the face, neck, breasts, and buttocks. With treatment, a boil can be cured in 5 to 10 days.

Causes
Boils are caused by bacteria. If a boil breaks open, the bacteria may spread to nearby skin, causing new boils to form.

Signs/Symptoms
A painful, pus-filled, red bump will appear. A boil can appear suddenly and become very painful within 24 hours.

Care
Often, a boil will go away without treatment. However, your doctor may need to open the boil to let the pus out; and antibiotics may be

needed to treat the infection. Keep your skin clean. Do not pick the boil. Warm soaks may help healing.

- Apply heat to help relieve the pain and get rid of the boil faster. Use warm, wet compresses or a heating pad set on low 4 to 6 times a day for 20 minutes.
- Do not pick the boil. Keep the skin clean.

Call Your Doctor If . . .
- The boil gets bigger or does not improve in 3 to 4 days.
- You develop a high temperature.
- You develop new boils, or other members of your family develop boils.

Bone Marrow Biopsy

WHAT YOU SHOULD KNOW

For a bone marrow biopsy (BYE-op-see), your doctor will remove a sample of your bone marrow, the substance inside your bones that manufactures most blood cells, and send it to a laboratory for testing.

Risks
There's a chance of infection when the sample is taken. There is also a very small chance that an organ could be hurt during the procedure.

IF YOU'RE HEADING FOR THE HOSPITAL . . .

Before You Go
- Tell your doctor if you are taking aspirin or a medicine to thin your blood.
- Tell your doctor if you have had surgery on your heart.
- Your doctor may want you to stop eating several hours before the biopsy.

What to Expect While You're There
You may encounter the following procedures and equipment during your stay.
- **Vital Signs:** These include your temperature, blood pressure, pulse (counting your heartbeats), and respirations (counting your breaths). A stethoscope is used to listen to your heart and lungs. Your blood pressure is taken by wrapping a cuff around your arm.
- **During the Bone Marrow Biopsy . . .**
  —You will lie on your stomach or back with a sheet covering you.

The biopsy is usually taken from the hip bone, but could be taken from your breastbone (sternum) or a leg bone.

—You will be asked not to move. Your doctor will give you numbing medicine, so you will feel little pain. The area where the biopsy is to be taken will be cleaned.

—Your doctor will advance a needle through your tissue and bone and into the marrow. You may feel pressure while the needle is passing into bone. A sample of the marrow will be taken.

—To stop the bleeding after the needle is removed, your doctor will apply pressure. A bandage will be put on the area to keep it clean. You may be asked to rest for a short period after the biopsy is done.

—The procedure will take about 30 to 45 minutes.

After You Leave
• Your doctor may prescribe medicine to ease any pain.
• Keep the area dry for 24 hours. When you shower or bathe, place a waterproof material, such as plastic, over the wound site.
• For the first 24 hours, apply an ice pack to the area to reduce pain and swelling. Put ice in a plastic bag and place a towel between the bag of ice and your skin or the bandage. Keep the ice pack on for 2 hours, then off for up to 2 hours.

Call Your Doctor If . . .
• You have severe pain in the area of the biopsy for more than 24 hours.
• You have any bleeding other than a small spot on the dressing.

Seek Care Immediately If . . .
• Your temperature goes higher than 101 degrees F (38.3 degrees C).

Boxer's Fracture

See Broken Hand

Breast Abscess Drainage

WHAT YOU SHOULD KNOW

An abscess is an infected area of tissue that contains pus. A breast abscess forms when germs enter the breast tissue through the nipple and infect the milk ducts and glands. This type of abscess is most likely to develop in women who are breast-feeding a new baby, especially if they have cracked nipples. The abscess needs to be opened (incised or cut) and the pus drained. This will reduce the pain and help clear up the infection. It takes about 3 weeks to recover.

WHAT YOU SHOULD DO

• After the abscess has been drained, take the following measures.
• If you are breast feeding, do not nurse your baby from the breast with the abscess for about 2 weeks. You may continue to nurse from the other breast. In the meantime, use a breast pump to remove milk from the infected breast. Do this as often as you normally nurse your baby, but do not feed this milk to the baby.
• You may use an electric heating pad (set on low), a heat lamp, or a warm, moist towel to help relieve pain at the incision.
• You may bathe and shower as usual. If there is a drain in the incision, wait until it is removed before washing the incision. Then you may wash the incision gently with mild, unscented soap.
• Change the dressing on the incision once a day, after bathing.
• You may restart normal activity and go back to work as soon as you feel up to it.
• Do not do strenuous exercise for 3 weeks.

Call Your Doctor If . . .
• You notice an increase in pain, swelling, redness, drainage, or bleeding in the area of the incision.
• You have a high temperature.

Breast Infection

See Mastitis

Breast Self-Exam

WHAT YOU SHOULD KNOW

Breast self-exam (BSE) is the process of checking your breasts monthly for lumps and other changes.

Why do it?
More women get breast cancer than any kind of cancer. The best way to beat it is to find it early. Learning how to check your breasts can save your life.

You may not do BSE because you are "too busy" or "don't know what you are looking for." Some women do not check their breasts because they are afraid of finding a lump. Don't let this possibility stop you. Most breast lumps or changes in your breasts are **not** cancer.

However, if a lump is cancerous, it's better to find it as soon as possible.

When to do it?
If you are 20 years of age or older you should check your breasts monthly.

WHAT YOU SHOULD DO

- The best time to check your breasts is about 1 week after your period ends. The breasts are not swollen, lumpy, or tender at this time. Check them the same day each month if you are not having periods because of pregnancy or menopause. Talk to your doctor if you have had a hysterectomy. He or she will tell you the best time to check your breasts. Even if you have breast implants, BSE should be done each month.
- At first, you will find it hard to know what feels normal and what does not in your breasts. Regular BSE's will help you learn the feel of your breasts.
- Use the following procedure to check your breasts:
  —Stand in front of a mirror with your arms at your sides. Look at each breast and nipple to check for swelling, lumps, dimpling, scaly skin, or other skin changes.
  —Join your hands behind your head and push your hands forward while looking at your breasts in the mirror. Repeat these steps again with your arms raised over your head.
  —Lie down and put a pillow or towel under your left shoulder. Put your left hand over your head. Gently press into the skin of your breast using the pads of the first 3 fingers of your right hand. Move your finger pads in a circle as you feel your breast tissue.
  —Start at the outer part of your breast and slowly move around it in a clockwise direction. Make small, round movements with your hands. Squeeze your nipple to check for liquid coming from it.
  —Check your other breast the same way. Gently use pressure as you move your fingers around your breasts. Feel the skin deep in your breasts and the skin near the top.
  —Raise your left arm and use the pads of your first 3 fingers of your right hand to feel in and around your armpit. Do the same thing with the other armpit.
- Your breasts can also be checked while you are bathing. Lumps can be felt more easily when your skin is wet. You should have your doctor check your breasts once each year.

Call Your Doctor If . . .
• You find **any** lumps or changes in your breasts.
• You have breast pain or liquid from your nipples.

Breast X-Ray

See Mammogram

Broken Ankle

WHAT YOU SHOULD KNOW

If you break one of the bones in your ankle, you're in for many weeks of discomfort and inconvenience. However, with the right treatment and care, you can expect a full recovery.

Causes
Common causes of ankle fractures include falls, car accidents, and sports injuries. They also can occur when you turn your ankle.

Signs/Symptoms
The fracture can be expected to cause pain, swelling, soreness, problems moving your leg and foot, weakness, numbness, tingling, and bruising.

Treatment
The doctor will take an x-ray of the break, set the bones in the correct position, and put a cast or splint around it to keep the bones from moving out of position. A bad or unusual break may require surgery and a period of recovery in the hospital.

WHAT YOU SHOULD DO

• Use your crutches to keep your weight off of the ankle until your doctor says you can stop.
• To lessen the swelling, raise your ankle above your heart. Keep the injured leg on pillows while lying down and on a stool when sitting.
• Apply ice to the injury for 15 to 20 minutes each hour for the first 1 to 2 days. Put the ice in a plastic bag and place a thin towel between the bag of ice and your cast.
• If you have a plaster or fiberglass cast:
　—Do not try to scratch the skin under the cast with a sharp or pointed object.
　—Check the skin around the cast every day. You may put lotion on any red or sore areas.

—If your fiberglass cast gets a little wet, you can dry it with a hair dryer.

• If you have a plaster splint:

—Wear the splint until your doctor says you no longer need it or until you are seen for a follow-up examination.

—You may loosen the elastic around the splint if you develop numbness or tingling in your toes.

• Do not put pressure on any part of your cast or splint. It may break.

• Keep your cast or splint dry. It can be protected during bathing with a plastic bag. Do not lower the cast or splint into water.

• You may use over-the-counter medicines, such as acetaminophen or ibuprofen to relieve the pain. Take all medications exactly as directed by your doctor.

Call Your Doctor If . . .

• You have continued severe pain or more swelling than you did before the cast was put on.

Seek Care Immediately If . . .

• Your cast gets damaged or breaks.

• Your skin or toenails below the injury turn blue or gray, or begin to feel cold or numb.

• There is a bad smell from your cast.

• There are new stains coming from under the cast.

Broken Arm

WHAT YOU SHOULD KNOW

A break can occur in any of several different bones and can take a variety of forms. Healing time depends on the location and nature of the fracture, and can take from weeks to months.

Causes

A fall or accident is almost always the cause.

Signs/Symptoms

You'll experience pain, swelling, bruising, and possibly bleeding. The arm may be weak or numb, or may tingle. It may look injured or out of alignment.

Care

The doctor will probably need to put a cast or a splint on the arm to keep the bones from moving. A serious fracture may need surgery.

WHAT YOU SHOULD DO

- To reduce the swelling, keep the injured arm above the level of your heart as much as possible.
- Apply ice to the injury for 15 to 20 minutes each hour for the first 1 to 2 days. Put the ice in a plastic bag and place a thin towel between the bag of ice and your cast.
- If you have a plaster or fiberglass cast:
  —Do not try to scratch the skin under the cast by pushing a sharp or pointed object down the cast.
  —Check the skin around the cast every day. You may put lotion on any red or sore areas.
  —If your fiberglass cast gets a little wet, it can be dried with a hair dryer.
- If you have a plaster splint:
  —Wear the splint until your follow-up examination unless your doctor has given you other instructions.
  —You may loosen the elastic around the splint if your fingers become numb or begin to tingle.
- Do not put pressure on any part of your cast or splint; it may break.
- Keep your cast or splint dry. While bathing, protect it with a plastic bag. Do not lower it into water.
- If your doctor prescribes pain medication, take no more than directed. If the medication makes you drowsy, don't drive. You may also use over-the-counter pain killers.

Seek Care Immediately If . . .
- The cast gets damaged or breaks.
- You have continued severe pain or increased swelling.
- The skin or fingernails of the casted arm turn blue or gray, or feel cold or numb.
- There is a bad smell coming from the cast.
- There are new stains coming from under the cast.

Broken Collarbone

WHAT YOU SHOULD KNOW

A broken collarbone can be painful, but usually heals completely without further problems. Medically, it's known as a clavicle (CLAV-ih-kul) fracture.

Causes
Clavicle fractures usually occur in a fall, a car accident, or a sports injury.

Signs/Symptoms
You're likely to experience pain, swelling, soreness, problems moving the shoulder and arm, weakness, numbness, tingling, and bruises.

Care
In many cases, a "figure-eight" bandage is used to hold the broken bone together. Alternatively, you may need to wear a sling.

WHAT YOU SHOULD DO

- To decrease pain and swelling, apply ice to the injury for 15 to 20 minutes each hour for the first 1 or 2 days. Put the ice in a plastic bag and place a towel between the bag of ice and your skin.
- After the first 1 or 2 days, you may apply heat to the injury to help relieve pain for the next 48 hours. You may use a warm heating pad, whirlpool bath, or warm, moist towels. Apply the heat for 15 to 20 minutes every hour.
- Wear a splint or sling constantly for several weeks, even at night. You may remove the splint or sling for bathing or showering. Be sure to keep your shoulder in the same place as when the splint was on. Do not lift your arm.
- If you are using a "figure-eight" splint, it must be tightened by another person every day:
  —Tighten it enough to keep the shoulders held back in a military posture.
  —Allow enough room to place the index finger between the body and the strap.
  —Loosen the splint IMMEDIATELY if you feel numbness or tingling in your hands.
- You may take over-the-counter medications such as acetaminophen or ibuprofen to ease the pain.

Call Your Doctor If . . .
- You have increased pain and swelling.

Seek Care Immediately If . . .
- Your arm is numb, cold, or pale even when the splint is loose.

Broken Elbow

WHAT YOU SHOULD KNOW

A bone fracture in your elbow can take weeks or months to heal.

Causes
Most broken elbows are sustained in a fall or accident.

Signs/Symptoms
You may have pain, swelling, bruising, or bleeding at the elbow. Your arm may feel weak, numb, or tingly, and it may be difficult or impossible to move.

Care
The doctor will order an x-ray of the broken bone. A splint or cast will usually be put on your arm to keep the bones from moving. Your doctor may give you pain medicine. Surgery may be necessary if you have a bad fracture. A second x-ray will probably be taken to make sure the elbow has healed.

WHAT YOU SHOULD DO

- To reduce the swelling, keep the injury raised above the level of your heart as much as possible. When lying down, place the elbow on pillows.
- Apply ice to the injury for 15 to 20 minutes each hour for the first 1 to 2 days. Put the ice in a plastic bag and place a thin towel between the bag of ice and your splint or cast.
- If you have a plaster splint:
  —Wear the splint until your doctor says you can take it off or until your follow-up examination.
  —You may loosen the elastic around the splint if your fingers become numb or tingling.
- Do not put pressure on any part of a plaster splint or cast; it could break.
- Keep the cast or splint dry. It can be protected during bathing with a plastic bag. Do not lower it into water.
- A sling may be used to support the arm.
- If the doctor prescribes pain medicine that makes you drowsy, don't drive. You also may use over-the-counter medicines for pain. Take all medications exactly as directed.
- If you are given a tetanus shot, your arm may get swollen, red, and warm to the touch at the site of the shot. This is a normal response to the medicine.

Seek Care Immediately If . . .

• Your splint or cast gets damaged or breaks.
• You have continued severe pain, or more swelling than you did before treatment.
• The skin or fingernails below the injury turn blue or gray, or become cold or numb.
• There is a bad smell coming from your cast.

Broken Facial Bones

See Facial Fracture

Broken Finger

WHAT YOU SHOULD KNOW

When you break a finger, fractures can occur in one or more of the bones. Healing usually takes 6 to 8 weeks. If you have a really bad break, your doctor may order an x-ray to see whether the break has healed.

Causes

Most broken fingers occur in a fall or accident.

Signs/Symptoms

Likely symptoms include swelling, pain, bruising, bleeding, numbness, or tingling of the injured finger. If the break has caused some bones to move out of place, the hand may look misshapen.

Care

You may need an x-ray. The doctor will probably apply a splint to keep the bones in place. If you have a serious fracture, surgery may be necessary. If you scratched or tore some skin, you may also need a tetanus shot.

WHAT YOU SHOULD DO

• Wear your splint until your doctor says you may take it off or until your follow-up examination. You may retape the splint if it gets wet. When retaping, make sure the splint stays in the same place and position.
• Apply ice to the injury for 15 to 20 minutes each hour for the first 1 to 2 days. Put the ice in a plastic bag and place a towel between the bag of ice and your skin.

- Keep your finger above the level of your heart whenever possible to reduce the swelling.
- To help ease the pain, you may take over-the-counter medicines. Take all medications exactly as directed by your doctor.
- If you are given a tetanus shot, your arm may get swollen, red, and warm to the touch at the site of the shot. This is a normal reaction to the medicine.

Call Your Doctor If . . .
- The pain or swelling gets worse.
- The injured finger is cold when the others are warm.
- The finger becomes swollen and very red.
- The finger turns white or blue.
- The finger is numb or tingling.

Broken Foot

WHAT YOU SHOULD KNOW

A break in one or more bones of the foot, including the injury known as a subtalar (sub-TAY-lar) fracture, can be very painful. Healing time ranges from several weeks to a couple of months. An x-ray will show when the fracture has healed and you can resume normal activity.

Causes
This type of fracture is usually caused by a fall or an object that lands on the foot.

Signs/Symptoms
You are likely to suffer pain, swelling, bruising and weakness of the foot. It may tingle or feel numb. If the bones are broken badly, they may look misshapen. You may be unable to walk.

Care
Your doctor will probably take an x-ray of the foot. You may need to wear a cast or splint on the foot, depending on how bad the break is, and will have to use crutches for a while. If you scraped or tore your skin and haven't had a tetanus shot in 5 to 10 years, you may need a booster.

WHAT YOU SHOULD DO

If you are not given a cast or splint:
- Use crutches and avoid putting any weight on the injured foot until

your doctor gives the okay. Then slowly increase the amount of time that you use the foot, stopping as soon as it begins to feel painful.
- After the first 1 to 2 days, you may apply heat to the injury to help relieve pain. Use a warm heating pad, whirlpool bath, or warm, moist towels for 15 to 20 minutes every hour for 48 hours.

If you are given a cast or splint:
- Use crutches until your doctor says they are no longer needed.
- To reduce swelling, keep your foot on pillows while lying down and on a chair or footstool when sitting. Keep the foot above the level of your heart, if possible.
- Apply ice to the injury for 15 to 20 minutes each hour for the first 1 to 2 days. Put the ice in a plastic bag and place a thin towel between the bag of ice and your cast.
- If you are given a plaster or fiberglass cast:
  —Do not try to scratch the skin under the cast by pushing a sharp or pointed object between the cast and your foot.
  —Check the skin around the cast every day. You may put lotion on any red or sore areas.
  —If you have a fiberglass cast and it gets a little wet, it can be dried with a hair dryer.
- If you are given a plaster splint:
  —Wear the splint until your doctor says you may remove it.
  —You may loosen the ace wrap around the splint if your toes become numb or start tingling.
- Do not put pressure or lean on any part of your cast or splint. It may break.
- Keep the cast or splint dry. It can be covered with a plastic bag during bathing. Do not lower it into water.

You may use acetaminophen or ibuprofen to relieve pain and swelling. Take all medicines as directed by your doctor. If you feel the medicine is not helping, call your doctor, but do not stop taking it on your own.

If you have been given a tetanus shot, your arm may be red, swollen, and painful at the site of the injection. This is a normal reaction to the medicine in the shot.

Call Your Doctor If . . .
- The cast gets damaged or breaks.
- The pain gets worse or you have more swelling than before the cast was put on.
- The skin or toenails below the injury turn blue or gray, or feel cold or numb.

• The cast develops a bad odor.
• There are new stains coming from under the cast.

Broken Hand

WHAT YOU SHOULD KNOW

Hand fractures can involve a single broken bone or several of them. When the bone next to the little finger is broken, the injury is sometimes called a "Boxer's fracture." This kind of damage is often seen in people who punch walls and those who fight without boxing gloves. Healing of the broken bone(s) usually takes 6 to 8 weeks. An x-ray will show when the fracture has completely mended.

Causes

The usual cause is sudden impact on the hand during a fall or accident. Boxer's fractures occur when the hand hits something while closed into a fist.

Signs/Symptoms

Likely symptoms include swelling, pain, bruising, or bleeding in the injured part of the hand. Your hand may feel weak, numb, or tingly. If the break pushes some bones out of place, the hand may look misshapen. If you scratched or tore some skin, you may need a tetanus shot.

Care

Your doctor may order an x-ray. You may also need a splint or a cast to keep the broken bone(s) in place. Surgery may be required for a bad fracture.

WHAT YOU SHOULD DO

• To reduce swelling, keep the injured hand above the level of your heart as much as possible.
• Apply ice to the injury for 15 to 20 minutes each hour for the first 1 to 2 days. Put the ice in a plastic bag and place a thin towel between the bag of ice and your cast.
• Move the fingers of your casted hand several times a day. This will reduce swelling and keep the hand from getting stiff.
• If you have a plaster or fiberglass cast:
  —Do not try to scratch the skin under the cast by pushing a sharp or pointed object down the cast.
  —Check the skin around the cast every day. You may put lotion on any red or sore areas.

—If your fiberglass cast gets a little wet, it can be dried off with a hair dryer.
- If you have a plaster splint:
  —Wear the splint until your doctor says you may take it off or until your follow-up examination.
  —You should loosen the elastic around the splint if your fingers become numb or tingling.
- Do not push down or lean on any part of your cast or splint. It may break.
- Keep your cast or splint dry. To protect it during bathing, cover it with a plastic bag secured with tape or a loose rubber band. Do not lower the cast or splint into water.
- Always take your medicine exactly as directed. If you feel it is not helping, call your doctor.
- If the doctor prescribes pain medicine that makes you drowsy, don't drive. You also may use over-the-counter medicines for pain. Take all medications exactly as directed.
- If you are given a tetanus shot, your arm may get swollen, red, and warm to the touch at the site of the shot. This is a normal reaction to the medicine.

Call Your Doctor If . . .
- Your cast gets damaged or breaks.
- You have really bad pain that does not go away.
- You have more swelling than you did before the cast was put on.
- The skin or fingernails of the casted hand turn blue or gray, or feel cold or numb.
- There is a bad smell coming from your cast.
- There are new stains coming from under the cast.

Broken Jaw

WHAT YOU SHOULD KNOW

Jaw fractures occur in the lower jaw, also known as the mandible (MAN-dih-bull). The jaw bone may take weeks or months to heal. An x-ray will show when the broken bone has knitted.

Causes
Most jaw fractures are sustained in accidents.

Signs/Symptoms
There will be swelling, pain, bruising, or bleeding in the area of the

break. You also may have pain in front of your ear and trouble opening your mouth.

Care

Your jaws will probably be wired together to keep the bones in place. Surgery may be necessary if you have a bad fracture.

WHAT YOU SHOULD DO

- If your jaws are wired together, learn how to cut the wire quickly in case you throw up or have a really bad coughing attack. Keep wire cutters handy at all times.
- Apply ice to the injury for 15 to 20 minutes each hour for the first 1 to 2 days. Put the ice in a plastic bag and place a towel between the bag of ice and your skin.
- After the first 1 to 2 days, you may put heat on the injury to help ease the pain. Use a warm heating pad (set on low), whirlpool bath, or warm, moist towels for 15 to 20 minutes every hour for 48 hours.
- You will be able to take nothing but liquids while your jaw is wired. Drink high-protein nutritional supplements until the jaw has healed.
- Do not push on your jaw or allow anything else to push on it. Sleep on your back.
- Do not exercise so hard that you must pant for breath.
- You may take over-the-counter medicines to ease the pain. Always take medications exactly as directed.

Call Your Doctor If . . .
- You develop a high temperature, a severe headache, or loss of feeling in your face.
- You have really bad jaw pain that does not go away with medicine.
- The wires or splints become loose.

Seek Care Immediately If . . .
- You have trouble breathing.

Broken Leg

WHAT YOU SHOULD KNOW

A break can occur in any of several different bones and can take a variety of forms. Healing time depends on the location and nature of the fracture, and can take from weeks to months.

Causes
A fall or accident is almost always the cause.

Signs/Symptoms

You'll experience pain, swelling, bruising, and possibly bleeding. The leg may be weak or numb, or may tingle. It may look injured or out of alignment. You may have difficulty moving it, or may not be able to move it at all.

Care

The doctor will probably need to put a cast or a splint on the leg to keep the bones from moving. A serious fracture may need surgery.

WHAT YOU SHOULD DO

- To reduce the swelling, keep the injured leg on pillows while lying down and on a stool when sitting.
- Apply ice to the injury for 15 to 20 minutes each hour for the first 1 to 2 days. Put the ice in a plastic bag and place a thin towel between the bag of ice and your cast.
- If you have a plaster or fiberglass cast:
  —Do not try to scratch the skin under the cast by pushing a sharp or pointed object down the cast.
  —Check the skin around the cast every day. You may put lotion on any red or sore areas.
  —If your fiberglass cast gets a little wet, it can be dried with a hair dryer.
- If you have a plaster splint:
  —Wear the splint for as long as directed or until your follow-up examination.
  —You may loosen the elastic around the splint if your toes become numb or begin to tingle.
- Do not put pressure on any part of the cast or splint; it may break.
- Keep the cast or splint dry. During bathing, protect it with a plastic bag. Do not lower it into water.
- If your doctor prescribes pain medication, take no more than directed. If the medication makes you drowsy, don't drive. You may also use over-the-counter pain killers.

Seek Care Immediately If . . .

- Your cast gets damaged or breaks.
- You have continued severe pain or more increased swelling.
- The skin or toenails below the injury turn blue or gray, or feel cold or numb.
- There is a bad smell coming from the cast.
- There are new stains coming from under the cast.

Broken Nose

WHAT YOU SHOULD KNOW

A small fracture of the bone in your nose will usually heal in about a month. A really bad break may need surgery after the swelling is gone.

Causes
Any blow to the nose can cause a break. The injury is typically sustained during athletics or in a fall.

Signs/Symptoms
Swelling, pain, bruising, and bleeding can be expected. Your face may feel numb or tingle. If the break has pushed the bones out of place, the nose may seem out of shape.

Care
If you have a bad break, you will probably need an x-ray, and surgery may be necessary. X-rays often fail to detect a nasal fracture, so the doctor may delay them for 1 to 4 days after the injury, or until the swelling has gone down. The nose is usually filled with cotton packing, and you may have to wear a splint over the top of your nose for protection during the healing process. If skin was scratched or torn during the accident, you may also have to get a tetanus shot.

WHAT YOU SHOULD DO

- Apply ice to the injury for 15 to 20 minutes each hour for the first 1 to 2 days. Put the ice in a plastic bag and place a towel between the bag of ice and your skin.
- When you lie down, rest your head on 2 or 3 pillows so it is above the level of your heart. This will help reduce pain and swelling.
- Always take your medicine as directed. Over-the-counter medications may be taken for pain.
- If you are given a tetanus shot, your arm may get swollen, red, and warm to the touch at the injection site. This is a normal reaction to the medicine.
- If you are given a splint for your nose, try to keep it dry and do not remove it until your doctor gives the go-ahead.
- You may be allowed to take the splint off to shower. Ask your doctor whether this is okay.

Call Your Doctor If . . .
- The pain gets worse or you keep having nosebleeds.

Seek Care Immediately If . . .
- You have bleeding from the nose that does not stop after 10 minutes with the nostrils pinched closed.
- You see clear fluid draining from the nose.
- You notice a grape-like swelling on the septum (the wall between the nostrils). This is a collection of blood that must be drained to keep the nose from becoming infected.

Broken Shoulder Blade

WHAT YOU SHOULD KNOW

The large, flat bones in your back known as shoulder blades (scapula) rarely get fractured. If a break does occur, it is usually accompanied by other injuries. The broken shoulder blade may take from 6 to 8 weeks to knit. At that time, your doctor may want to take an x-ray to see if the bone is healed.

Causes
An accident is usually to blame—especially a car or motorcycle accident.

Signs/Symptoms
Typically, you'll have swelling, pain, bruising, or bleeding in the injured area. Your shoulder or arm may feel weak, numb, or tingly. The break may push some bones out of place and make the shoulder look misshapen.

Care
Your doctor may order an x-ray, and you may need a splint or sling to prevent you from moving your shoulder and twisting the bones out of place. Surgery may be necessary if you have a bad fracture. If you scratched or tore some skin, you may also need a tetanus shot.

WHAT YOU SHOULD DO

- Apply ice to the injury for 15 to 20 minutes each hour for the first 1 to 2 days. Put the ice in a plastic bag and place a thin towel between the bag of ice and your skin or the splint.
- After the first 1 to 2 days, you may put heat on the injury to help lessen the pain. Use a heating pad (set on low), whirlpool bath, or warm, moist towels for 15 to 20 minutes every hour for 48 hours.
- Wear your sling until your doctor says you may take it off or until your follow-up examination.

—You may take off the sling to dress or bathe, but be careful not to move your arm.

—Never lift your arm.

• If the doctor prescribes pain medicine that makes you drowsy, don't drive. You also may take over-the-counter medicines for pain. Take all medications exactly as directed.

• If you are given a tetanus shot, your arm may get swollen, red, and warm to the touch at the site of the shot. This is a normal reaction to the medicine.

Call Your Doctor If . . .

• Pain and swelling gets worse.

• Your arm becomes numb, pale, or cold.

Seek Care Immediately If . . .

• You have pain in your chest, trouble breathing, cough, or fever.

Broken Toe

WHAT YOU SHOULD KNOW

When you break a toe, fractures can occur in one or more of the bones. Healing usually takes 3 to 6 weeks. If you still have pain at this time, you may need an x-ray to see how the toe is healing.

Causes

These injuries are almost always the result of an accident or fall.

Signs/Symptoms

It will probably hurt to walk. Other possible symptoms include swelling, pain, bruising, bleeding, weakness, numbness, or tingling of the injured toe. Because the break may move some bones out of place, the toe may look misshapen.

Care

Your doctor may order an x-ray and may give you a splint or a cast shoe to keep the bones of the toe in place. A cast shoe should make it easier to walk. Surgery may be necessary if you have a bad fracture. If you scratched or tore some skin, you may also need a tetanus shot.

WHAT YOU SHOULD DO

• If your toes are taped together, leave them that way until your doctor says you can remove the tape, or until your follow-up examination.

You can change the tape after bathing. Always use a small piece of cotton between the toes when taping them together.

- To reduce swelling, keep your foot lifted above the level of your heart as much as possible. Lie down and prop your foot up on some pillows.
- Apply ice to the injury for 15 to 20 minutes each hour for the first 1 to 2 days. Put the ice in a plastic bag and place a thin towel between the bag of ice and your cast.
- Your doctor may have you wear a cast shoe if your foot is very swollen. If not, wear sturdy, supportive shoes.
- You may use over-the-counter medicines to relieve the pain. Always take medications exactly as directed.
- If you are given a tetanus shot, your arm may get swollen, red, and warm to the touch at the site of the shot. This is a normal reaction to the medicine.

Call Your Doctor If . . .
- The pain or swelling gets worse.
- The injured toe is cold when the others are warm.
- The toe becomes very swollen or red.
- The toe turns white or blue.

Seek Care Immediately If . . .
- The toe feels numb or tingly.

Bronchiolitis

WHAT YOU SHOULD KNOW

Bronchiolitis (bronk-ee-o-LIE-tis) is an infection of the airways in the lungs. The infected airways swell and cause trouble breathing. The disease is common in winter and early spring. Children less than 18 months old are more likely to get bronchiolitis.

Antibiotics will not work, but other medicines can be given to help the child feel better. The child may be sick for 2 to 7 days and get better in 10 to 14 days. Most children won't get bronchiolitis more than once.

Causes
Bronchiolitis begins with a cold—sneezing and a runny nose.

Signs/Symptoms
The child may have fever, cough, and trouble breathing. He or she may wheeze (a noise heard when breathing in and out) for 7 days and cough for 14 days. The child may seem more tired than usual.

Ear infections are common with bronchiolitis. Signs of an ear infection are ear tugging, ear pain, and fever. Call your doctor if any of these occur.

Risks

Children can die from bronchiolitis. But the risks of serious illness or death are very small if you follow your doctor's directions.

WHAT YOU SHOULD DO

- If you have a humidifier, run it in the child's room, out of reach of the bed. Fill it with cool water. Direct the mist stream towards your child's face. Using the humidifier will help loosen the sputum in your child's throat, making it easier to breathe.
- Hanging wrung-out wet towels or sheets in your child's room will also add moisture to the air.
- Extra bed pillows will raise your child's head and make breathing easier.
- Once the breathing is easier, keep the child warm and give clear liquids (water, apple juice, lemonade, tea, or ginger ale). The liquids should be room temperature. Giving plenty of liquids will keep the child's sputum thin.
- Keep the child's nose mucus-free. Gently use a rubber bulb suction device to remove the mucus.
- You should try to stay calm and have your child rest as much as possible. If children are afraid and crying, their breathing problems and coughing will get worse. It may help to have the child sleep in the same room with you, where he or she will feel safer.
- Do not let anyone smoke near the child. Smoke can make the child's coughing and breathing problems worse.
- If the child has a high fever, give acetaminophen, **Not** aspirin.

Call Your Doctor If . . .

- Your child is more sleepy than usual, is urinating less, has a dry mouth and cracked lips, cries without tears, or is dizzy. These are signs of dehydration.
- The child has a high temperature.
- The child is tugging his or her ears, has ear pain, or fever.

Seek Care Immediately If . . .

- **Call 911 or 0 (operator)** for help if your child has any of the following signs: trouble breathing or swallowing, the skin between the ribs is being sucked-in with each breath, or the lips or fingernails are turning blue or white.

What to Expect While You're There

You may encounter the following procedures and equipment during your child's stay.

- **Taking Vital Signs:** These include the child's temperature, blood pressure, pulse (counting heartbeats), and respirations (counting breaths). A stethoscope is used to listen to the heart and lungs. Blood pressure is taken by wrapping a cuff around the child's arm.
- **Pulse Oximeter:** The child may be hooked up to a pulse oximeter (ox-IM-uh-ter). It is placed on the ear, finger, or toe and is connected to a machine that measures the oxygen in your child's blood.
- **Oxygen:** The child will probably be placed in a clear plastic mist tent. This will help make breathing easier. Oxygen also may be given using nasal prongs or a face mask.
- **Breathing Treatments:** A machine will be used to help the child inhale medicine that keeps the airways open. A doctor will assist with these treatments. At first, they may be needed quite often. Later, they may be needed only if the child is having trouble breathing.
- **IV:** A tube placed in your child's veins for giving medicine or liquids. It will be capped or have tubing connected to it. Encourage your child to drink liquids when the IV is removed.
- **Chest X-ray:** This is a picture of the heart and lungs. The doctor uses it to see how your child's heart and lungs are handling the illness.
- **Blood:** Is usually taken from a vein in your child's hand or from the bend in the elbow. Tests are done on the blood.
- **Blood Gases:** Blood is taken from an artery in your child's wrist, elbow, or groin. It is tested to see how much oxygen it contains.
- **ECG:** Also called a heart monitor, an electrocardiograph (e-lec-tro-CAR-dee-o-graf), or EKG. The patches on your child's chest are hooked up to a TV-type screen. This screen shows a tracing of each heartbeat. Your child's heart will be watched for signs of injury or damage that could be related to the illness.
- **Visiting:** You may stay with the child to give comfort and support. Your child will feel safer in the hospital with you nearby.

After You Leave

- Little can be done to keep your child from getting a cold that can cause bronchiolitis, but try to avoid anyone who has a cold. Wash your hands often with soap to try to avoid spreading infection.
- If the child does get a cold, use a cool mist humidifier in his or her room.

• If the child develops another case of bronchiolitis, follow the guidelines under "What You Should Do," above.

Bronchitis, Acute

See Acute Bronchitis

Bronchitis, Chronic

See Chronic Bronchitis

Bronchoscopy

WHAT YOU SHOULD KNOW

Your doctor can examine the inside of your windpipe and bronchial tubes by passing a soft instrument through your nose or mouth into your lungs. This procedure is called a bronchoscopy (bron-KOS-ko-pee). Tissue may be removed through the instrument for tests in the lab.

Risks
There is a chance of injury to your throat, windpipe, or bronchial tubes. You might also bleed (hemorrhage), get an infection, or develop heart or lung problems. However, these problems are unlikely if you follow your doctor's directions.

IF YOU'RE HEADING FOR THE HOSPITAL . . .

Before You Go
• Your doctor will tell you when you must stop eating or drinking. Follow these directions exactly.
• You will need to remove earrings, necklaces, and other jewelry before the test.
• If you wear glasses, contact lenses, or false teeth, take them off just before the test.

What to Expect While You're There
You may encounter the following procedures and equipment during your stay:
• **Taking Your Vital Signs:** These include your temperature, blood pressure, pulse (counting your heartbeats), and respirations (counting your breaths). A stethoscope is used to listen to your heart and lungs. Your blood pressure is taken by wrapping a cuff around your arm.
• **Pulse Oximeter:** You may be hooked up to a pulse oximeter (ox-

IM-uh-ter). It is placed on your ear, finger, or toe and is connected to a machine that measures the oxygen in your blood.
• **IV:** A tube placed in your vein for giving medicine or liquids. It will be capped or have tubing connected to it.
• **During the Bronchoscopy . . .**
   —The test will take about an hour. You will be asked to lie down with a pillow under your head. Your doctor will put numbing medicine in your throat to prevent coughing or gagging.
   —Your doctor will gently pass the bronchoscope (BRON-ko-scope)—a small tube with a light and lenses on the tip—through your mouth or nose and down your throat and windpipe.
   —You may need to breathe through your nose if the tube is in your mouth. If the tube is in your nose, breathe through your mouth. You will get oxygen to help you breathe. Your throat may get dry. You will not be able to talk during the procedure.
   —Your doctor will look closely at your windpipe and the small tubes leading to your lungs. A sample of your tissue or sputum may be sent to the lab for tests.
   —You will be carefully watched for complications for a while after the test.

After You Leave
• The medicine given during the test will make you sleepy; do not drive for 12 hours after your test.
• You may resume normal activities as soon as you feel up to it.
• You may begin drinking or eating approximately 4 hours after the procedure.
• Take throat lozenges or gargle with salt water if your throat is sore. Taking liquids will help eliminate any dryness in your mouth or throat.

Call Your Doctor If . . .
• You have a high temperature.

Seek Care Immediately If . . .
• You begin to cough up blood.
• You have breathing problems or start wheezing.
• You develop chest pain.

Brown Recluse Spider Bite

WHAT YOU SHOULD KNOW

The brown recluse spider, sometimes called a "fiddle back" spider, is light tan to dark brown in color and has a dark violin-shaped mark on its back. It is about the size of a quarter; walks on long, thin legs; and hides in dark, dry, warm places like a closet or woodpile. When it gets trapped under bed sheets or in your clothing, it can deliver a serious bite.

Signs/Symptoms

You're likely to suffer itching, redness, rash, blister, pain, or swelling in the area of skin where you were bitten. You may also become nauseated; vomit; perspire; and develop a headache, chills, or fever.

Care

Unless the bite area gets worse or other symptoms arise, follow the directions below. You may also need medicine for an infection, pain, swelling, or itching.

WHAT YOU SHOULD DO

- Wash the skin where you were bitten with soap and water.
- Apply an ice pack or cool compress several times a day for 24 to 48 hours. To help reduce redness and swelling, keep the bite area raised above the level of your heart. DO NOT use heat.
- Soak the area daily in Burow's solution (available in drug stores without a prescription).
- Do not scratch the bite area. Keep it clean and covered with an adhesive or sterile gauze bandage.
- To avoid another spider bite:
  —Remove wood piles and other rubbish from outside areas.
  —Thoroughly clean closets, sheds, and attics.
  —Wear gloves, shoes, and long sleeves and pants when doing such chores.
  —Shake out clothing (especially old clothing) and shoes before putting them on.
  —Look for spiders under the sheets before getting into bed.
  —To frighten spiders away, make noise when entering attics or other spaces where they may be living.
  —Chemical pest control may be necessary. However, it doesn't always work.
- If you have been given a tetanus shot, your arm may get swollen, red, and warm to the touch at the site of the injection. This is a normal response to the medicine in the shot.

Call Your Doctor If . . .

- Your symptoms do not improve in a few hours.

• You have increasing pain to the bite area (even though it may not look worse).

Seek Care Immediately If . . .
• The bite area appears to be getting bigger (more than 1/4 inch) or growing deeper.
• You have a high temperature; chills; nausea; vomiting; muscle aches; weakness; extreme tiredness; seizures; or a measles-like or red, raised rash.
• You have blood in your urine or any other unusual bleeding.
• Your skin turns yellow.

Bruises

WHAT YOU SHOULD KNOW

A bruise, known medically as a contusion (cun-TOO-shun) or hematoma (HE-muh-TOE-muh) is an injury that does not break the skin. A bruise may take 2 or 3 weeks to heal.

Causes
A blow that breaks small blood vessels under the skin.

Signs/Symptoms
Bleeding under the skin causes it to turn black and blue. As the bruise heals the skin color changes from purple to green to yellow. Bruises may be accompanied by pain or swelling.

Care
Wrapping the injury with an ace wrap may slow the bleeding under the skin. If the bruise is really bad, you may need a splint to keep the area from moving during the healing process.

WHAT YOU SHOULD DO

• You may continue your normal daily activities, but you should rest the injured area for a few days.
• Apply ice to the injury for 15 to 20 minutes each hour for the first 1 to 2 days. Put the ice in a plastic bag and place a towel between the bag of ice and your skin.
• After the first 1 to 2 days, you may put heat on the injury to help ease the pain. Use a heating pad (set on low), a whirlpool bath, or warm, moist towels for 15 to 20 minutes every hour for 48 hours.
• For 48 hours, keep the injury lifted above the level of your heart whenever possible to reduce pain and swelling.

- If you have a splint, wear it until your doctor says you may take it off or until your follow-up visit. If the fingers or toes near the bruise become numb or tingly, you may need to loosen the splint. Call your doctor for instructions if you are not sure how.
- You may use over-the-counter medicines to relieve the pain. Always take as directed.

Call Your Doctor If . . .
- The pain becomes worse.
- You develop a high temperature.
- The swelling around the bruise gets worse.
- You see redness or red lines near the bruise.

Burn Care

WHAT YOU SHOULD KNOW

You can sustain a burn from heat, electricity, chemicals, or radiation —including sunlight. Most burns heal in 1 to 3 weeks.

Signs/Symptoms
There are three degrees of severity, each with distinctive symptoms:
- First-degree burns are mild and injure only the outer layer of skin. The skin becomes red, but will turn white when touched. The area may also be painful to the touch.
- Second-degree burns are deeper, more severe, and very painful. Blisters may form on the burned area. This type of burn takes about 2 weeks to heal.
- Third-degree burns are the deepest and most serious kind. The skin becomes white and leathery, but it does not feel very tender when touched.

There may be swelling in the burned area. Serious burns may be accompanied by headache, fever, and dizziness.

Care
Your doctor may prescribe an antibiotic ointment. Use it as directed, and follow the first-aid steps outlined below. If the burn is severe, you may need to be hospitalized to avoid infection and receive special care.

WHAT YOU SHOULD DO

- Soak the burned area in cold water for 10 minutes.
- Gently wash the burn with warm, soapy water. Pat it dry with a clean towel, and cover it with a clean, dry bandage.

- You will need to clean the burn and put on new bandages several times a day. Be sure that everything that touches the burn is clean. Only use the burn medicine prescribed by your doctor. When changing bandages:
  —Wash your hands well with soap and water. Dry them with a clean towel.
  —Remove the outer bandage by cutting it off with a pair of scissors. Do not pull off the bandage if it is sticking to the burn. Instead, soak it in warm water for a few minutes and then remove it slowly.
  —Gently wash the burn with warm, soapy water. Use a clean, soft washcloth to help remove any old cream, blood, and loose skin. Do not break blisters. This may increase the pain.
  —Rinse the burn with clear warm water. Pat dry with a clean towel.
  —With a clean tongue depressor, apply the antibiotic ointment prescribed by your doctor to a gauze pad in a thin layer. Throw the tongue depressor away when you're done. Do NOT put it back in the container of ointment.
  —Cover the burn with the gauze. Be careful not to touch the gauze that comes in contact with the burn. Carefully rewrap the burn with a clean bandage as directed by your doctor.
- Keep the bandage clean and dry. Change it if it gets wet.
- If the burn is on your arm or leg, keep it raised or propped up for the first 24 hours to help reduce swelling.
- You may use aspirin, acetaminophen, or ibuprofen for pain.
- Do not bump or overuse the burned area.
- Drink plenty of water or juice to prevent dehydration.
- To avoid getting burned, follow these guidelines:
  —Wear sunscreen when you are out in the sun.
  —Wear protective clothing and follow safety rules when you are working with heat or radiation.
  —Teach your children not to play with matches or touch the stove (even when it is not on).
  —Throw away frayed electrical cords. Have an electrician fix all faulty or bad electrical wiring in your house.
  —Do not touch uncovered electrical wires or outlets.
  —Test bath water before getting into a bathtub or putting your child in one.
  —Do not set your hot water heater too high. Usually the dial should be set in the middle between hot and cold.
  —Do not smoke in bed.

Call Your Doctor If . . .

- You have increasing pain and redness in the burned area or bad-smelling drainage from the burn. These are signs of infection.
- You develop a high temperature.

Seek Care Immediately If . . .

- You develop swelling, numbness, or tingling below a burn on your arm or leg.

Burn Prevention

WHAT YOU SHOULD KNOW

Burns can result from contact with heat, chemicals, electricity, or radiation. They can damage not only the skin, but other organs. They are most common in young children.

WHAT YOU SHOULD DO

Here are some tips and reminders that will protect your children from burns:

- Don't hold a baby when you are cooking or drinking anything hot. The baby may grab for it and get burned if it spills.
- Keep coffee pots, irons, hot foods, and boiling water away from the edge of the table or stove.
- Turn pot handles toward the back of the stove so children can't reach them.
- Never open the oven door with a child nearby.
- Before putting your child into the bathtub, check the water temperature with your wrist.
- Don't let children touch the faucet handles in the bathtub. They may turn on the hot water and get burned. **Never** leave a baby or young child alone in a tub.
- Lower your hot water heater setting to low or medium (130 degrees F).
- Use a cool mist humidifier instead of a steam vaporizer.
- Put fireplace screens or guards around fireplaces, furnaces, or radiators. Keep space heaters out of your child's reach. Don't leave a child alone around fires of any kind.
- Make sure your child's pajamas are flame-resistant.
- If you smoke, don't leave lit cigarettes unattended. Dispose of them properly. Keep cigarette lighters and matches in a safe place where children can't reach them.
- Install smoke detectors. Check them on a regular basis to make sure

they are still working. Teach your children the best way to get out of the house in a fire.

- Lock up liquids that may catch on fire, such as gasoline or kerosene. Leave them in the container that they came in and label them.
- Before putting a child in a car seat, check the temperature of the seat, especially any metal parts. Cover the car seat with a towel when you park in the sun.
- Allow only older children to use fireworks and only with adult supervision.
- Keep children away from electrical cords. Replace frayed cords. Cover unused electrical outlets with childproof covers (available in hardware stores and baby departments).
- Test the temperature of infant food heated in a microwave oven before feeding it to a baby.
- To prevent sunburn, always apply sunscreen to children before going out in the sun.

Burns, Corneal

See Corneal Flash Burns

Burns, Electrical

See Electrical Burns

Bursitis

WHAT YOU SHOULD KNOW

Bursitis (bur-SIGH-tis) is swelling and irritation of a bursa—one of the fluid-filled sacs that act as shock absorbers between the tendons and bones. The joints most likely to be affected are the knees, hips, shoulders, and elbows. With treatment, symptoms disappear in 7 to 14 days.

Causes
Injury and overuse of the joint are the most common causes. The problem can also stem from infection, arthritis, or gout. Sometimes the cause is unknown.

Signs/Symptoms
Typically, you'll suffer pain, swelling, tenderness, and loss of movement in the affected joint. These symptoms are sometimes accompanied by fever.

Care

Your doctor may prescribe medication. Use it as directed and follow the guidelines listed below.

WHAT YOU SHOULD DO

- Apply ice to the injury for 10 to 20 minutes each hour for the first 1 to 2 days. Put the ice in a plastic bag and place a towel between the bag of ice and your skin.
- After the first day or two, you may apply heat to the joint to help relieve pain. Use a warm heating pad, whirlpool bath, or warm, moist towels for 10 to 20 minutes every hour for 48 hours.
- Rest the injured joint as much as possible. When the pain decreases, begin normal, slow movements.

Call Your Doctor If . . .

- Your pain increases during treatment.
- You develop a high temperature.

CAD

See Coronary Artery Disease

Candidiasis

WHAT YOU SHOULD KNOW

Also known as a yeast infection, vaginal candidiasis (can-dih-DYE-ah-sis) is a very common infection of the vagina that causes discharge, itching, and swelling. It is not serious and, with treatment, usually goes away in about 2 weeks. Many women get more repeated yeast infections.

Causes

The infection is caused by a type of yeast or fungus called Candida. This yeast lives in your mouth, vagina, and rectum all the time; but it sometimes gets out of control and causes an infection. Women who are pregnant or have trouble with their blood sugar (diabetes) can easily get a yeast infection. Medicines like birth control pills or antibiotics also make the infection more likely.

Signs/Symptoms

The main symptom is a thick white discharge from the vagina that may look like cottage cheese and may have a bad smell. Swelling, redness, and itching around the vagina are common. Some women may feel burning when they urinate.

Care

Your doctor will examine you and take a sample of the discharge. You will probably need medicine to kill the yeast. If you are given yeast medicine, use it until it is all gone, even if the condition improves. The medicine is usually given as a cream or suppository that you put inside your vagina.

WHAT YOU SHOULD DO

- Always use your medicine as directed by your doctor. If you feel it is not helping, call your doctor. Do not quit using it on your own.
- If you are using medicine to kill the yeast, it may be messy. Use a thin sanitary pad to protect your clothing.
- Wear clean cotton underpants or pantyhose with a cotton crotch.
- Keep the vaginal area clean and dry.
- Don't have sex until your symptoms are gone.
- Take showers instead of tub baths. Use plain, unscented soap.
- Don't use feminine hygiene sprays or powders or bubble bath. Don't douche during treatment unless your doctor tells you to. After the infection is cleared up, don't douche more often than once a week.
- To help keep from getting more yeast infections, don't eat a lot of sweets or drink alcohol. Don't take antibiotic medicine unless you have to. Wipe from front to back after urinating or having a bowel movement.

Call Your Doctor If . . .

- Your symptoms get worse or last more than a few days.
- You have vaginal bleeding that is not during your period.
- Your symptoms come back after treatment.

Canker Sores

WHAT YOU SHOULD KNOW

Canker sores, also called aphthous (AF-thus) ulcers, may appear singly or in groups on your inner lips, gums, inner cheeks, or tongue. Although they are painful, they are not harmful. They usually heal within 2 weeks, but they often come back.

Causes

The cause of canker sores is unknown. However, an infection, stress, changes before a woman's monthly period (PMS), food (such as pickles or potato chips), rough dentures, braces, or tooth brushing may bring on an attack.

Signs/Symptoms

The sores are small, painful, gray-colored spots that are circled in red. For 2 or 3 days, you may experience pain when you eat or speak.

Care

There is no cure for canker sores. Some medicines can ease the pain. Follow your doctor's advice for caring for your mouth. You may need to have your dentures or braces adjusted if they are causing the sores.

WHAT YOU SHOULD DO

- The following nonprescription medicines may help reduce the pain.
  - **Medicines and lozenges** to numb and protect the sores. Follow the directions on the label.
  - **Milk of magnesia.** 3 or 4 times a day, swish a small amount in your mouth for several minutes, then spit it out.
  - **Aspirin or acetaminophen.**
- Keep your mouth clean by brushing your teeth and rinsing your mouth after meals and at bedtime. Rinse with a mixture of 1/2 water and 1/2 hydrogen peroxide.
- You may clean the sore spots with a cotton swab dipped in a solution of 1/2 water and 1/2 hydrogen peroxide.
- Cold or cool liquids may be soothing and help numb pain. Do not drink citrus and carbonated drinks (for instance, orange juice, grapefruit juice, lemonade, soda). Drinking through a straw may be helpful.
- Soft foods such as gelatin, ice cream, yogurt, custard, applesauce, pudding, and mashed potatoes will irritate the mouth less than salty, spicy, or acidic foods (such as tomatoes).
- Avoid hard-edged foods such as potato chips. If the hard edges touch the sores, it could be painful.

Call Your Doctor If . . .

- You develop a high temperature.
- The pain is unbearable and none of the above suggestions helps.
- You get more than 4 canker sores at a time.
- The sores are not better in 5 to 6 days.
- You cannot eat or drink because of the pain.

Carbon Monoxide Poisoning

You cannot see, taste, or smell carbon monoxide gas, yet prolonged exposure to it can be deadly. Carbon monoxide can build up without warning in closed spaces like your house, car, tent, camper, or garage, and may be present at indoor automobile events like a tractor pull.

Causes
Carbon monoxide is produced by kerosene heaters, broken furnaces, auto engines, and gas fireplaces. It can also come from charcoal, Sterno, wood, or coal stoves, and is found in smoke from any kind of fire. It works its damage by preventing oxygen from moving from your lungs into the red blood cells.

Signs/Symptoms
Symptoms of carbon monoxide poisoning include headache, upset stomach, vomiting, chest pain, and heart palpitations. You may feel confused, sleepy, dizzy, or faint. You also could begin stumbling or slurring your speech. Blurred vision, trouble breathing, and seizures are also possible.

Care
Get into fresh air as soon as possible. Call your local Poison Control Center, doctor, or emergency department. The doctors there can tell you if you need to see someone for special care. You may also need extra oxygen and medicine to relieve your headache.

• If there is carbon monoxide in your home, do not go back into the house until the source of the gas is repaired. Air out the house before you go back in, no matter how cold it is outside.
• If your car is the source of carbon monoxide, have the exhaust fixed immediately.
• Have your gas company check your furnace every year before you turn it on for the season. If it stays on all the time, have it checked every year anyway.
• Before starting up a kerosene heater, gas fireplace, or charcoal, wood, or coal stove, have it checked to make sure it's working properly. When using a heater or stove, be sure to keep a window slightly open to let fresh air in.
• Do not allow your children to ride in the back of a pickup truck that

has a cover (cap) over the truck bed. Carbon monoxide can build up to deadly levels under these caps.

• Buy several carbon monoxide detectors and install them in your home.

Seek Care Immediately If . . .

• You think you're developing symptoms of carbon monoxide poisoning.

Caries, Dental

See Toothache

Carpal Tunnel Syndrome

WHAT YOU SHOULD KNOW

Carpal tunnel syndrome occurs when the median nerve leading from the arm to the hand gets pinched as it passes through the carpal tunnel, a narrow, hollow area in the wrist. One or both hands can be affected.

Causes

Pressure on the median nerve is often the result of the swelling caused by a wrist injury, arthritis, diabetes, or water retention during pregnancy and menopause. Repetitive action such as using power tools may make the problem worse.

Signs/Symptoms

You'll experience loss of feeling in part of the hand, usually in the thumb, index, and middle fingers. Pain in the wrist and palm is sometimes accompanied by a sharp pain that shoots from the wrist up the arm, especially at night. Other symptoms include stiffness of the wrist in the morning, cramping of the hands, inability to make a fist, weakness in the thumb, a feeling of burning in the fingers, and a tendency to drop things.

Care

The problem may clear up on its own. Wearing a splint on the wrist will help; and your doctor can prescribe medications to reduce the pressure on the nerve. Sometimes, however, surgery is needed to free the pinched nerve.

WHAT YOU SHOULD DO

- If your doctor prescribes medication to help reduce swelling, take it exactly as directed.
- If your doctor recommends a splint to keep your wrist from bending, it is especially important to leave it on at night. Wear it as long as you have pain and numbness in your hand—from 1 to 2 months.
- If you have pain at night, it may help to rub or shake your hand, or to hang your hand over the side of the bed.
- To speed healing, you must give your wrist a rest and stop the activity that caused the problem. If your symptoms are work-related, you may need to talk with your employer about changing to a job that doesn't require as much wrist action.

Call Your Doctor If . . .
- There is no improvement after 2 weeks of care.
- You develop new, unexplained symptoms.

Car Seats

See Safety Seats

Cast Care

WHAT YOU SHOULD KNOW

Casts are used to keep an injured part of the body from moving so it can heal. A cast can be made of plaster or fiberglass. Plaster looks and feels smooth, while fiberglass looks like woven cloth and feels rough on the outside. Fiberglass also comes in many different colors.

The cast feels hard 10 to 15 minutes after it is applied. However, it takes 24 hours to dry completely, so be careful with it for the first day, while it still can easily crack.

WHAT YOU SHOULD DO

- Put ice on the injury for 15 to 20 minutes each hour for the first 1 or 2 days. Put the ice in a plastic bag and place a towel between the bag of ice and your cast.
- If you can, keep the injury above the level of your heart for 48 hours. This will help relieve the pain and swelling.
- Keep the cast dry. Cover it with a plastic bag or plastic wrap while bathing. Do not lower the cast into the water.
- Do not try to scratch the skin under the cast by pushing a sharp or pointed object down inside the cast.

- Check the skin around the cast every day. You may put lotion on any red or sore areas.
- Do not push or lean on any part of your cast; it may break. You may need to use crutches if you have a cast on your leg, ankle, or foot. A sling may be necessary to support a cast on an elbow, arm, wrist, or hand.

Call Your Doctor If . . .
- The cast gets damaged or breaks.
- You have really bad pain that is getting worse.
- You have more swelling than you did before the cast was put on.
- The skin or the nails below the cast turn blue or gray.
- The skin below the cast feels cold or numb.
- There is a bad smell from the cast.
- There are new stains coming from under the cast.

Cat Scratch or Bite

WHAT YOU SHOULD KNOW

Cats carry plenty of germs on their claws and in their mouths, so there is a danger of contracting rabies, cat-scratch disease, or lockjaw (tetanus). It's important to clean the wound thoroughly and, if possible, have the cat checked for disease. How long it takes the wound to heal depends on how deep it is.

Signs/Symptoms
You may have bleeding, pain, swelling, redness, and bruising in the area of the bite.

Care
Clean the wound with soap and water immediately. You may need a tetanus shot if you have not had one in a long time. You may also need to take an antibiotic medicine to keep the wound from developing an infection.

WHAT YOU SHOULD DO

- If you have stitches, keep them clean and dry for several days. Then you can clean the wound. Make an appointment with your doctor to have your stitches taken out.
- Keep the area of the scratch or bite clean. Wash the wound with soap and water 3 to 4 times a day.
- If you have a bandage, keep it clean and dry. Change it whenever it

gets dirty. To loosen the bandage if it sticks to the wound, put a little water on it, then gently pull it off the wound.

- Try to raise the site of the bite or scratch above the level of your heart to keep the swelling down.
- If you have been given a tetanus shot, your arm may get swollen, red, and warm to the touch at the shot site. This is a normal reaction to the medicine.
- If you are taking antibiotics, continue to take them until they are all gone, even if you feel well. If you feel they are not helping, call your doctor. Do not quit taking them on your own.
- Find out who owns the cat and ask whether the animal has had its shots. Your doctor may need to send a report to the animal control officer, and the cat may have to be checked for disease.

Call Your Doctor If . . .
- You have signs of infection (redness, red streaking or pus coming from the wound, or warmth or swelling around the area of the scratch).
- You have a high temperature.
- You are tired or dizzy, have a headache or a cough, or just don't feel well.
- You get tender lumps in your groin or under your arm.

Seek Care Immediately If . . .
- You get numbness or tender lumps at the site of the scratch.
- You have trouble talking, walking, or breathing.
- You get tingling near the scratch area, have trouble swallowing, and develop stiffness in your jaw and neck.

Cavity, Dental

See Toothache

Cellulitis

WHAT YOU SHOULD KNOW

Cellulitis (SELL-u-LIE-tis), also called soft tissue infection, is an inflammation of the skin or underlying tissue. It can appear anywhere on the body, but is most commonly found on the face, arms, or lower legs. The infection is not contagious. With treatment, cellulitis can be cured in 7 to 10 days; left untreated, the infection can get into your blood.

Causes

Bacteria—particularly strep—that get into the skin from a cut or a sore.

Signs/Symptoms

The infection causes tenderness, redness, and swelling in an area of the skin. Other possible symptoms are fever, chills, and sweats.

Care

You may need an antibiotic to fight the infection. If the infection becomes severe, you may require hospitalization.

WHAT YOU SHOULD DO

- If your doctor prescribes an antibiotic, finish all the medication, even if you are feeling better. If you stop treatment too soon, some of the bacteria may survive and re-infect you.
- Rest in bed until the fever is gone, and pain and redness have subsided.
- If the infection is on your arm or leg, keep the limb elevated by placing it on a pillow or chair.
- Use warm water soaks to relieve pain and help healing. Soak a clean cloth in warm water, wring it out a little, and apply it to the affected area. Resoak the cloth often to keep it warm. Apply soaks for about 1 hour and repeat the soaking several times during the day.
- Make an appointment to have your doctor recheck the infected site.

Call Your Doctor If . . .

- You develop a high temperature or your fever does not disappear with treatment.
- You find a blister on the infected area, see the area of redness spreading, or notice red streaks coming from the infected site.
- The joint or bone underneath the infected skin becomes painful after the skin has healed.
- You develop new, unexplained symptoms.

Seek Care Immediately If . . .

- You feel drowsy and lethargic, or develop vomiting or diarrhea.

Cerebrovascular Accident

See Stroke

Cerumen Impaction

See Earwax Buildup

Cervical Spine Strain

See Whiplash

Cervicitis

WHAT YOU SHOULD KNOW

Cervicitis (sir-vi-SIGH-tis) is swelling and irritation of the cervix (the bottom part of the uterus). It is a common female problem, and is usually not serious. Treatment depends on the cause.

Causes

Often the cause of cervicitis is an infection acquired while having sex. An IUD (intrauterine device) or a forgotten tampon is sometimes at fault. Chemicals in douches also can cause the problem.

Signs/Symptoms

Yellow discharge from the vagina that may or may not have a bad smell is frequently a symptom. Others include bleeding, itching, pain during sex, or a burning feeling when you urinate. You may have belly or lower back pain.

Care

If the cause is an infection, the doctor will prescribe antibiotic medicine to eliminate the germs. Your partner(s) may also need to be treated.

WHAT YOU SHOULD DO

• If you have an infection:
  —Be sure to take the prescribed medication for as long as directed. If the germs aren't completely eliminated, the infection may spread up into the pelvic area. This can cause damage that may make it hard for you to get pregnant.
  —Your sexual partner(s) must be examined and treated.
  —Don't have sex while you are being treated.
• During treatment, use sanitary pads instead of tampons.
• Do not use a douche during treatment.

Call Your Doctor If . . .

• Your discomfort lasts longer than a few days.

- Your symptoms get worse.
- During or after treatment, you have vaginal bleeding between periods.

Cesarean Section

WHAT YOU SHOULD KNOW

A Cesarean (suh-ZAIR-e-un) section—also called a C-section—allows safe, quick delivery of a baby when a vaginal delivery is not possible. In a C-section, the doctor makes a cut in the lower belly and into the uterus. The baby is delivered through this cut (often called an incision). After the procedure, it will take about 4 weeks for you to feel like your old self.

There are many reasons for doing a C-section: The baby may be in the wrong position, the baby's head may be too large to pass through the birth canal, your contractions may not be strong enough to deliver the baby, the placenta (afterbirth) may not be in the right place, or you may have had a C-section before.

IF YOU'RE HEADING FOR THE HOSPITAL . . .

Remember These Pointers After You Leave
- A hard ridge may form along your incision. It will slowly go down as the incision heals.
- Use an electric heating pad (set on low) or a warm, moist towel to relieve the pain in your incision.
- You may shower as usual. Gently wash your incision with a mild, unscented soap.
- Do not douche unless your doctor tells you to.
- Resume your normal activities as soon as you are able.
- You may drive a car after you have been home for 3 weeks.
- You may have sex when your doctor tells you it is okay and when you are able.
- For comfort when you are feeding your baby, rest the baby on a pillow over the incision area.

Call Your Doctor If . . .
- Bleeding from the incision soaks more than one pad every hour or turns bright red.
- The feeling that you need to urinate right away lasts longer than 1 month.
- Your vaginal discharge (bleeding) lasts longer than 1 month.
- You have pain, red streaks, or warmth on the lower part of one of your legs.

Chalazion

A chalazion (kuh-LAY-zee-un) is a lump on the eyelid that may become infected. It rarely produces eye pain or changes in your sight. With care, it should be gone in 1 to 2 months.

Causes
A chalazion develops when blockage in an oil gland causes it to swell.

Signs/Symptoms
Swelling of the eyelid and eye irritation are the typical symptoms.

Care
Warm packs on the eyelid will ease discomfort. Have the problem checked by your doctor. Medicine or surgery may be needed if the chalazion is infected.

WHAT YOU SHOULD DO

- To avoid spreading any possible infection, don't touch the chalazion and wash your hands often, drying them with a clean towel.
- If the chalazion is infected:
  —Apply a warm, clean washcloth to the eyelid several times a day for 10 to 20 minutes to help ease pain and bring pus to the surface.
  —Return to your doctor to have the pus removed.
  —Do NOT try to remove the pus yourself by squeezing the chalazion or sticking it with a pin or needle.
- If the chalazion is not infected, applying a warm, clean washcloth will still ease discomfort and speed healing.
- You may use nonprescription medicines such as acetaminophen or ibuprofen to reduce the swelling and ease the pain.

Call Your Doctor If . . .
- Your eye becomes painful or your vision changes.
- A head of pus does not develop on an infected chalazion after 2 days of applying warm compresses.
- The chalazion becomes painful, red, or swollen; grows larger; or does not start to disappear after 2 weeks.

Change of Life

WHAT YOU SHOULD KNOW

Menopause (MEN-o-paws) is the time in your life when menstrual periods stop. It is also called the "change of life" or "the change." It begins around age 50, but it can happen from age 35 to 59. Going through menopause usually takes 1 to 2 years.

Causes
During menopause your ovaries slowly stop making hormones. The main hormones are called estrogen (ES-troh-jen) and progesterone (pro-JES-ter-own). These hormones play a large part in your monthly periods. Many of the changes during menopause are due to loss of estrogen and progesterone.

Signs/Symptoms
Your periods will become irregular and then stop. You may have hot flashes, night sweats, vaginal dryness, and bone changes. You could also feel nervous, moody, tired, or depressed. These signs vary from woman to woman.

WHAT YOU SHOULD DO

Menopause is a normal part of life. You will learn to deal with the changes in your own way. Discuss any unpleasant symptoms with your doctor. Some can be treated with medicine. Keep the following points in mind.
- **Menstrual Period:** One of the first signs of menopause is a change in your period. You may skip periods or they may come closer together. Your flow may be lighter or heavier than normal.
- **Hot Flashes:**
  —This is the most common sign of menopause. Hot flashes can last for a few seconds or for an hour. They are more common at night. Layer your clothing if you are having hot flashes and sweating. Wear cotton clothing if sweating at night is a problem.
  —They may continue for a year, but not longer than 5 years. Medicine may help ease hot flashes if they bother you.
- **Changes in the Vagina:** Vaginal dryness may make sex uncomfortable. Your doctor may give you an estrogen cream to put in and around your vagina. You can also use a water-based jelly.
- **Urine Problems:** After menopause you may have urinary tract infections or problems with your kidneys. You may go to the bathroom more often, have pain when you urinate, or have to get up at night to urinate.
- **Bone Changes:** During menopause, your bones lose calcium, which is a mineral in your body. This causes your bones to become thinner. There is a greater problem with bones breaking as you age.

- **Body Changes:**
  - —You may notice your hair is thinner and feels different. You may lose hair between your legs and get some hair on your face. Your breasts may not be as full and nipples not as raised.
  - —Headaches, night sweats, trouble sleeping, and tiredness are other signs.
- **Pregnancy:** It is possible for you to get pregnant while going through menopause. You are not free from possible pregnancy until you have gone a year without a menstrual period. Keep using birth control during this time if you do not want to get pregnant.
- **Exercise:** You should exercise regularly. This will slow down bone loss and keep your weight and appetite under control. It will also make you feel better.
- **Food:** Eating foods that are high in calcium helps slow down bone loss. Calcium is found in milk and dairy foods, nuts, seafood, and green leafy vegetables. Your doctor may want you to take calcium pills.
- **Mood Changes:** You may go through menopause with no mood changes. But you could feel nervous, irritable, tired, or have mild depression. These are usually not serious problems, but you should talk to your doctor about them. Talking to your partner or a close friend or relative may also help.
- **Heart Disease:** This is more common in women after menopause. Eating good foods, exercising regularly, quitting smoking, and watching your weight are ways to keep your heart healthy.
- **Health Checkups:** Visit your doctor each year for routine checkups. If you are taking estrogen, you should have a Pap smear every 12 months. Talk with your doctor about concerns or problems you are having with menopause
- **Medicine:** Your doctor may want you to take medicine to help with the changes caused by menopause. Call your doctor before you stop taking any medicines.

Call Your Doctor If . . .

- You have heavy vaginal bleeding.
- You have bleeding that lasts longer than what is normal for you.
- You have spotting (blood) between periods.
- You have a period 6 months or more after your last period.
- You have burning when you pass urine.
- You have trouble passing your urine.

Chemical Eye Burns

WHAT YOU SHOULD KNOW

If certain chemicals get in your eye, they can cause a great deal of damage. Both acid burns and alkali burns from substances such as lye, lime, and ammonia can be extremely serious.

Signs/Symptoms
Typically, you'll suffer pain, redness, and swelling of the eye, as well as blurred vision.

Care
Rinse the eye right away as outlined below and call your doctor immediately. You may need medicine to reduce the pain and swelling.

WHAT YOU SHOULD DO

• Rinse the eye with tap water or saline for 15 to 30 minutes. You may find it easier to rinse the eye if you stand in the shower and hold the eye open to the water.
• Your doctor may put an antibiotic eye ointment in the eye and cover it with a patch to ease the pain and keep windblown material out of it. Do not loosen or remove the eye patch until your doctor gives the go-ahead.
• Do not drive while the eye is patched; you will be unable to judge distances very well.
• You may use aspirin, acetaminophen, or ibuprofen to ease the pain.
• To prevent chemical eye burns, always wear protective eyeglasses when working with chemicals.

Call Your Doctor If . . .
• The pain in your eye gets worse.
• Your vision changes.
• You develop a high temperature.
• You see any new discharge coming from your eye.

Chemical Pneumonia

WHAT YOU SHOULD KNOW

Chemical pneumonia is swelling and irritation of the lungs caused by breathing in fumes from such chemicals as bug sprays, pool cleaners, or gasoline. This kind of pneumonia cannot be spread to other people.

Causes

Inhaling any type of irritating fumes can result in this problem. You can also get pneumonia if you breathe in when vomiting.

Signs/Symptoms

Common symptoms include coughing, choking, gagging, trouble breathing, or fast breathing. You also might have bluish fingernails, toenails, or skin; a fast heartbeat; headache; fever or upset stomach; vomiting; diarrhea; and convulsions. Other possible symptoms include fatigue, dizziness, and difficulty walking.

Care

If you are not having too much trouble breathing, you can recover at home. You may need medicine for pain, swelling, fever, or infection. If you need extra oxygen or medicines to help you breathe more easily, a hospital stay may be required.

WHAT YOU SHOULD DO

- Take any medicine the doctor prescribes exactly as directed. If you feel it is not helping, call your doctor. Do not quit taking it on your own.
- For pain and fever, you may take over-the-counter medicines such as acetaminophen or ibuprofen.
- Use a cool-mist humidifier or vaporizer to increase air moisture. This will make it easier for you to breathe. Do not use hot steam.
- Rest in bed until your temperature is normal (98.6 degrees F or 37 degrees C) and your chest pain and breathing problems are gone.
- Drink 6 to 8 glasses of liquids (soda-can size) to keep mucus thin and easy to cough up.
- If you have muscle pain from coughing, put a heating pad or warm wet cloth on the achy muscles. Do this for 10 to 20 minutes 3 to 4 times a day to lessen the pain.
- To keep your lungs free of infection, take deep breaths, then cough. Do this often during the day. If your chest hurts when you cough, hugging a pillow tightly while you cough may reduce the pain.
- Do not smoke until you are better. Quit smoking if possible. It harms the heart and lungs. If you have trouble quitting, ask your doctor for help.
- To keep from getting this type of pneumonia again:
  —Open a window when you use cleaning products, especially when you are in a small room.
  —Do not spray or use chemicals outside when it's windy.
  —If you must work in the wind, make sure the chemicals are

blowing away from you instead of toward you. Also wear a mask over your mouth and nose, and wear clothing that protects your skin.

Call Your Doctor If . . .

• You have a high temperature.
• Your chest pain does not get better in a few days.
• You get an upset stomach, start throwing up, or have diarrhea.
• You are coughing up bloody sputum.
• You have any problems that may be related to the medicine you are taking (for example, a rash, itching, swelling, or stomach pain).

Seek Care Immediately If . . .

• You have a lot of trouble breathing or have dark or bluish fingernails, toenails, or skin.
• You have a really bad headache, neck stiffness, or feel confused.
• You continue to have a fever and chills and feel worse.

Chest Pain

WHAT YOU SHOULD KNOW

Chest pain can result from diseases in many different parts of the body, including the heart, lungs, stomach, and bowel. The muscles and bones of the chest wall may be involved. Anxiety, rapid breathing, and gas also can produce chest pain. The cause can be very dangerous, or no danger at all.

Signs/Symptoms

Any kind of pain or discomfort (such as burning or pressure) felt in the chest.

Care

Because chest pain can be caused by something serious, your doctor will usually first do tests to check for life-threatening problems. You will have a complete exam, and will probably have to give a sample of your blood. You will have an electrocardiogram (e-LEK-tro-CAR-dee-o-gram) to check your heart. A chest x-ray may also be done.

You may need other tests, x-rays, or scans if a cause cannot be found. You may be given different medicines to see if they help relieve the pain. Other care will depend on what your doctor decides is causing the pain.

Do's and Don'ts

Never drive yourself to the hospital when you are having chest pain. Good rules of health are to quit smoking, lose weight if you weigh too much, and try to exercise every day.

Risks

Without treatment, the cause of your chest pain may get worse, and possibly become life-threatening.

WHAT YOU SHOULD DO

Call Your Doctor If . . .

• You have questions or concerns about your illness or medicine.
• You think your medicine is causing you problems such as a rash, itching, or swelling.

Seek Care Immediately If . . .

• You have severe chest pain, especially pain that is crushing or pressure-like and spreads to the arms, back, neck, or jaw; or if you also have sweating, nausea, or difficulty breathing. **THIS IS AN EMERGENCY**. Get medical help at once. Dial **0 (operator) or call 911**. Do **NOT** drive yourself to the hospital.
• Your chest pain gets worse or does not get better within 24 hours.
• You have attacks of really bad pain lasting more than 15 minutes at a time.
• Your skin, fingers, or toes appear blue or gray.
• You feel dizzy or you faint.
• You have tingling or numbness in your arms or legs, or cannot move them.
• You breathe very rapidly at rest or find that you are gasping for air.
• You start to sweat and look pale.
• You have a high temperature.
• You are having trouble breathing, and get swelling, itching, or a rash after taking your medicine.

IF YOU'RE HEADING FOR THE HOSPITAL . . .

What to Expect While You're There

You may encounter the following procedures and equipment during your stay.

• **Taking Vital Signs:** These include your temperature, blood pressure, pulse (counting your heartbeats), and respirations (counting your breaths). A stethoscope is used to listen to your heart and lungs. Your blood pressure is taken by wrapping a cuff around your arm.
• **Pulse Oximeter:** You may be hooked up to a pulse oximeter

(ox-IM-uh-ter). It is placed on your ear, finger, or toe and is connected to a machine that measures the oxygen in your blood.

- **Oxygen:** Your body may need extra oxygen at this time. It is given either by a mask or nasal prongs. Tell your doctor if the oxygen is drying out your nose or if the nasal prongs bother you.
- **ECG:** Also called a heart monitor, an electrocardiograph (e-LEK-tro-CAR-dee-o-graf), or EKG. The patches on your chest are hooked up to a TV-type screen or a small portable box (telemetry unit). This screen shows a tracing of each heartbeat.
- **12 Lead ECG:** This test makes tracings from different parts of your heart. It can help your doctor decide whether there is a heart problem.
- **Activity:** You may need to rest in bed. Once you are feeling better, you will be allowed out of bed.
- **Blood:** Usually taken from a vein in your hand or from the bend in your elbow. Tests will be done on the blood.
- **Blood Gases:** Blood is taken from an artery in your wrist, elbow, or groin. It is tested for the amount of oxygen in your blood.
- **Chest X-ray:** This picture of your lungs and heart helps the doctor determine the source of the pain.
- **IV:** A tube placed in your vein for giving medicine or liquids. It will be capped or have tubing connected to it.
- **CT Scan:** Also called a "CAT" scan, this is an x-ray using a computer. It is used to make pictures of the part of your body that may be causing the pain.
- **Upper GI:** This is an x-ray of your stomach and intestines. You will need to drink a chalky liquid before the x-rays.
- **Medicines:**
  - **Nitroglycerin** (ny-tro-GLIS-er-in): Reduces the amount of oxygen your heart needs. Also opens the arteries to your heart so that it gets more oxygen. As a result, the pain usually diminishes or goes away. However, the "nitro" may also give you a headache or make you dizzy. It is taken by placing it under your tongue or attaching a medicine-filled patch to your chest, arm, or back.
  - **Pain Medicine:** May be given in your IV, as a shot, or by mouth. If the pain does not go away or comes back, tell a doctor right away.

After You Leave

- Return immediately to your doctor if you start having any of the symptoms listed in the section entitled "Seek Care Immediately If . . ." above. These are signs of serious diseases that need immediate medical care.

- You need to return later or make an appointment with another doctor to find the exact cause of your pain.
- Always take your medicine as directed by your doctor. If you feel it is not helping, call your doctor. Do not quit taking it on your own.
- Quit smoking. It harms the heart and lungs. If you are having trouble stopping, ask your doctor for help.
- Since it is hard to avoid stress, learn to control it. Learn new ways to relax (deep breathing, relaxing muscles, meditation, or biofeedback). Try to talk to someone about things that upset you.
- Weighing too much can make the heart work harder. If you need to lose weight, ask your doctor for a weight-loss plan.

CHF

See Congestive Heart Failure

Chickenpox

WHAT YOU SHOULD KNOW

Chickenpox, also known as varicella, is a common childhood infection. In the United States, most children between 3 to 9 years old get chickenpox. A shot (vaccination) to prevent the disease is now available.

Causes
Chickenpox is caused by the varicella virus. The disease is spread by close contact with an infected person. It may be 14 to 16 days after exposure before the child gets sick.

Signs/Symptoms
Fever, headache, and tiredness are the first signs. Many small, red bumps then appear and turn into water blisters. These itchy blisters break and crust over. New blisters keep forming for 3 or 4 days.

Your child can give the disease to others until all the sores are crusted over. This can take about 1 week. It takes about 2 weeks for all the scabs to fall off.

Care
There is no cure for chickenpox. Antibiotics do not help. The child needs plenty of rest and liquids. Lukewarm baths and calamine lotion may help the itching.

WHAT YOU SHOULD DO

- **For fever:** DO NOT GIVE ASPIRIN to a child with chickenpox who is under 18 years of age. This could lead to brain and liver damage (Reye's syndrome). Instead, give the child acetaminophen. Carefully check for aspirin on the label of any over-the-counter medicines.
- **For itching:**
  —Your doctor can prescribe medicine for itching. You also may use an over-the-counter antihistamine product.
  —You may use calamine lotion on the sores. Follow the directions on the label. Do not use on sores in the mouth.
  —Give the child baths in lukewarm water for the first few days. Add 1/2 cup of baking soda to the water. Let your child bathe for about 30 minutes. Do this several times a day. You also may use an oatmeal bath product that you can buy at a drug store.
- Try to keep your child from scratching the rash or picking off the scabs. Keep the child's fingernails cut short. Put socks on the child's hands at night. Use a soap that kills germs for handwashing.
- If your child has painful sores in the mouth, make tea twice as strong as usual, add a little sugar, and use for a mouthwash or gargle.
- Keep the child quiet and cool. Sweating and becoming warm makes itching worse. Keep the child out of the sun.
- Give plenty of fluids. Good choices are cool liquids such as water, milk, and apple juice. Avoid salty foods and orange juice.
- Keep your child home from school or daycare for about 1 week. The child should stay away from babies and pregnant women.

Call Your Doctor If . . .
- The child has sores in the eyes.
- The sores get bigger or have pus in them.

Seek Care Immediately If . . .
- The child starts vomiting, acts confused or too sleepy, or has seizures.
- The child has trouble breathing or is breathing very fast.

Chlamydia Infection

WHAT YOU SHOULD KNOW

Chlamydia (klah-MID-ee-uh) is a germ that causes a common infection in the sex organs of both men and women. It is spread through vaginal, rectal, or oral sex. Women who don't know they have chlamydia can pass the infection to their babies during childbirth.

Causes
Chlamydia infection is caused by microscopic bacteria.

Signs/Symptoms
Possible symptoms include fever, stomach pain, and discharge from the penis, anus, or vagina. Other signs are painful urination and redness or itching around the penis or vagina. Sometimes the infection causes no symptoms at all.

Care
A sample of your discharge may be tested. You will need to take antibiotic medicine to get rid of the infection.

WHAT YOU SHOULD DO

• It is important to follow your doctor's instructions for treatment. Take your medicine until it is all gone, even if you feel well. Not completing the treatment can result in serious problems. The infection may spread into a woman's uterus and fallopian tubes and can cause damage that may make it difficult for her to get pregnant.
• Tell all partners with whom you had sex before treatment that you have a chlamydia infection. They also may be infected and need treatment.
• Don't have sex while you are being treated. After that, use a condom. This helps protect against catching or spreading chlamydia and other infections.
• Women should not douche during treatment.
• Wash your hands often, especially after urinating or having a bowel movement. Don't touch your eyes with your hands.
• If you are pregnant, be sure to tell you doctor that you have a chlamydia infection. It may cause labor to begin too early. Also, babies born to infected mothers may get an eye or lung infection.

Call Your Doctor If . . .
• Your symptoms last longer than one week or get worse during treatment.
• Your symptoms return after treatment.
• You have any problems that may be related to the medicine you are taking.

Seek Care Immediately If . . .
• You have stomach pain that gets worse.
• You develop a high temperature and chills.

Cholecystitis

See Gallstones

Chronic Bronchitis

WHAT YOU SHOULD KNOW

Chronic bronchitis is one of the lung disorders classified as chronic obstructive pulmonary disease (COPD). In bronchitis, tissue in the airways leading to the lungs swells up, making the passages narrower. Chronic bronchitis affects the larger airways first, later reaching the rest of them.

Causes

Cigarette smoking is the leading cause. Others are air pollution, allergies, and infections. Dust or chemical-filled air at work can cause bronchitis. The disease becomes more likely as we get older.

Signs/Symptoms

The main sign is a cough that lasts for at least 3 months, 2 years in a row. Other signs are trouble breathing, coughing up thick sputum, wheezing, and chest tightness.

As chronic bronchitis worsens, the skin and nailbeds become pale or a bluish color. You may also have repeated lung infections and swelling in your hands and feet.

Care

Chronic bronchitis can be controlled and even reversed with medicine and treatments to help make breathing easier. By avoiding the things that cause the disease, you can keep your bronchitis from getting worse.

Risks

If you don't follow your doctor's directions, this disease will get worse, ending in death. However, the illness can be controlled with medicine, exercise, and diet.

WHAT YOU SHOULD DO

• You will breathe easier if you take your medicine exactly as directed. If you feel it is not helping, call your doctor. Do not quit taking it on your own.

- If you are prescribed antibiotics, continue to take them until they are all gone—even if you feel well.
- If your medicine makes you drowsy, do not drive or use heavy equipment.
- Quit smoking. It's probably the cause of your bronchitis, and will certainly make it worse. If you are having trouble quitting, ask your doctor for help.
- Try to avoid anything that makes your breathing harder, such as things that you're allergic to and polluted air.
- Try to avoid people who have colds or the flu. Get shots to prevent the flu and pneumonia.
- Eat foods that have plenty of protein, vitamins, and minerals in them. Your doctor can give you some suggestions.
- If you are coughing up sputum, do not eat or drink foods that contain milk. They can make sputum thicker.
- If you do not have to limit the amount of liquids you drink, drink 8 to 10 (soda-can size) glasses of water each day. This helps thin the sputum so it can be coughed up more easily.
- To help keep your lungs free of infection, take 2 or 3 deep breaths and then cough. Do this often during the day.
- A humidifier will help keep the air moist and your sputum thin, making it easier to cough up. Be sure to keep your humidifier free of fungus. Clean it every day.
- Stay inside during very cold or hot weather, or on days when the air pollution is high. If you work in a polluted area, you may need to change jobs.
- When you are active, you may feel short of breath. Here are some breathing exercises that may relieve the problem:
  —Breathe with pursed or puckered lips (as if you are playing the trumpet).
  —Breathe using your diaphragm. Put one hand on your abdomen and breathe in so that the hand moves outward or up. Breathing this way allows your lungs more room to expand and take in air.
- If you use medicine that you inhale, follow these steps:
  —First, shake the inhaler.
  —Breathe out slowly, all the way.
  —Put the mouthpiece of the inhaler in your mouth or 2 inches away (about half a finger's length), or use the spacer (a piece of plastic-like tubing that attaches to the inhaler).
  —Breathe in and push down on the inhaler at the same time (to create the mist).
  —Hold your breath for about 10 seconds.
  —Breathe out slowly through puckered lips or through your nose.

—If you need to take 2 puffs, wait 2 to 5 seconds before taking the second one.

—Gargling after using your inhaler may help relieve burning in your throat.

Call Your Doctor If . . .

• Your sputum gets thicker even though you're taking your medicine and drinking water as directed.

• You cough up sputum that is bloody, yellow, or green.

• Your nail beds stay gray or blue even after you are breathing easier.

• You have nausea, vomiting, sweating, or a headache.

• You have a high temperature.

IF YOU'RE HEADING FOR THE HOSPITAL . . .

What to Expect While You're There

You may encounter the following procedures and equipment during your stay.

• **Activity:** At first you will need to rest in bed, with a few pillows to keep you sitting up a little. This will help your breathing. Do not lie flat. Once you are breathing easier, you will be allowed to increase your exercise.

• **Oxygen:** You may need extra oxygen at this time. It is given either by a mask or nasal prongs. Tell your doctor if the oxygen is drying out your nose or if the nasal prongs bother you.

• **Pulse Oximeter:** While you are getting oxygen, you may be hooked up to a pulse oximeter (ox-IM-uh-ter). It is placed on your ear, finger, or toe and is connected to a machine. It measures the oxygen in your blood.

• **IV:** A tube placed in your vein for giving medicine or liquids. It will be capped or have tubing connected to it.

• **Medicines:** The drugs below will help you breathe easier. They can be taken by mouth or given in your IV.

—**Antibiotics:** If you have an infection in the lungs, you'll be given antibiotics to clear it up.

—**Bronchodilators** (bronk-o-DIE-lay-tors): The medicines may be needed to help open your lung's airways.

—**Steroids** (STAIR-oids): You may be given one of these drugs to decrease the swelling and inflammation of the tissue in your lungs.

• **Breathing Treatments:** A machine will be used to help you inhale medicine. A therapist will help with these treatments. They will help open your airways so you can breathe easier. At first you may need

them frequently. As you get better, you may only need them when
you are having trouble breathing.

- **Postural Drainage:** A nurse may tap your back briskly with his or
  her hands. This helps loosen the sputum in your lungs so you can
  cough it up more easily.
- **Taking Vital Signs:** These include your temperature, blood pressure, pulse (counting your heartbeats), and respirations (counting
  your breaths). A stethoscope is used to listen to your heart and lungs.
  Your blood pressure is taken by wrapping a cuff around your arm.
- **ECG:** Also called a heart monitor, an electrocardiograph (e-lec-tro-
  CAR-dee-o-graf), or EKG. The patches on your chest are hooked up
  to a TV-type screen or a small portable box (telemetry unit). This
  screen shows a tracing of each heartbeat. Your heart will be watched
  for signs of injury or damage.
- **12 Lead ECG:** This test makes tracings from different parts of your
  heart. It can help your doctor decide whether there is a heart
  problem.
- **Chest X-ray:** This picture of your lungs and heart will be used to
  monitor your condition.
- **Blood Gases:** Blood taken from an artery in your wrist, elbow, or
  groin is tested for oxygen.
- **Blood:** Usually taken for testing from a vein in your hand or from
  the bend in your elbow.

Chronic Obstructive Pulmonary Disease

See Chronic Bronchitis and Emphysema

Chronic Renal Failure

See Kidney Failure, Chronic

Circumcision

WHAT YOU SHOULD KNOW

During a circumcision (SIR-come-SIH-shun), the doctor removes the
foreskin on the penis. Immediately after the procedure, the area will
be red and tender, but the tenderness should be almost gone by the
third day. The scab on the incision will come off in 7 to 10 days. If
your doctor uses a Plastibel® ring, it should fall off in 14 days.

Risks

A circumcision could cause infection, bleeding, or injury to your child's penis or urinary duct (urethra). If you follow the doctor's directions, however, there is little chance of a problem.

IF YOU'RE HEADING FOR THE HOSPITAL . . .

Before You Go

• Your doctor will examine the child's penis to see whether it is all right to perform the circumcision at this time.

• Your doctor may not want your child to eat for a few hours before the circumcision.

What to Expect While You're There

You may encounter the following procedures and equipment during your stay:

• **Taking Your Child's Vital Signs:** These include your son's temperature, blood pressure, pulse (counting heartbeats), and respirations (counting breaths). A stethoscope (steth-uh-scope) is used to listen to his heart and lungs. His blood pressure is taken by wrapping a cuff around his arm. The procedure is painless.

• **During the Circumcision . . .**
—The child will lie on a padded board and straps will be put around him to keep him from moving.
—The doctor will clean the area around the head of the penis. He or she may give the baby numbing medicine so he will feel little pain.
—The foreskin is removed after a special instrument or plastic ring is applied. Your child should have little bleeding. Ointment and a bandage will be put on the child's penis to help keep it from rubbing against a diaper.
—The entire circumcision will take about 20 to 30 minutes.

After You Leave

• If the Plastibel® ring was used:
—Gently clean the area with warm water 3 times a day or whenever necessary. You do not need to use soap.
—After washing, apply the jelly or ointment suggested by your doctor to the area where the cut was made to keep it soft during healing. A black rim around the plastic ring is normal.
—Do not pull the ring off; this could cause bleeding.

• If your baby has a gauze bandage: first wet it thoroughly with warm water and then gently remove it. After the bandage is off, clean the area as instructed above.

Call Your Doctor If . . .
• The ring does not fall off as quickly as your doctor said it would.
• The area where the cut was made is bleeding freely.
• The baby acts sick.

Seek Care Immediately If . . .
• The baby's urine comes out in dribbles or the urine stream is weak.
• The penis turns blue or black.
• The normal skin of the penis is tender or red.
• There is any pus on the penis.
• The baby develops a high temperature.

Clavicle Fracture

See Broken Collarbone

Cluster Headache

WHAT YOU SHOULD KNOW

Cluster headaches cause pain on one side of the head, behind or around one eye. The pain usually starts near one eye and shoots up to the top of the head on that side. These headaches frequently occur in "clusters," often starting at the same time each day over a period of time. They may also come and go for several days, weeks, or months. Each headache can last from 15 minutes to 2 hours. Cluster headaches occur most often in the spring and fall. They are more common among men than among women.

Causes
The cause is not known.

Signs/Symptoms
The headaches are typically sudden and severe, and may be accompanied by watery eyes or a runny nose. You may feel sweaty, restless, or nauseated. The headaches often start at night and may wake you up.

Care
There is no cure for cluster headaches, but there are ways to help relieve the pain. Prescription medications are available. Some must be taken in a shot, breathed in by mouth, or put in the rectum to get them into the bloodstream quickly.

WHAT YOU SHOULD DO

- If your doctor has prescribed any medicine, take it exactly as directed. Ask your doctor whether it is safe to drive or operate heavy machinery while you are taking this medication.
- An attack may be triggered by:
  —Smoking or drinking alcohol.
  —Napping in the daytime.
  —Breathing in solvents, gasoline, or oil-based paints for long periods of time.
  —Traveling to high-altitude areas (above 5,000 feet) or in airplanes.
- When you have a headache, avoid bright lights, alcohol, and stressful situations that cause you to become angry or excited; they can worsen the pain.
- Your doctor can recommend preventive medication to take before airplane travel. Using oxygen during the flight may help relieve a headache.
- A cold pack to your head may bring relief.
- Supervised exercise often helps prevent cluster headaches. Be sure to talk to your doctor, however, before starting an exercise program.
- Biofeedback therapy may help reduce the pain. Ask your doctor about this type of program.

Call Your Doctor If . . .
- You have any problem that may be related to the medicine you are taking.

Seek Care Immediately If . . .
- You have a headache that gets worse or lasts more than 2 hours despite treatment.
- You develop a high temperature.
- You faint or develop weakness, numbness, double vision, difficulty with talking, or neck pain or stiffness.

Cocaine Abuse

WHAT YOU SHOULD KNOW

Cocaine is highly addictive. One weekend of heavy use turns some people into cocaine addicts. Crack is even more addictive because it provides a stronger and faster "high."

Once addicted, you will find yourself spending more and more of your time and money assuring a supply. Heavy use of cocaine can lead to death from overdose or heart attack, so breaking the habit can truly be a matter of life and death. Going "cold turkey" can make you sick; but medical help is available, and you *can* quit successfully.

Causes
Snorting, smoking, or shooting cocaine or crack all can quickly lead to addiction. Pregnant women who use crack or cocaine pass the addiction to their babies. These children often have trouble thinking and learning later in life.

Signs/Symptoms
At first, a cocaine "high" will make you excited and full of energy. Continued use of the drug, however, will lead to unpleasant symptoms such as rapid heartbeat, chest pain, nose bleeds, insomnia, and trouble thinking or paying attention. You're likely to become very nervous or begin believing that everyone is out to get you. Ultimately, you may suffer hallucinations, seizures, and heart attack.

Withdrawal symptoms, such as depression, lack of energy, sore muscles, sweating, and shaking, are likely to occur if you suddenly stop using the drug without medical help.

Care
You may need a hospital stay during the withdrawal period so that your doctors can watch you more closely and deal with any possible problems. You may also be given medicines to help reduce withdrawal symptoms. Counseling and support groups are an important part of therapy.

WHAT YOU SHOULD DO

- The first step to quitting is to admit you have a problem. Be honest and open with family and close friends. Ask for their help.
- Tell your doctor exactly how much of the drug you have been taking. Also tell your doctor if you are taking any other medications. Don't hesitate to be honest. Doctors are familiar with the problem.
- Stay away from people who use drugs and who encourage others to use them.
- Support-group meetings and counseling can help you quit. Take advantage of both.
- Eat a healthy diet, drink 6 to 8 glasses of water a day, and get plenty of rest.
- Don't smoke or drink coffee or alcohol. They can make you nervous and increase your withdrawal symptoms.
- Don't dwell on the problem. Find new things to do. Get out of the house every day. Go for walks outside.

Call Your Doctor If . . .
• You cannot fight the need to take more drugs. Call your doctor, a counselor, friend, or family member you trust RIGHT AWAY.
• You feel as though your problems are getting the best of you, and you can't deal with them on your own.

Seek Care Immediately If . . .
• You have chest pain, sweating, or trouble breathing.
• You get a severe headache, pass out, and lose control of your bladder.
• You feel confused, very nervous, or suicidal.
• You have pain, a numb or prickly feeling, or burning in your arms or legs.

Coccyx Injury

WHAT YOU SHOULD KNOW

A bruise in the area of the tail bone, or coccyx, is usually not serious, though it may make it painful to sit or to walk.

Causes
The injury is usually the result of a fall or an accident.

Signs/Symptoms
There will be pain or bruising. It may hurt to have a bowel movement.

Care
There is no treatment other than measures to relieve the pain.

WHAT YOU SHOULD DO

• Apply ice to the sore area for 15 to 20 minutes each hour for the first 1 to 2 days. Put the ice in a plastic bag and place a towel between the bag of ice and your skin.
• After the first 1 to 2 days, you may apply heat to the injury to help relieve pain. Use a warm heating pad (set on low), whirlpool bath, or warm, moist towels for 15 to 20 minutes every hour for 48 hours. Lie on your stomach, DO NOT lie on the heating pad.
• Sitting on a large rubber ring or a cushion may ease the pain. Some people feel more comfortable sitting on a hard surface.
• You may increase your activity as the pain allows.
• You may use over-the-counter medicines to ease the pain. Take stool softeners if bowel movements are painful. Take all medications exactly as directed by your doctor.

Call Your Doctor If . . .
• Your pain becomes worse.
• Bowel movements cause a lot of discomfort.
• You are unable to move your bowels.

Cold Sores

WHAT YOU SHOULD KNOW

Cold sores, also known as fever blisters, are caused by herpes (HER-peez) simplex 1 virus (HSV-1). This common virus can create painful blisters on the lips, gums, and mouth. It sometimes affects the sex organs, and in rare cases affects the eyeball.

Causes
The virus usually spreads through person-to-person contact. It can also be caught through contact with saliva, bowel movements, urine, or fluid from an infected eye. The blisters carry infection until they heal.

Signs/Symptoms
Typically, painful blisters develop around the mouth (and sometimes the sex organs). The blisters are yellowish in the middle with a thin red ring around them. If the eye is infected, it becomes red and painful, and may feel as though there is a foreign object in it. The eye may also be sensitive to light and produce copious tears.

Care
Use acetaminophen for pain. You may be given medicine to take by mouth or an antibiotic cream to put on your blisters if they become infected with bacteria.

WHAT YOU SHOULD DO

• You may use acetaminophen to help relieve pain, but DO NOT TAKE ASPIRIN.
• Don't touch the blisters or pick at the scabs. Until the blisters heal, don't touch your eyes without washing your hands first. Wash your hands often.
• To help reduce discomfort, apply an ice cube or ice pack to your lip for 30 minutes or suck on frozen juice bars.
• Apply rubbing alcohol to the blisters to reduce swelling and to help the sores dry up. Do this for 2 minutes, 4 times a day.
• Protect your lips from the sun by using a sunscreen when you go outdoors.

- Avoid close contact with other people, especially kissing or oral sex, until the blisters heal. The virus that causes cold sores usually is different from the one that causes sores on the genitals. However, cold sores may occur in persons who have oral sex with a partner who has genital herpes.
- Hot or cold foods may hurt your mouth, and you may want to use a straw. Eating a well-balanced diet will help healing.
- If an eye gets infected, don't use any type of eyedrops without first checking with your doctor. Certain eyedrops can make the herpes virus grow in the cornea.
- To lessen the chance of getting blisters again, avoid direct sunlight and stress, and don't let yourself get run-down.

Call Your Doctor If . . .
- Your eye feels irritated, or you feel like you have something in your eye.
- You develop a fever, feel achy, or see pus instead of clear fluid in the sores. These are signs of a bacterial infection.
- You get blisters on your genitals.
- You develop new, unexplained symptoms.

Colic

WHAT YOU SHOULD KNOW

A colicky infant cries for hours for no known reason. The cry is often a fussy screaming. Colic begins in infants about 2 to 4 weeks old and can last 5 months. It is more common in boys and first-born children.

Causes
The exact cause of colic is unknown. Tiredness, food allergy, overly warm milk, or overfeeding your baby may play a part. Stress in the home, loneliness, and pain may also have a role. Your colicky infant may simply want to be held or to go to sleep.

Signs/Symptoms
Your infant may cry once or twice a day for 1 to 2 hours. Between these crying spells, the baby may seem fine. Crying often starts in late afternoon or early evening and frequently stops when you hold the child. The crying does no harm.

Care
It is hard to treat colic since its cause is unknown. Holding, cuddling, and rocking your baby usually works best.

WHAT YOU SHOULD DO

- Burp your infant after each ounce of formula. If you are breast-feeding, burp the baby every 5 minutes. Always hold the child while feeding, and allow at least 20 minutes for each session.
- Do not give a feeding every time the baby cries. Wait at least 2 hours between feedings. Check to see if the baby is in a cramped position, is too hot or cold, has a soiled diaper or an open diaper pin, or needs to be cuddled.
- When trying to comfort a crying infant, use soothing gentle motions. Use a rocking chair or cradle, put the baby in a wind-up swing, or carry the child in a front-pack. If the crying continues after more than 20 minutes of gentle motion, let the baby cry himself to sleep.
- When your baby is having an attack of gas, hold him or her securely and gently massage the lower part of the stomach. You may also apply a heating pad set on *low* or a warm water bottle to the stomach. Be very careful not to burn the baby. Do not lay the infant on the heating pad.
- Try not to let your baby sleep more than 3 hours at a time during the day.
- The baby's constant crying can be very stressful. Try to be patient and stay calm. Ask someone to care for the infant so you can get out for an hour or two. Remember, you did not cause your infant's colic, so don't blame yourself.

Call Your Doctor If . . .
- Your baby seems to be in pain or acts sick.
- Your baby has been crying constantly for more than 3 hours.
- Your baby develops a high temperature and is less than 3 months of age.

Seek Care Immediately If . . .
- You are afraid that you will hurt the baby.

Colitis

WHAT YOU SHOULD KNOW

Colitis (co-LIE-tis) is an irritation of the colon, also known as the bowel or large intestine. Colitis occurs most often in people 15 to 30 years old.

Causes
The underlying reasons for colitis are unknown, but it does appear to run in families. It can be triggered by certain foods and medicines, infections, and stress.

Signs/Symptoms

Colitis is marked by frequent loose stools that may be blood-specked, abdominal pain, fever, chills, nausea, weight loss, and tiredness. These signs may come and go from day to day.

Care

The doctor will run tests on your blood and your stools. You will need medicine, rest, and a special diet. A bad attack may require hospital care. There is no cure for most types of colitis, but you should feel better with treatment.

Risks

Colitis can cause long-term problems and even death. To reduce your chances of developing serious problems, you must follow your doctor's advice carefully.

WHAT YOU SHOULD DO

- Colitis can increase the risk of cancer. For this reason, it is important to keep it under control.
- Rest often. When you feel better, you can begin normal activities.
- Avoid raw vegetables and fruit, spicy foods, alcohol, chocolate, nuts, and drinks that have caffeine in them (coffee, tea, cola). Milk, cheese, and ice cream may also upset your colon.
- Drink 8 to 10 (soda-can size) glasses of water each day. This replaces some of the liquid you lose in watery stools.
- For pain relief, take acetaminophen. Do not take aspirin or ibuprofen; they may irritate the colon.
- Take any medicine your doctor prescribes exactly as directed. If you feel it is not helping, call your doctor, but do not quit taking it on your own.
- Since it is hard to avoid stress, control it by learning new ways to relax (deep breathing, relaxing muscles, meditation, or biofeedback). Talk to someone about things that upset you.

Call Your Doctor If . . .

- You go for several days without a bowel movement.

Seek Care Immediately If . . .

- You have a high temperature.
- Your stool is black or has blood in it.
- You have severe pain in your abdomen.
- You develop a skin rash.

IF YOU'RE HEADING FOR THE HOSPITAL . . .

What to Expect While You're There

You may encounter the following procedures and equipment during your stay.

• **Medicine:**

—**Pain medicine** may be given in your IV, as a shot, or by mouth. If the pain does not go away or comes back, tell a doctor right away.

—**Anti-diarrheal medicine** may be given to stop loose stools.

—**Steroids** may be used to decrease the swelling and redness of the tissue in your colon.

—**Antibiotics** may be prescribed to fight infection. They may be given by IV, in a shot, or by mouth.

• **Abdominal X-ray:** This picture of your abdomen will help the doctor judge the severity of your condition.

• **Barium X-ray:** In this procedure, your rectum and colon are filled with barium (a white chalky liquid). When the x-ray is taken, the barium outlines the colon.

• **Colonoscopy** (co-lun-OSS-co-pee): A soft tube with a lighted tip is gently passed through your rectum so that your doctor can inspect the interior of your colon.

• **Sigmoidoscopy** (sig-moyd-OSS-co-pee): The sigmoid (SIG-moyd) is the lowest end of your colon. A soft tube with a lighted tip is gently passed through your rectum to inspect this area.

• **Cold/Heat:** Putting a cool towel or heating pad (set on low) on your abdomen may relieve your pain.

• **Activity:** You may need to rest in bed until you are feeling better.

• **Taking Vital Signs:** These include your temperature, blood pressure, pulse (counting your heartbeats), and respirations (counting your breaths). A stethoscope is used to listen to your heart and lungs. Your blood pressure is taken by wrapping a cuff around your arm.

• **Blood:** Usually taken from a vein in your hand or from the bend in your elbow. Tests will be done on the blood.

• **Blood Transfusion:** If you are losing too much blood, a transfusion may be needed.

• **Other Care:** Your rectal area may be sore from loose stools and rough toilet paper. Your doctor can prescribe an ointment.

• **Surgery:** If your colitis is serious, you may need surgery.

Collapsed Lung

The collapse or caving-in of all or part of a lung occurs when air gets into the area between the lung and the chest wall. If this happens, the lung cannot fill up with air as you take a breath. It may occur spontaneously without a known cause, often in healthy people. Medically, the condition is known as a pneumothorax (nu-mo-THOR-ax).

Causes
Often, collapsed lung is due to rupture of an air pocket or bleb (fluid filled sac) in the lung. Changes in pressure during diving, flying, or even stretching can cause a bleb to break. Asthma or infections in the lung also can cause a rupture.

Signs/Symptoms
Usually, the bigger the collapse of the lung, the worse the signs. Common signs are sudden, sharp pain located on the side of the affected lung; trouble breathing; fast breathing; or coughing. When you breathe in, there's a possibility that your chest may appear lop-sided or asymmetrical.

Care
Whether you are in the hospital or not, you will need a chest x-ray. If the lung collapse is small, it may go away on its own, and you may be allowed to go home. If it is larger or causing breathing problems, you will be admitted to the hospital.

Risks
If only a small part of the lung is collapsed, it may heal by itself. But if a large collapse is not treated, your lungs may fail or become infected.

Call Your Doctor If . . .
• You have a high temperature.
• You have increased chest pain or trouble breathing.
• You have pain when you cough.
• You cough up sputum that is yellow, green, or gray.

Seek Care Immediately If . . .
• You have sharp, sudden chest pain and trouble breathing. You may

also have a dry cough with these signs. Have someone drive you to the nearest hospital immediately, or **call 911 or 0 (operator)**.

IF YOU'RE HEADING FOR THE HOSPITAL . . .

What to Expect While You're There

You may encounter the following procedures and equipment during your stay.

- **Chest X-ray:** This picture of the lungs will show the location and size of the collapse.
- **Chest Tube:**
  —A tube may be placed in the side of your chest to let out the air surrounding the lung. The tube may be hooked up to underwater drainage or gentle suction. Removing the air outside the lung allows it to re-expand.
  —If the tubing is kinked, the tape becomes loose, or the tube comes apart from the rest of the system, call a nurse at once.
- **Medicine:** You may need pain-killing medicine. This will allow you to breathe more easily and take deeper breaths, which will help prevent a lung infection. You may also need cough medicine.
- **Coughing and Deep Breathing:** It is important to do this often because it helps keep your lungs from getting infected.
  —To ease your pain during coughing and deep breathing, you may need to loosely wrap your rib cage with a 6-inch elastic bandage.
  —Holding a pillow tightly against your chest when you cough can help reduce the pain. Lying on the side that is hurting may also help ease the pain.
- **Cold/Heat:** A cool towel or heating pad (set on low) may be placed on the chest to help relieve the pain.
- **Sputum Sample:** If you are coughing up sputum, your doctor may need to send a sample to the lab. This sample may reveal an infection. It will also help the doctor choose the medicine you need.
- **Other Care:** You may need surgery if your lung keeps collapsing. Another possible treatment is injection of a substance that will harden the tissue of the collapsed part of the lung.
- **Taking Vital Signs:** These include your temperature, blood pressure, pulse (counting your heartbeats), and respirations (counting your breaths). A stethoscope is used to listen to your heart and lungs. Your blood pressure is taken by wrapping a cuff around your arm.
- **Oxygen:** Your body may need extra oxygen at this time. It is given either by a mask or nasal prongs. Tell your doctor if the oxygen is drying out your nose or if the nasal prongs bother you.
- **Pulse Oximeter:** While you are getting oxygen, you may be hooked up to a pulse oximeter (ox-IM-uh-ter). It is placed on your ear,

finger, or toe and is connected to a machine that measures the oxygen in your blood.

- **ECG:** Also called a heart monitor, an electrocardiograph (e-lec-tro-CAR-dee-o-graf), or EKG. The patches on your chest are hooked up to a TV-type screen or a small portable box (telemetry unit). This screen shows a tracing of each heartbeat. Your heart will be watched for signs of injury or damage that could be related to your illness.
- **12 Lead ECG:** This test makes tracings from different parts of your heart. It can help your doctor decide whether there is a heart problem.
- **Blood:** Usually taken from a vein in your hand or from the bend in your elbow. Tests will be done on the blood.
- **Blood Gases:** Blood is taken from an artery in your wrist, elbow, or groin. It is tested for the amount of oxygen it contains.
- **IV:** A tube placed in your vein for giving medicine or liquids. It will be capped or have tubing connected to it.

After You Leave

- Try not to cough, sing, talk loudly, or laugh for several days. This causes increased pressure in your lungs and may result in another collapse during this healing period.
- Rest until you feel better. You may then return to your normal activities.
- If you have chest soreness, apply ice, a heating pad (set on low), or warm cloths to the sore area for 10 to 20 minutes, 2 to 3 times a day. It's important to ease the pain so that you can breathe more easily.
- Take medicines only as directed by your doctor. If you feel they are not helping, call your doctor.
- If you are taking antibiotics, continue to take them until they are gone—even if you feel better.
- If you are taking medicine that makes you drowsy, do not drive or use heavy equipment.

Collarbone Fracture

See Broken Collarbone

Colonoscopy

WHAT YOU SHOULD KNOW

A colonoscopy (co-lun-OS-co-pee) is a procedure that lets your doctor inspect the inside of your colon (also called the bowel, gut, or large intestine) with a soft tube inserted through your rectum.

Risks
It's possible that your colon could be injured during the test. To avoid problems, be sure to follow your doctor's instructions very carefully.

IF YOU'RE HEADING FOR THE HOSPITAL . . .

Before You Go
• You will need to clean out your colon to get ready for this test. To do this, you will be given medicine and allowed to drink only liquids before the test.
  —For 1 or 2 days before your test, drink only clear liquids (Jell-O, broth, juice).
  —On the day of your test, do **not** eat or drink anything. This includes **no** water. Your doctor will tell you exactly when to stop eating and drinking.
  —To help clean out the colon, you may be given a laxative to take the night before, or the day of your test.
  —You may also need to have an enema before the test.

What to Expect While You're There
• **Taking Vital Signs:** Before the test, a nurse will take your temperature, blood pressure, pulse (counting your heartbeats), and respirations (counting your breaths). A stethoscope is used to listen to your heart and lungs. Your blood pressure is taken by wrapping a cuff around your arm.
• **Pulse Oximeter:** You may be hooked up to a pulse oximeter (ox-IM-uh-ter). It is placed on the ear, finger, or toe and connected to a machine that measures the oxygen in your blood.
• **Electrocardiograph** (e-lec-tro-CAR-dee-o-graf): This machine is also called an EKG. The patches on your chest are hooked up to a TV-type screen or a small portable box (telemetry unit) that shows a tracing of each heartbeat. Your heart is being watched for signs of irritation that could be related to the test or another problem.
• **Pain Medication:** The test can be uncomfortable, so you may be given medication before it begins.
• **During the Colonoscopy**
  —You will be asked to roll over on your side or stomach. You may have to raise one or both knees toward your chest. A sheet will cover your lower body.
  —A soft tube with a light and camera lenses on its tip will be gently inserted through your rectum. The camera will take pictures of your colon that show up on a TV-like screen. To improve the view, air may be pumped into the colon.

—A sample of the tissue inside your colon and, perhaps, a stool sample will be taken.

—The test will take about an hour to an hour and a half.

After You Leave

• If pain medication has made you drowsy, do not drive when you leave.

• You may resume normal activities and begin drinking or eating when you feel up to it.

Call Your Doctor If . . .

• You have a generally ill feeling, headache, chills, or muscle aches.

• You have a high temperature.

Seek Care Immediately If . . .

• You begin to have bright red bleeding from your rectum.

• You feel dizzy or short of breath, or you faint.

• You have vomiting and sharp pain in your abdomen.

Colposcopy

WHAT YOU SHOULD KNOW

During a colposcopy (kol-POS-kuh-pea), your doctor uses an instrument called a colposcope (KOL-po-scope) to examine your cervix and vagina. The colposcope magnifies the area to give the doctor a detailed view. The test is usually done when your Pap smear shows some possible problems. The doctor may take a small piece of tissue (biopsy) from your cervix or vagina to be tested.

After the Exam

• If a biopsy sample was taken, you may have slight vaginal bleeding or spotting for a couple of hours. Wear a sanitary pad or use a tampon until the bleeding stops.

• Do not have sex until your doctor gives you the go-ahead.

• If your doctor does not call you, call him or her to get the results of your tests. They should be ready in a few days.

Call Your Doctor If . . .

• You have bleeding from your vagina for several days.

Common Colds

Colds (known medically as upper respiratory infections) affect the air passages in the head, neck, and chest. The nose, throat, sinuses, ears, windpipe (trachea) and airways of the lung (bronchi) all can be involved. Without treatment, a cold will improve in a week or two.

Colds are the most common illness among children. Although youngsters often feel better within 3 or 4 days of developing the infection, they may continue coughing for 2 to 3 weeks. Many children have 6 colds a year.

Causes
Colds are caused by viruses. They can spread easily, especially during the first 3 or 4 days of illness. You can catch a cold at home, work, school, or day care by touching someone who has one, or by being nearby when an infected person coughs or sneezes. You are most likely to get a cold in the winter, and are most susceptible if you are tired, under stress, or plagued with allergies (especially hay fever).

Signs/Symptoms
Typical symptoms include sneezing, runny nose, stuffy nose, headache, cough, sore throat, trouble breathing, fatigue, muscle aches, and red, watery eyes. Some people develop a fever.

Care
Over-the-counter medications, such as acetaminophen or ibuprofen may relieve a headache, runny nose, or fever. However, antibiotics cannot cure the common cold.

WHAT YOU SHOULD DO

- Use over-the-counter medicines exactly as directed.
- Be careful not to blow your nose too hard, or you might have a nosebleed.
- To keep a young child's nose free from mucus, soak a cotton ball with warm water and put 3 drops into each nostril. Wait about 1 minute, then have the youngster blow his or her nose. If the child is too young for this, use a soft rubber suction bulb. Close one nostril, squeeze the bulb, insert it into the open nostril, and release the bulb so that it sucks up the mucus.
- Use a cool-mist humidifier (vaporizer) to increase air moisture so that you can breathe more easily. Do not use hot steam.
- Rest as much as possible and get plenty of sleep.

- Wash your hands often, especially after you blow your nose. Cover your mouth and nose with a tissue when you sneeze or cough.
- Drink 8 to 10 (soda-can size) glasses of clear liquids, such as water, fruit juice, tea, clear soups, and soda, every day.
- To avoid catching another upper respiratory infection, wash your hands after touching someone who has a cold; avoid crowded places, especially in the winter; and eat a balanced diet.
- Keep children at home until any fever has gone.

Call Your Doctor If . . .
- You develop a high temperature or your fever lasts more than a couple of days.
- You have a sore throat that gets worse, or you see white or yellow spots in your throat.
- Your cough gets worse or lasts more than 10 days.
- You develop a rash.
- You feel large and tender lumps in your neck.
- You develop an earache or a bad headache.
- You have a thick, green or yellow discharge from your nose.
- You cough up thick yellow, green, gray or bloody mucus.
- Your child's eyes grow red and become coated with a yellow discharge.

Seek Care Immediately If . . .
- You have trouble breathing or develop chest pain.
- Your skin or nails look gray or blue.
- A youngster with a cold seems sleepier than usual, urinates less than normal, has a dry mouth and cracked lips, cries without tears, or seems dizzy. These are signs of dehydration.

Concussion

WHAT YOU SHOULD KNOW

A concussion (con-CUH-shun) is a mild injury to the tissues of the brain. It can result from a blow to any part of the head, including the face, scalp, or skull. Some concussions lead to slow bleeding in the head and other problems.

Causes
Generally, concussions follow a blow to the head sustained in a fall, a car accident, or a sports mishap.

Signs/Symptoms

Immediately after a blow to the head, victims of concussion usually suffer a temporary loss of consciousness. Later, you may develop headache, dizziness, or fatigue. You also may have cuts, bruises, and swelling. Other possible symptoms are numbness, nausea, vomiting, large pupils (black center of eye), mental confusion, and memory problems. You may not see clearly or be fully awake.

Treatment

Your doctor may order a CT scan (computerized x-ray) to see whether you have serious brain damage. Blood tests and other tests may be done.

You may need to rest in bed for a few days and limit your diet to liquids. Do not take ANY medication without first checking with your doctor. If your doctor thinks it is necessary, you may be put in the hospital, where you can be carefully monitored.

Risks

A blow to the head can cause long-term injury or even death. However, the risk of serious problems is small if you follow your doctor's advice carefully.

WHAT YOU SHOULD DO

Seek Care Immediately If . . .

• You experience any of the following:
  —Inability to answer simple questions (What day is it? What happened to you?)
  —Inability to wake up completely.
  —Increased headache that is not relieved by acetaminophen.
  —Changes in behavior, including ability to recognize family or friends.
  —Vomiting that continues after 8 hours or starts later than the first few hours after injury.
  —Pupils that are different sizes.
  —Stumbling or other problems with walking.
  —Weakness of the arms or legs.
  —Double vision.
  —Slurred speech.
  —Seizures.

IF YOU'RE HEADING FOR THE HOSPITAL . . .

What to Expect While You're There

You may encounter the following procedures and equipment during your stay.

- **Taking Vital Signs:** These include your temperature, blood pressure, pulse (counting your heartbeats), and respirations (counting your breaths). A stethoscope is used to listen to your heart and lungs. Your blood pressure is taken by wrapping a cuff around your arm.
- **Oxygen:** Your body may need extra oxygen at this time. It is given either by a mask or nasal prongs. Tell a doctor if the oxygen is drying out your nose or if the nasal prongs bother you.
- **Pulse Oximeter:** While you are getting oxygen, you may be hooked up to a pulse oximeter (ox-IM-uh-ter). This is a clip placed on your ear, finger, or toe and connected to a machine that measures the oxygen in your blood.
- **Neuro Signs:** The doctor will check your eyes, test how easily you awaken, and check your memory. These important signs tell the doctor how well your brain is handling the injury.
- **CT Scan:** This procedure, also called a "CAT" scan, is used to take a computerized x-ray of your brain.
- **IV:** A tube placed in your vein for giving medicine or liquids. It will be capped or have tubing connected to it.
- **Blood:** Usually taken from a vein in your hand or from the bend in your elbow and used for testing.
- **Blood Gases:** Blood is taken from an artery in your wrist, elbow, or groin. It is tested for its oxygen content.
- **ECG:** Also called a heart monitor, an electrocardiograph (e-LEK-tro-CAR-dee-o-graf), or EKG. Patches on your chest are hooked up to a TV-type screen or a small portable box (telemetry unit). This screen shows a tracing of each heartbeat. Your heart will be watched for signs of problems that could be related to your head injury.
- **EEG:** This brain wave study is also called an electroencephalogram (e-LEK-tro-n-SEF-uh-lo-gram). Doctors use it to detect hidden damage to the brain.
- **Activity:** You may need to rest in bed. When you feel better, you will be allowed to get up.

After You Leave

- Your doctor will allow you to leave the hospital as soon as you can be watched safely at home. Remember, though, that it is possible for more serious symptoms to develop later.
- You MUST have someone with you at home for the next 24 hours in

case you get worse. This person must wake you up every few hours for the first 24 hours to see if you have any of the symptoms listed under the "Seek Care Immediately If . . ." section above.

- Rest in bed for 24 hours. You may begin normal activities again after you feel better.
- Drink only clear fluids (water, soft drinks, or apple juice) until any vomiting you have suffered has stopped for at least 6 hours. Do not drink any alcoholic beverages for 24 hours.
- You may use over-the-counter medicines, such as acetaminophen. Your doctor should tell you which medicines to take and how to take them. Follow directions exactly.
- If you normally take other medications, ask your doctor if you should continue to take them while recovering from this injury.

Condom Use

WHAT YOU SHOULD KNOW

Condoms (CON-dums) are used by men during sex to prevent infections and pregnancy. A condom is a tube-shaped piece of thin latex (rubber) that is closed at one end. It fits all the way over the penis and catches semen and sperm.

Some condoms are made of an animal membrane instead of latex. These condoms will help prevent pregnancy but do not protect against sexually transmitted diseases such as HIV infection.

WHAT YOU SHOULD DO

- Practice using a condom a few times when you are alone before using one for the first time with a partner.
- Put the condom on as soon as your penis is hard. Do NOT go inside your partner unless you are wearing a condom. Put the condom over the tip of your penis, then unroll it all the way to the base. Handle the condom carefully so you don't tear or puncture it. Leave about 1 inch of space at the tip of the condom. This leaves room to catch semen and sperm so the condom doesn't break.
- If the condom breaks or tears during sex, pull your penis out right away and put on a new condom.
- After sex, hold on to your penis and the top edge of the condom. Pull both out of your partner at the same time. Remove the condom carefully. Do NOT wait until your penis gets soft to pull it out. This can cause the condom to leak or slip off.
- Use a condom only once. Then throw it away. Use a new condom every time you have sex.
- If you need to wet the condom, use a lubricant with a water base.

Don't use lubricants such as petroleum jelly, cooking oil, shortening, lotion, or saliva. These may weaken the rubber.

• For better protection from diseases and pregnancy, use a condom with a sperm-killing chemical called nonoxynol-9 or use birth control jelly or foam. Some condoms come already coated with spermicidal lubricant.

• Store condoms in a cool, dry place. Heat will weaken the rubber and can cause the condom to break. Don't keep them in your pocket, purse, wallet, or inside a car for long periods of time.

• Don't use condoms that are old, cracked, sticky, brittle, or discolored.

• Try talking with your partner about what both of you like and don't like about condoms. This may make them easier to use.

Condyloma Acuminata

See Genital Warts

Congestive Heart Failure

WHAT YOU SHOULD KNOW

Congestive heart failure, also called CHF, occurs when the heart muscle is weak and has trouble pumping blood through the body. As a result, blood collects in the lungs or other parts of the body.

Causes
This condition may be the result of a heart attack, heart disease, high blood pressure, problems with the heart valves, infections of the heart, or a disease of the heart muscle.

Other causes may include severe physical or emotional stress, drugs, or lung or thyroid disease.

Signs/Symptoms
A typical symptom is trouble breathing, especially during exercise or when lying down. Other signs are swollen legs and feet, feeling tired or weak, weight gain, and loss of appetite.

Treatment
May include medicine to get rid of the extra fluid in your lungs and body, and drugs that help to make your heartbeat stronger. You may also need oxygen to help you breathe easier, and have tests to find out why you have CHF.

Do's and Don'ts

To control your heart failure, quit smoking, get lots of rest, shorten your work day, avoid getting upset, don't gain weight, keep out of very hot or cold temperatures, exercise, and eat a diet low in salt.

Risks

The disease can be controlled with medicine, but without care the condition can get worse, eventually leading to death.

WHAT YOU SHOULD DO

- Always take your medicine as directed by your doctor. If you feel it is not helping, call your doctor. Do not quit taking it on your own.
- If you take aspirin regularly, continue to take it. Aspirin helps thin the blood so blood clots don't form. Do not take acetaminophen or ibuprofen instead.
- If you have other illnesses like diabetes or high blood pressure, you need to control them. Take medicines as directed. Because of these illnesses, you have a higher chance of getting a heart attack.
- Exercise daily. It helps make the heart stronger, lowers blood pressure, and keeps you healthy. If your exercise plan seems too hard or too easy, speak with your doctor.
- Get at least 7 hours of rest each night. Take a nap during the day if you are tired.
- Since it is hard to avoid stress, learn to control it. Learn new ways to relax (deep breathing, relaxing muscles, imagery). Don't hesitate to talk to someone about things that upset you.
- Quit smoking. It harms the heart and lungs. If you are having trouble quitting, ask your doctor for help.
- Weigh yourself before breakfast daily. Weight gain can be a sign of worsening CHF. Call your doctor if you have gained 2 to 3 pounds in a day. Your doctor also will ask you to take your blood pressure and pulse regularly.
- Weighing too much makes the heart work harder. If you need to lose weight, talk to your doctor about a plan that is good for you.
- A diet low in fat, salt, and cholesterol is very important. It keeps your heart healthy and strong. Ask your doctor what you should and should not eat.
- It may take time getting used to a new diet. Special cookbooks may help you and the cook in your family find new recipes.
- Avoid really hot or cold temperatures. In hot weather, do activities during the cool part of the day. In cold weather, dress warmly in loose fitting clothes. Make sure to cover your head and mouth for warmth and for easier breathing.

- Ask your doctor how often you may have sex and whether you may drive.
- Do not lift or push or pull anything heavy or work with your arms above shoulder level until your doctor says you may.

Call Your Doctor If . . .
- You are light-headed, dizzy, sweaty, or nauseated after you take your medicine.
- You have gained several pounds in 1 or 2 days.
- Your blood pressure is higher or lower than usual.
- Your pulse is faster or slower than usual.
- You cough up yellow, green, or pink frothy sputum.
- You are wheezing (a high pitched noise when breathing in or out).
- You have trouble breathing, swelling in your feet or ankles, or are more tired than usual.
- You have a high temperature, muscle aches, headache, and dizziness. These are signs of an infection.
- You have chest pain during exercise that doesn't go away with rest.

Seek Care Immediately If . . .
- You have the following signs of worsening heart failure:
  —You have more trouble breathing than usual, are weak, cannot sleep or rest because of trouble breathing, or have a fast or uneven heartbeat.
  —You have increased swelling in your legs and feet and torso, and you feel dizzy. **THIS IS AN EMERGENCY.** Call for help immediately, or **call 911 or 0 (operator)** to get you to the nearest medical clinic or hospital. **Do not drive yourself!**

IF YOU'RE HEADING FOR THE HOSPITAL . . .

What to Expect While You're There
You may encounter the following procedures and equipment during your stay.
- **Taking Vital Signs:** These include your temperature, blood pressure, pulse (counting your heartbeats), and respirations (counting your breaths). A stethoscope is used to listen to your heart and lungs. Your blood pressure is taken by wrapping a cuff around your arm.
- **Pulse Oximeter:** While you are getting oxygen, you may be hooked up to a pulse oximeter (ox-IM-uh-ter). It is placed on your ear, finger, or toe and is connected to a machine that measures the oxygen in your blood.
- **ECG:** Also called a heart monitor, an electrocardiograph (e-lec-tro-CAR-dee-o-graf), or EKG. Patches on your chest are hooked up to

a TV-type screen or a small portable box (telemetry unit). This screen shows a tracing of each heartbeat. Your heart will be watched for signs of injury or damage that could be related to your illness.

- **12 Lead ECG:** This test makes tracings from different parts of your heart. It can help your doctor evaluate the problem.
- **Oxygen:** Your body may need extra oxygen at this time. It is given either by a mask or nasal prongs. Tell your doctor if the oxygen is drying out your nose or if the nasal prongs bother you.
- **IV:** A tube placed in your vein for giving medicine or liquids. It will be capped or have tubing connected to it.
- **Blood:** Usually taken from a vein in your hand or from the bend in your elbow. Tests will be done on the blood.
- **Blood Gases:** Blood is taken from an artery in your wrist, elbow, or groin. It is tested for the amount of oxygen it contains.
- **Chest X-ray:** This is a picture of your lungs and heart. The caregivers use it to see how your heart and lungs are handling the illness.
- **ECHO:** Also called an echocardiogram (e-ko-CAR-dee-o-gram). This uses sound waves to view your heart while it is beating. It can help caregivers decide what is causing your heart failure.
- **Other Tests:** May be needed to find out what is causing your chest pain.
  - **Stress Test:** Used to watch your heart during exercise.
  - **Cardiac Catheterization** (cath-uh-ter-i-ZAY-shun): A test used to study the arteries sending blood to your heart.
- **Medicine:**
  - **Diuretics (di-your-ET-ics):** Also called "water pills." They should make you pass urine more often and thus get rid of any extra fluid your body or lungs may have collected. Diuretics can be given as a pill or in your IV.
  - **Heart Medicine:** May be given to make your heartbeat stronger. You may also need medicine to make your arteries open up more so blood can flow easily.
- **Weight:** You will be weighed daily. This is one way to find out how much extra fluid is in your body. If you gain too much weight, you may need diuretics to get rid of the extra fluid.
- **Rest:** You will need a lot at first. Resting with your head on 2 or 3 pillows will help you breathe easier.
- **Exercise:** As you feel better, you may slowly start to exercise. Stop when you feel tired, have trouble breathing, or have chest pain. Remember, it will take time to build up your strength.
- **Angioplasty:** May be needed to open up a blocked artery to your heart.

- **Surgery:** May be needed if the arteries to your heart are severely blocked.

Conjunctivitis

See Pinkeye

Constipation

WHAT YOU SHOULD KNOW

Constipation—difficulty with bowel movements—occurs when stools become too hard or cause pain.

Causes

Constipation can result if you don't eat enough fiber (fruits, vegetables, bran, whole-grain cereals) or fail to drink 6 to 8 glasses (soda-can size) of liquid daily. It also can develop when you go for a longer time than normal without a bowel movement. Other possible causes include lack of exercise, depression, and certain illnesses.

Signs/Symptoms

You may feel the need for a bowel movement, but can't follow through—or feel as though you aren't moving your bowels as frequently or as much as usual. You may need to strain hard, or experience pain or bleeding.

WHAT YOU SHOULD DO

- You may use certain over-the-counter medicines for constipation; but take them only as recommended by your doctor.
  - —Stool softeners will make the stool easier to pass. Follow the directions on the label.
  - —Do NOT use laxatives or enemas regularly. You can become dependent on them and make the constipation worse. If a laxative is advisable, your doctor will recommend how often to take it.
- Set aside a regular time for a bowel movement each day. The best time is after meals, especially breakfast. Bending forward so your chest touches your thighs helps move the stool out. Wait at least 10 minutes, even if nothing happens.
- Eat a well-balanced, high-fiber diet. Fiber makes stools larger, softer, and easier to pass. Good choices for fiber are fresh fruits and vegetables, whole-grain breads, oatmeal and bran cereal, and brown rice. Avoid constipating foods such as dairy products and foods high in sugar.

- Drink plenty of fluids. Drink fruit juice at least once a day and at least 6 to 8 glasses (soda-can size) of water a day.
- Exercise regularly. Walking is a good choice.

Call Your Doctor If . . .
- Constipation lasts longer than 2 weeks.
- You have fever and abdominal pain with the constipation.
- There is bright red blood in the stool.

Constipation in Children

WHAT YOU SHOULD KNOW

It is not unusual for children to grunt, strain, draw up their legs, and become red in the face when having a bowel movement. Constipation means the bowel movement is hard and dry, making it painful and hard to push out.

Some children have two or three movements daily. Others may have a normal movement only every 5 to 7 days. Breastfed children can have large, soft movements without pain every 7 days. Formula-fed children will have firmer stools.

Constipation is generally not a serious problem. But it can make the child uncomfortable.

Causes
Adding new foods, such as chocolate, to your child's diet can cause constipation. Eating or drinking too much milk, cheese, yogurt, ice cream, or other milk products can cause the problem. Certain medicines, such as iron, also can cause constipation.

Constipation can also result from waiting too long to go to the bathroom. School-age children can become constipated because they are afraid of using the school bathroom.

Family problems such as a new baby or a family death also can cause some children who are being toilet trained to become constipated.

Signs/Symptoms
Pain while having a bowel movement is a sign of constipation. Your child may cry while trying to pass the movement or say that it hurts.

The child may go many days without having a bowel movement. He or she may want to have one, but even with pushing and straining, can't pass the stool.

Constipation can cause small tears that bleed near the rectum. These tears will heal without medicine. You may notice small amounts of bright red blood on the toilet tissue or on the bowel movement.

A diaper rash can also cause pain during a bowel movement. The child will not want to have a bowel movement because of the pain on his or her bottom.

Care

Most cases of constipation can be treated at home as long as the child does not have a lot of belly pain.

WHAT YOU SHOULD DO

- Constipation is usually not a serious problem. It can cause your child to be uncomfortable without proper care.
- If your baby is less than four months of age, twice a day give fruit juices such as apple, grape, or prune juice.
- When your baby is four months of age you can begin strained baby foods such as cereal, apricots, peaches, plums, pears, prunes, beans, peas or spinach. Squash, carrots, apples, and bananas may make the constipation worse. Feed your baby solid food two to three times daily.
- If your child is one year or older, he or she should eat fruits and vegetables three times daily. Encourage the child to eat raw unpeeled fruits and vegetables. Cut the food into small pieces to prevent choking. Avoid food that can't be chewed easily.
- Some foods can make your child's constipation worse. Limit the amount of milk, ice cream, cheese, white rice, bananas, cooked carrots, and applesauce in your child's diet.
- Babies need to drink water each day. The amount depends on their age. Ask your doctor how much your child needs.
- It can be hard for babies to have a bowel movement lying down. You can help by gently holding the knees against his or her chest. This is a more natural way to push out a stool.
- Put the child in a warm water tub several times a day. This may relax the rectal area and make it easier to pass a bowel movement.
- Tell the child not to wait too long to go to the bathroom if he or she has the urge to have a bowel movement.
- Encourage your child to be more physically active. This will reduce constipation.
- Toilet training or family problems can cause a child to be constipated. If this happens, you may want to stop the toilet training for a while and go back to using diapers.
- Your child's diaper rash may cause constipation because of pain

while having a bowel movement. Talk to your child's doctor for information about caring for the diaper rash.
• If your child develops small tears near the rectum from trying to have a bowel movement, let him or her sit in warm salt water three times daily (your doctor will tell you how much salt to add to the tub water). Do not leave your child alone in the bathroom. After the bath you can rub 1/2 percent hydrocortisone cream on the area. This cream can be bought over-the-counter at a drug store.
• Do not give your child an enema, suppository (medicine put into the rectum), or a stool softener (medicine to soften the stool) without talking to your doctor.

Call Your Doctor If . . .
• Your child has not had a bowel movement in several days.
• Your child has bowel movements that are very hard or painful to pass.
• You see blood in the diaper or bowel movement.
• The rectal area has tears that are not healing.

Seek Care Immediately If . . .
• Your child has constant, severe abdominal pain that has lasted for more than 2 hours.

Contact Dermatitis

WHAT YOU SHOULD KNOW

Contact dermatitis (DER-muh-TIE-tus) is a skin reaction to an irritating substance. People with allergies often have this condition. It frequently affects the hands, feet, and skin folds such as those found in the groin. The problem may come and go, but can usually be treated effectively.

Causes
In people predisposed to this problem, a wide variety of substances may cause irritation. Typical culprits include sprays, jewelry, soaps, some medicines, and makeup. The condition tends to run in families.

Signs/Symptoms
The exposed area becomes dry, red, cracked, and itchy, and develops what looks like a rash. The skin may blister and become sore.

Care

Try to find out what is causing the problem and stay away from it. Medication may relieve the itching and irritation.

WHAT YOU SHOULD DO

- Keep the area of skin that is affected away from hot water, soap, sunlight, chemicals, acidic substances, or anything else that you think would irritate it. Do not rub the skin.
- You may use over-the-counter medications such as topical steroids (which reduce inflammation) and lubricants (which keep moisture in your skin). Burow's solution will reduce inflammation. Mix one packet or tablet in 2 cups of cool water. Dip a clean washcloth in the mixture, wring it out a bit, put it on the affected area, and leave it in place for 30 minutes. Then resoak the washcloth and apply again. Do this as often as possible throughout the day. If the area is too large to cover with a washcloth, take several cornstarch, baking soda, or colloidal oatmeal baths daily.
- Do not use any other creams, lotions, or ointments. Many of these products may make your dermatitis worse.
- If your doctor prescribes medicine to use on the irritated area, apply it exactly as directed. Certain strong medicines can cause side effects even when applied only to the skin.
- You may want to rest the affected area until it is less sore.

Call Your Doctor If . . .

- You develop a high temperature
- You see signs of infection, such as swelling, tenderness, redness, or warmth, at the affected area.
- Treatment does not relieve your symptoms within a few days.
- You have any problems that may be related to the medicine you are using.

Contusions

See Bruises

Convulsions

See Seizures

COPD

See Chronic Bronchitis and Emphysema

Cord Care

WHAT YOU SHOULD KNOW

The stump of a baby's umbilical (um-BILL-uh-cul) cord (at the belly button or navel) usually falls off after 1 to 3 weeks.

Signs/Symptoms

Watch for infection. If the area near the stump is reddened, swollen, or drains green or yellow liquid, call the doctor.

WHAT YOU SHOULD DO

- Your baby's umbilical cord should be kept clean and dry until it falls off. Using a cotton ball or cotton tip applicator, put rubbing alcohol on the area where the stump attaches to your baby's skin. The rubbing alcohol prevents infection and helps dry the stump. Do this twice a day, and continue for a week after the stump falls off.
- Keep your baby's diaper folded down below the stump area. The air will help dry the stump. Give your baby a sponge bath instead of a tub bath until the stump has fallen off and the area is healed.
- The stump may bleed slightly when it begins to fall off. This is normal and should not cause concern. Your baby's belly button should be healed in 5 to 10 days. No special care is needed after this time.

Call Your Doctor If . . .

- The belly button is draining bad-smelling green or yellow liquid.
- The belly button has a bad smell after it is cleaned.
- The skin around the belly button is red or swollen.
- Your baby's temperature is rising.

Seek Care Immediately If . . .

- Your baby has a high temperature.

Corneal Abrasion

WHAT YOU SHOULD KNOW

A corneal abrasion is simply a scratch on the cornea, the clear area that covers the front part of your eye. A small scratch may heal in 1 to 2 days; deeper or larger scratches may take up to a week.

Causes

Contact lenses that do not fit well or are worn too long can cause an abrasion. Abrasions are also sustained in accidents.

Signs/Symptoms
Typically, there will be eye pain, redness, blurred vision, or tearing. The eyes may become sensitive to light. The eyelid may twitch.

Care
The doctor will probably prescribe medicine for the eyes and ask you to wear a protective eye patch.

WHAT YOU SHOULD DO

• If you are wearing an eye patch, do NOT loosen or remove it until your doctor gives the go-ahead. If the tape comes loose, retape it just as it was before.
• Do not drive or operate machinery while your eye is patched; your ability to judge distances will be impaired. In some states, driving with one eye patched is against the law.
• Do not wear contact lenses until your doctor says it is safe to do so.

Call Your Doctor If . . .
• Your eye pain gets worse.
• You have any problems with your eye patch.

Corneal Flash Burns

WHAT YOU SHOULD KNOW

If your eye is not protected, your cornea (the clear layer covering the eyeball) can be burned by a powerful light. Mild flash burns heal in a few days. There usually is no lasting eye damage.

Causes
Welding arcs, sun lamps, and even reflected sunlight can sometimes burn the eye.

Signs/Symptoms
Typically, you'll experience pain, swelling, and blurred vision.

Care
The doctor may prescribe antibiotics for infection and eye patches to ease pain and speed healing. You may also need pain medication.

WHAT YOU SHOULD DO

• If you are wearing one or two eye patches:
   —Do not remove or loosen the patches.

—If both of your eyes are patched, make arrangements for someone
to assist you until the patches are removed.

—Do not drive or operate machinery until both patches are
removed.

• You may use aspirin, acetaminophen, or ibuprofen for pain.

• To prevent corneal flash burns:

—Always wear sunglasses that filter ultraviolet (UV) rays when you
are outdoors in intense sunlight. This is especially important
around bright, reflective surfaces such as snow, water, sand, or ce-
ment, and at high altitudes. Never look right into the sun.

—Always cover your eyes when you use a sun lamp or tanning machine. Closing your eyes or wearing ordinary sunglasses or cotton
eye patches will not protect against eye damage.

Call Your Doctor If . . .

• Your eye pain gets worse.

• You have any problems with your eye patches.

• You have any problems that may be related to the medicine you are
taking.

Corneal Foreign Body

See Foreign Body in the Eye

Corneal Ulcer

WHAT YOU SHOULD KNOW

A corneal ulcer is an open sore in the cornea, the thin, colorless covering of the eye. With treatment, it is usually cured in 2 to 3 weeks;
without treatment, it may lead to long-term vision problems.

Causes

Corneal ulcers are the result of an infection that takes hold after an
eye injury or overuse of contact lenses. In some cases they are caused
by failure of the eyelid to close as it should.

Signs/Symptoms

You can expect severe eye pain, blurred vision, tearing, twitching of
the eyelid, redness in the white of the eye, or discharge from the eye.
The eyes may become sensitive to bright light.

Care

Do not touch or rub your eye. Your doctor will prescribe medicine to treat the ulcer.

WHAT YOU SHOULD DO

- Follow your doctor's orders carefully. Otherwise, the ulcer may penetrate the cornea and allow the infection to enter the eyeball. This could cause permanent loss of vision.
- Applying a clean, cool or warm washcloth to your eye may help ease the discomfort.
- Wash your hands often and dry them with a clean towel. Do not touch your eyes with your fingers.
- Rest your eyes as much as possible until the infection is gone. Do not read or watch television for long periods of time. Wear dark glasses to protect your eyes from bright light.
- For pain, you may use over-the-counter medicines such as acetaminophen or ibuprofen.

Call Your Doctor If . . .

- Your eye is still painful after several days of treatment.
- You develop a high temperature.
- You have new or unexplained symptoms.

Seek Care Immediately If . . .

- The pain in your eye gets worse.
- You notice changes in your vision.

Coronary Artery Disease

WHAT YOU SHOULD KNOW

Coronary Artery Disease, also called CAD, occurs when the arteries in the heart get narrower and harder or become blocked. It is one of the leading causes of death in America. It can lead to angina, a heart attack, or congestive heart failure.

The odds of dying from CAD today are much less than they were 40 years ago. This is because we have learned about the factors that increase risk of the disease. Some of these factors can be prevented.

Causes

When fat collects inside the arteries leading to the heart muscle, the arteries get narrow or become blocked, and can no longer supply the oxygen the heart muscle needs.

Risk Factors

The risk of CAD increases as you get older. You are also at greater risk if you have a family history of heart disease. These risks cannot be changed, but others can be eliminated. Needless risks include cigarette smoking, stress, high blood pressure, a fat-filled diet, excess weight, and lack of exercise.

Do's and Don'ts

You can decrease your chances of getting CAD by not smoking and by exercising regularly; decreasing stress; and controlling other illnesses (such as diabetes or high blood pressure). You should also eat a diet low in fat and salt, and high in fiber (from such sources as fruit, wheat, and grains).

Care

If you are admitted to the hospital, it will be to receive treatment for problems caused by the CAD, not to treat the CAD itself. You may also be admitted to the hospital to see how badly your heart vessels are blocked.

WHAT YOU SHOULD DO

- Check your blood pressure and pulse as directed by your doctor.
- Always take your medicine exactly as prescribed. If you feel it is not helping, call your doctor. Do not quit taking it on your own.
- If you take aspirin regularly, continue to take it. Aspirin helps thin the blood so blood clots don't form. Do not take acetaminophen or ibuprofen instead.
- If you are using nitroglycerin (ni-tro-GLIS-er-in), continue to use it. It may give you a headache and make you feel a little dizzy, so take it while sitting or lying down.
- A diet low in fat, salt, and cholesterol is very important. It keeps your heart healthy and strong. Ask your doctor for guidelines.
- Getting used to a new diet may take time. Special cookbooks may help the cook in your family find new recipes.
- Quit smoking. It causes less oxygen to get to your heart. If you have trouble stopping, ask your doctor for help.
- Exercise daily. It helps make the heart stronger, lowers blood pressure, and keeps you healthy. If your exercise plan seems too hard or too easy, talk to your doctor.
- Excess weight can make the heart work harder. If you need to lose weight, ask your doctor for a plan.
- Since it is hard to avoid stress, learn to control it. Ways to relax

include deep breathing, relaxing the muscles, and imagery. Don't hesitate to talk to someone about things that upset you.

• If you have other illnesses like diabetes or high blood pressure, you need to control them. Take medicines as directed. Because of these illnesses, you have a higher chance of getting a heart attack.

• For more information about the heart, call the **American Heart Association at 1-800-AHA-USA1 (1-800-242-8721)** or call your local **Red Cross**.

Call Your Doctor If . . .

• You have chest pain anytime that doesn't go away with rest.

Seek Care Immediately If . . .

• You have chest pain that spreads to your arms, jaw, or back, and you are sweating, sick to your stomach, and have trouble breathing. These are signs of a heart attack. **THIS IS AN EMERGENCY. Call 911 or 0 (operator) to get to the nearest hospital or clinic. Do not drive yourself!**

Corynebacterium Vaginalis

See Bacterial Vaginosis

Costochondritis

WHAT YOU SHOULD KNOW

Costochondritis (COS-to-kon-DRY-tis) is an irritation and swelling of the joints that connect the ribs to the breastbone. It is most common in young adults. It may take 3 to 6 weeks to disappear.

Causes

Often, no cause can be found.

Signs/Symptoms

The problem is marked by chest tightness and sharp pain that worsens when you move or breathe deeply. The pain may spread to the arm and may occur in more than one place.

Care

No special care is needed.

WHAT YOU SHOULD DO

- Avoid exhausting physical activity and try not to bump your ribs as you move around.
- Applying heat to the injury may help relieve pain. Use a warm heating pad, whirlpool bath, or warm, moist towels for 10 to 20 minutes every hour for 48 hours.
- Nonprescription medications such as aspirin, acetaminophen, and ibuprofen may ease the pain.

Call Your Doctor If . . .
- The pain increases or you are very uncomfortable.
- You develop a high temperature.
- You develop worse chest pains.
- You develop new, unexplained symptoms.

Crabs

WHAT YOU SHOULD KNOW

Crab lice, also known as pubic lice, are tiny, light brown insects that live in hairy areas of the body or in clothing. The lice lay eggs, called nits, which cling so tightly to body hair that they cannot be removed with normal washing. The problem is easily spread from person to person. With treatment, however, the lice should be gone in 5 days.

Causes
Pubic lice are often spread during sex. You can also catch them by sharing combs, hats, clothing, or bed linens.

Signs/Symptoms
You'll first notice itching in the hairy areas of your body, such as the genital area, scalp, or eyebrows. You may see red marks and bumps (called hives) where the insects have bitten your skin. You may even see the lice themselves on your hair.

Care
Lice-killing shampoos and lotions will eliminate the problem.

WHAT YOU SHOULD DO

- Be careful to apply medication exactly as directed.
- Lice-killing medicine does not always destroy all the nits. You must remove them from your hair with a fine-toothed comb. A special comb may come with the medicine. If not, you can buy one at a

drugstore. Comb the lice-infested hair completely, from the skin outward, once a day until treatment is complete. You do not have to shave or cut the hair in the affected area.
- Avoid close contact with anyone until your doctor tells you the lice are all gone.
- All the clothes, towels, sheets and blankets you use during treatment and the 3 days before must be machine washed. Use hot water, then dry them for at least 20 minutes in a hot dryer. If you do not have a washer and dryer, iron the items, seal them up in a plastic bag for 10 days, have them dry cleaned, or hang them outside for 2 days.
- Tell all sexual partners about the problem, so that they can be checked for lice and treated.

Call Your Doctor If . . .
- The bites become pus-filled or crusty, and your hair becomes matted or foul-smelling. These are signs of infection.
- Itching or red, swollen bite marks return after treatment.
- You have any problems that may be related to the medicine you are using.

CRF

See Kidney Failure, Chronic

Croup

WHAT YOU SHOULD KNOW

Croup, known medically as laryngotracheobronchitis, is an infection of the voice box. It is a common illness in infants and children from 3 months to 3 years of age. Croup usually occurs during late fall, winter, and early spring. Antibiotics will not work, but other medicines can be given to help your child feel better. A child may get croup more than once.

Causes
Croup usually starts with a cold, cough, and sore throat.

Signs/Symptoms
Often the child has a barky cough, noisy breathing, and a hoarse voice. Other signs are fast breathing, problems swallowing, and restlessness.

Croup attacks usually occur during the evening or night. The attacks are worst during the first 2 to 3 days.

Risks

Children can die from croup, but the chances of this are very small if you follow your doctor's suggestions.

WHAT YOU SHOULD DO

- You can help the child's breathing by sitting with him or her in a steamy bathroom. Turn on the hot water in the sink, shower, or bathtub and close the windows and bathroom door. When the room is steamed up, bring the child into the room and sit with him or her on your lap for at least 15 minutes. Do not leave the child alone.
- Call your doctor if the steam does not improve the child's breathing within 10 to 15 minutes.
- If it is cool outside, taking the clothed child outside in the cool air for 5 minutes may help make breathing easier.
- If you have a humidifier, place it out of reach by the child's bed. Fill it with cool water. Direct the mist stream towards the child's face. The humidifier will loosen the mucus in the child's throat, making it easier to breathe.
- Keep your child warm and give clear liquids (water, apple juice, lemonade, tea, or ginger ale) once breathing has improved. The liquids should be room temperature. They are important for keeping the child's mucus thin.
- Do not let anyone smoke around the child. The smoke can make his or her breathing and coughing worse.
- Do **not** give your child aspirin. Give acetaminophen for fever and comfort. Ask your doctor before giving ibuprofen.
- You should try to stay calm and see that the child gets as much rest as possible. His or her breathing and coughing will become worse if the child is afraid and crying.
- Most cases of croup can be treated at home as long as breathing problems and coughing don't increase. It could be 5 to 6 days before the child feels better.

Call Your Doctor If . . .

- The child is sleepier than usual, is urinating less, has a dry mouth and cracked lips, cries without tears, or is dizzy. These are signs of dehydration.
- The child has a high temperature.
- The child's breathing does not get better after 10 to 15 minutes in a steamy bathroom.
- The child cannot rest because the coughing won't stop.
- The cough lasts more than a few days.

Call Your Doctor Immediately If . . .

• **Call 911 or 0 (operator)** for help if your child has any of the following signs: trouble breathing or swallowing, the skin between the ribs is being sucked-in with each breath, the lips or fingernails are turning blue or white, or the child is leaning over and drooling.

IF YOU'RE HEADING FOR THE HOSPITAL . . .

What to Expect While You're There

You may encounter the following procedures and equipment during your child's stay.

• **Taking Vital Signs:** These include the child's temperature, blood pressure, pulse (counting heartbeats), and respirations (counting breaths). A stethoscope is used to listen to the heart and lungs. Blood pressure is taken by wrapping a cuff around the child's arm.

• **Pulse Oximeter:** The child may be hooked up to a pulse oximeter (ox-IM-uh-ter). It is placed on the ear, finger, or toe and is connected to a machine that measures the oxygen in your child's blood.

• **Oxygen:** The child will get moist cool air either from a mask, tent, or high humidity room. This will make breathing easier.

• **Breathing Treatments:** A machine will be used to help the child inhale medicine that keeps the airways open. A doctor will assist with these treatments. At first, they may be needed quite often. Later, they may be needed only if the child is having trouble breathing.

• **IV:** A tube placed in your child's veins for giving medicine or liquids. It will be capped or have tubing connected to it.

• **Chest X-ray:** This is a picture of the heart and lungs. The doctor uses it to see how your child's heart and lungs are handling the illness.

• **Blood:** Is usually taken from a vein in your child's hand or from the bend in the elbow. Tests are done on the blood.

• **Blood Gases:** Blood is taken from an artery in your child's wrist, elbow, or groin. It is tested to see how much oxygen it contains.

• **ECG:** Also called a heart monitor, an electrocardiograph (e-lec-tro-CAR-dee-o-graf), or EKG. The patches on your child's chest are hooked up to a TV-type screen. This screen shows a tracing of each heartbeat. Your child's heart will be watched for signs of injury or damage that could be related to the illness.

• **Visiting:** You may stay with the child to give comfort and support. Your child will feel safer in the hospital with you nearby.

After You Leave

• Little can be done to keep your child from getting a cold, which can cause croup; but try to avoid anyone who has a cold.

- If the child does get a cold, use a cool mist humidifier in his or her room.
- If the child develops another case of croup, follow the guidelines under "What You Should Do," above.

Crutches

WHAT YOU SHOULD KNOW

Crutches are often needed when you have an injured leg, foot, or hip. They are also used to provide extra balance. When using crutches, it is important to put your weight on your arms and hands rather than on your underarms. This could damage the nerves in your armpits.

Moving around on crutches is a slow process; so be patient. You will get the hang of it in time. The length of time you will need to use crutches depends on your illness or injury.

Usually, the doctor will fit you with new crutches and show you how to use them so you won't fall or develop nerve damage under your arms. Use your crutches only on firm ground that has no snow or ice. Make sure the rubber tips are not split or loose.

WHAT YOU SHOULD DO

- Walking:
  —Begin by placing both crutches in front of you at the same time. Put them about 1 inch in front and 6 to 8 inches to the side of your toes.
  —Lean on your hands, not your underarms. The top of the crutches should hit about 2 inches (3 fingers side by side) below your underarm.
  —Keep your elbows bent as you use the crutches. Keep your injured leg off the floor by bending your knee.
  —Move both crutches forward. Then swing your uninjured foot between the crutches landing heel first. Repeat with each step.
  —If you are using your crutches for balance, move your right foot and left crutch forward. Then move your left foot and right crutch forward. Continue walking this way.
- Going Up Stairs:
  —Face the stairs. Put the crutches close to the first step.
  —Push on the crutches with your elbows straight and put your uninjured leg on the first step.
  —Bring both crutches up to the first step at the same time. Repeat.
  —When using a railing, put both crutches under the arm opposite the railing.

- Going Down Stairs:
  —Stand with the toes of your uninjured leg close to the edge of the step.
  —Bend the knee of your uninjured leg. Slowly lower both crutches onto the next step.
  —Lean on your crutches. Slowly lower your uninjured leg on to the same step.
  —When using a railing, put both crutches under the arm opposite the railing.
- Sitting In A Chair:
  —Back up to the chair until you feel the edge of it against the back of your legs. Keep your injured leg forward.
  —Take your crutches out from under your arms. Sit while bending your uninjured knee.
- Getting Up From A Chair:
  —Sit on the edge of your chair. Put your uninjured foot close to the chair.
  —Push up with your hands using the crutches or arms of the chair. Put your weight on your uninjured foot as you get up.
  —Keep your injured leg bent at the knee and off the floor.

Cryosurgery, Skin

See Skin Cryosurgery

C-Section

See Cesarean Section

Cutting Teeth

See Teething

CVA

See Stroke

Cystoscopy

A Cystoscopy (cis-TOSS-co-pee) enables the doctor to examine the lower urinary tract visually. During the procedure, a thin fiberoptic instrument (a tube with a light and lenses on the end) is passed through the urinary duct (urethra) into the bladder.

Risks
The bladder or urethra could be injured during a cystoscopy. You could also develop a bladder infection. However, if you follow your doctor's directions, you are not likely to have problems.

IF YOU'RE HEADING FOR THE HOSPITAL . . .

Before You Go
• Your doctor will set a time after which you MUST NOT eat or drink. Be sure to follow these directions exactly.
• If your doctor says you need to clear your bowel before the cystoscopy, you may have to take a laxative.

What to Expect While You're There
You may encounter the following procedures and equipment during your stay:
• **Taking Your Vital Signs:** These include your temperature, blood pressure, pulse (counting your heartbeats), and respirations (counting your breaths). A stethoscope is used to listen to your heart and lungs. Your blood pressure is taken by wrapping a cuff around your arm.
• **During the Cystoscopy . . .**
  —You will lie on your back with a sheet covering you. You will need to bend your knees and slide your feet into metal stirrups. The area around the urethra will be washed with soap and water.
  —A soft tube will be gently inserted in the urethra and threaded into the bladder. The tube has a light and camera lenses on its tip. Pictures of the bladder and urethra will appear on a TV-like screen. You may feel the urge to urinate during this procedure.
  —To see how much your bladder can hold, the doctor may run liquid through the tube. A sample of bladder tissue and urine may be taken for study.
  —The entire procedure will take about 20 to 30 minutes.

After You Leave
• Avoid vigorous exercise for 2 weeks.
• Do not have sexual relations until your doctor tells you that healing is complete.
• You may notice a small amount of blood in your urine. This should go away in 24 hours.
• Drink 6 to 8 glasses (soda-can size) of water a day.

Call Your Doctor If . . .
• Urinating becomes painful or difficult.

• You develop a temperature of more than 101 degrees F (38.3 degrees C).

Seek Care Immediately If . . .
• You have blood specks in your urine or your urine turns a bright or dark red color.

D & C

See Dilatation and Curettage

Damaged Teeth

WHAT YOU SHOULD KNOW

Damage to the teeth ranges from a small chip on the edge of a tooth to a break at the gum line or a crack that reaches the roots.

Causes
Most tooth injuries occur in an accident or fall.

Signs/Symptoms
If you lose a small chip from a tooth, you may have no pain; but if a tooth cracks down to the soft tissue inside, the pain can be severe.

Care
Some injuries heal without treatment (see below). However, a broken tooth can easily become infected and should be seen by a dentist right away.

WHAT YOU SHOULD DO

• If a tooth is chipped or cracked, but there is no other damage, you may wish to see a dentist who does cosmetic work to have the tooth restored to its natural appearance. Regular follow-up visits are important to make sure there are no complications developing in the injured tooth.
• If there is damage to the inner parts of the tooth, you must see a dentist within 24 hours. If not treated, the tooth can become infected, and you could lose it. Until your dental visit, drink only cool or warm liquids (the tooth will be sensitive to cold and heat).
• If the tooth is injured below the gum line, but there is no injury to the enamel, the only symptom may be tenderness when biting or chewing for a few days. Apply a piece of ice to the injured gum area (unless that increases pain) several times a day for 2 or 3 days. No

immediate dental treatment is necessary, but you should make an appointment for a regular checkup to make sure there are no problems developing in the tooth.

- If a tooth is slightly loosened or pushed inward by the injury, eat only soft foods for 1 to 2 weeks, making sure to keep your diet as well-balanced as possible. Soft foods include gelatin, cooked cereal, baby food, ice cream, applesauce, bananas, eggs, pasta, cottage cheese, soups, and yogurt. A mildly displaced tooth usually returns to its normal position within a few weeks without treatment.
- If you have a mouth or lip wound, rinse your mouth with warm salt water (1/2 teaspoon salt in 8 ounces of water), or a half-and-half mixture of water and hydrogen peroxide, 3 or more times daily after eating. Do NOT swallow the solution. Apply hydrogen peroxide to the wounds with a cotton-tipped swab several times a day.

Call Your Dentist If . . .
- The injured tooth becomes more sensitive to cold, heat, air, sweetness, or sourness.
- Tooth pain develops or increases.
- The tooth gets darker in color.
- You develop any new symptoms, including a headache.

Deep Vein Thrombophlebitis

WHAT YOU SHOULD KNOW

Deep vein thrombophlebitis (throm-bo-fleh-BITE-is) or thrombosis is also called DVT for short. It develops when a blood clot forms inside a vein. The clot may block part or all of the blood flow. It may also break away from the vein wall and lodge in a lung.

DVT usually occurs in the lower legs (calves) or lower pelvis. Rarely does it occur elsewhere in the body.

Causes
The clots usually develop when blood pools or sits in a vein for an extended period. Resting in bed for a long time because of surgery or a long illness (such as a heart attack or stroke) may cause the blood to pool.

Signs/Symptoms
Swelling, pain, and redness in the area of the clot (usually in the ankle, calf, or thigh). Walking may be painful.

Risk factors

Being over 60 years old, weighing too much, smoking, or using birth control pills.

Do's and Don'ts

To keep from getting blood clots:
- Move your legs as soon as possible after surgery or during long periods of bed rest.
- Exercise your legs every 1 or 2 hours while on long car or airplane trips.
- Do not smoke if you are taking birth control pills.

Care

You will be put in the hospital and given blood thinners to keep clots from forming. This also allows the body to break up clots. You may also need tests to find out where and how big the clot is. The earlier you are treated the less likely you are to get a clot in your lung.

Risks

A blood clot in the leg is not dangerous, though it can lead to long-term problems. But if the clot breaks off and floats into the lung, it can be deadly if left untreated. Early care can keep this from happening.

WHAT YOU SHOULD DO

Call Your Doctor If . . .

- You are bruising easily and often.
- You are bleeding from your gums or nose, or have blood in your urine or stools. This may be due to blood thinners given to prevent new clots.
- You have increased swelling or pain in the calf of your leg. This may be a sign of a leg clot.

Seek Care Immediately If . . .

- You have sudden chest pain, trouble breathing, or are coughing-up blood. **Call 911 or 0 (operator)** to get to the nearest hospital or clinic. **Do not drive yourself!**

IF YOU'RE HEADING FOR THE HOSPITAL . . .

What to Expect While You're There

You may encounter the following procedures and equipment during your stay.
- **Taking Vital Signs:** These include your temperature, blood pressure, pulse (counting your heartbeats), and respirations (counting

your breaths). A stethoscope is used to listen to your heart and lungs. Your blood pressure is taken by wrapping a cuff around your arm.

- **Pulse Oximeter:** If you are getting oxygen, you may be hooked up to a pulse oximeter (ox-IM-uh-ter). It is placed on your ear, finger, or toe and is connected to a machine that measures the oxygen in your blood.
- **Blood:** Usually taken from a vein in your hand or from the bend in your elbow. Tests will be done on the blood.
- **Other Tests:** Sometimes special tests are needed to find the clot. One test is an x-ray of the veins after injecting dye. Another is ultrasound. This test uses sound waves to draw a picture of the vein and clot on a TV-type screen.
- **IV:** A tube placed in your vein for giving medicine or liquids. It will be capped or have tubing connected to it.
- **Medicine:**
  —**Heparin:** Keeps the blood thin so no other clots form. It is given in an IV.
  —**Other Blood Thinners:** Blood thinners that can be taken by mouth include aspirin and warfarin. These also keep the blood from forming clots.
  —**Clot Busters:** These drugs break apart clots. They are given in your IV, usually at the same time as heparin. This medicine can make you bleed or bruise easily.
  —**Pain Medicine:** May be given in your IV, as a shot, or by mouth. If the pain does not go away or comes back, tell a doctor right away.
- **Activity:**
  —At first you will need to rest in bed. Your feet may be raised a little. Elastic wraps and warm packs may be placed on the area of the clot.
  —You may be asked to slowly move your legs and ankles, and wiggle your toes a few minutes out of every hour that you are awake. This keeps blood from settling in your legs and causing more blood clots. You'll be warned to avoid crossing your legs or ankles.
  —Once you are allowed to walk, you will need to wear tight knee socks. This keeps the blood from pooling in your legs.
- **Surgery:** If the clot does not dissolve using medicine, it may have to be removed surgically.

After You Leave

- If you are taking a blood thinner (such as warfarin):

—Wear a medic-alert bracelet that says you are taking a blood thinner. Ask your doctor how to get one.

—Tell your dentist that you are taking it.

—Watch for bleeding from your gums, nose, or in your urine or stools.

—Avoid sports that can cause injury since you will bruise more easily.

—Keep your stools soft so you do. not strain. You can do this by eating a high fiber diet (breads and cereals) or taking stool softeners (as directed by your doctor).

• Always take your medicine as directed by your doctor. If you feel it is not helping, call your doctor. Do not quit taking it on your own.

• If you take aspirin regularly, continue to take it. Aspirin helps thin the blood so blood clots don't form. Do not take acetaminophen or ibuprofen instead.

• To keep blood from pooling in your legs and forming more clots:

—When you are on bedrest for a long time, move your legs, bend your ankles, and wiggle your toes for a few minutes every hour that you are awake.

—Wear special elastic knee socks, especially when you are in bed for a long time. Ask your doctor for them.

—Don't cross your ankles or legs for long periods of time.

—When you are sick or have surgery, start walking as soon as possible.

—When you travel, stand and walk every 1 to 2 hours.

—Do not wear tight garters, girdles, or knee-hi hose.

Dehydration in Adults

WHAT YOU SHOULD KNOW

Dehydration (dee-hi-DRAY-shun)—excessive loss of water and salt from the body—can become very dangerous if you allow it to go uncorrected.

Causes

Prolonged vomiting, diarrhea, or high fever can deplete the body's fluids. Other causes include staying in the sun or heat for too long and sweating a lot. An overdose of medicines that cause you to lose water and salt, such as diuretics (di-u-RET-ics) or "water pills," also can cause dehydration.

Signs/Symptoms

Typical symptoms include a dry tongue and mouth, great thirst, and less urination. Other symptoms include sunken eyes, wrinkled skin, dizziness, confusion, and a fast heartbeat and breathing.

Care
You may need to have your blood tested. You also may need a stay in the hospital, where you can be given IV fluids. If you think you are dehydrated, you should weigh yourself daily and write down the number. Also keep track of how much and how often you are vomiting and having diarrhea. Get lots of rest.

Risks
Without treatment, your blood pressure could fall too low, leading to shock and even death.

WHAT YOU SHOULD DO

- It is important to drink plenty of liquids to replace the water your body has lost. Drink a small amount of fluid every 30 to 60 minutes. Large amounts may upset your stomach.
- Drink clear liquids for the first 24 hours.
  - You can buy a special ready-made liquid called a rehydration or electrolyte solution at a drug or grocery store. It has the exact amounts of water, salts, and sugar your body needs to replace the lost water and salts. Follow the directions on the label.
  - You also can make your own fluid replacement mixture. Be sure to measure carefully. Add 1 level teaspoon of sugar and 1/2 level teaspoon of salt to 1 pint (2 measuring cups) of water.
  - Do not use liquids such as apple juice, soft drinks, tea, chicken broth, or sport drinks. They have the wrong amounts of water, salts, and sugar.
- If you have been vomiting and can't keep liquids down, suck on ice chips or flavored ice until the throwing up stops. You may drink more liquids as your vomiting lessens.
- Keep drinking liquids until your urine is pale yellow. You may need to drink 8 to 12 glasses (soda-can size) of liquids a day to bring your water level back to normal.
- If you are not vomiting, you may slowly return to your normal diet over the next 2 to 3 days.

Call Your Doctor If . . .
- You are having trouble keeping liquids down.
- You develop a high temperature.
- You do not feel better after drinking liquids for several hours.

Seek Care Immediately If . . .
- You pass very little urine or none at all after a few hours of treatment.
- You feel dizzy or faint.
- You have a fast heartbeat.
- Your skin looks wrinkled or your mouth feels very dry.
- You lose several pounds in a few days.

IF YOU'RE HEADING FOR THE HOSPITAL . . .

What to Expect While You're There
You may encounter the following procedures and equipment during your stay.
- **IV:** A tube placed in your vein for giving medicine or liquids. It will be used to get fluid back into your system. When not in use, it will be capped.
- **Strict Intake/Output:** Caregivers will carefully watch how much liquid you are getting and how much you are urinating.
- **Daily Weight:** Since severe fluid loss shows up in your weight, you will be weighed daily.
- **Taking Vital Signs:** These include your temperature, blood pressure, pulse (counting your heartbeats), and respirations (counting your breaths). A stethoscope is used to listen to your heart and lungs. Your blood pressure is taken by wrapping a cuff around your arm.
- **Pulse Oximeter:** You may be hooked up to a pulse oximeter (ox-IM-uh-ter). It is placed on your ear, finger, or toe and is connected to a machine. It measures the oxygen in your blood.
- **Blood:** Usually taken from a vein in your hand or from the bend in your elbow. Tests will be done on the blood.

Dehydration in Children

WHAT YOU SHOULD KNOW

Dehydration (dee-hi-DRAY-shun) is a loss of water and other important body salts. It can happen to any child; but it's most serious in newborns and infants. Your child should return to normal when the cause of the dehydration is found and body fluids are replaced.

Causes
Severe vomiting or diarrhea, usually caused by an infection, can drain the body of fluid. Fever, sweating, and prolonged exposure to the sun are other possible causes.

Signs/Symptoms

A dehydrated child may be sleepier than usual, urinate less, have a dry mouth and cracked lips, cry without tears, or seem dizzy. With babies less than one year old, the soft spot on top of their head may become sunken.

Care

Lost liquids must be replaced. The child may need to be put in the hospital for care and treatment.

WHAT YOU SHOULD DO

- For the first 24 hours give the child only clear fluids. Electrolyte solutions can be bought at the grocery store, or you can give gelatin water (a 3-ounce package in a quart of water), or a mixture made by adding 1/4 teaspoon salt and 1 tablespoon sugar to 1 pint of water.
  —If the child is vomiting, give fluid very slowly, starting with 1 or 2 teaspoons every 10 minutes.
  —If there is no vomiting and the child is less than 1 year old, you may give 1 tablespoon every 20 minutes.
  —If there is no vomiting and the child is over 1 year old, give 2 tablespoons every 30 minutes.
- If there is no vomiting, you may gradually return the child to his or her normal diet over the next 2 or 3 days.
  —If a baby is taking only formula, dilute it to 1/2 strength for the next 24 hours.
  —If you are breastfeeding, give the baby clear liquids for 2 feedings, then start breastfeeding again.
  —If your child is taking solid food, begin with bland foods such as applesauce or bananas and add other foods as tolerated. If the child is over 1 year old, do not include milk, ice cream, butter, or cheese in the diet for the next 3 days.
- Keep a record of how often you change your baby's diaper and how wet it is each time.

Call Your Doctor If . . .

- For children less than 3 months old, call if the child's temperature goes above 100 degrees F (37 degrees C).
- For children over 3 months, call if the child's temperature goes above 102 degrees F (39.4 degrees C).

Seek Care Immediately If . . .

- Your child has signs of worsening dehydration, including listlessness, excessive thirst, little or no urination in more than 6 hours, no tears, wrinkled skin, dizziness, irritability, weight loss, or, if the child is a baby, a sunken soft spot on the top of the head.

Dental Abscess

WHAT YOU SHOULD KNOW

A dental abscess (AB-sess) is an infection around the root of a tooth or in the gums or jawbone. The infection causes pus to collect, and a lump can appear.

Causes

Dental abscesses often get their start when bacteria invade a decayed tooth; the decay may then travel to the gums or jawbone. Decay can also begin in the mouth when teeth are not brushed or flossed properly.

Signs/Symptoms

Typically, you'll develop fever, redness and swelling of the gums or cheek. If you have a lump, it may feel hot. Other signs include tooth or mouth pain, a loose tooth, or inability to close your mouth all the way. If the abscess spreads, your face, neck, or chest may swell.

Care

Your dentist may need to drain the pus from the abscess. During this procedure, you're likely to be given gas or numbing medication to help you relax and to minimize the pain. You'll probably be given antibiotics to treat the infection, and pain medicine to ease your discomfort.

WHAT YOU SHOULD DO

- Rinse your mouth with warm water every hour or as needed to ease the pain. This will help draw the infection from the abscess.
- For pain, you may take over-the-counter medications, such as acetaminophen or ibuprofen.
- To help ease the pain, avoid chewing on the affected side for at least 2 days; you may need to limit yourself to a liquid diet.
- Putting ice on your face over the affected area may also relieve the pain. Apply the ice for 10 to 20 minutes out of every hour, as necessary.
- If the abscess is drained, the dentist may leave a small hole or drain. Keep the area free of food by rinsing with water after eating. You'll need to return to the dentist to have the drain removed.
- If an antibiotic is prescribed, take it as directed until you have fin-

ished all the medication. Do not stop taking it when you begin to feel better. If you end treatment too soon, some bacteria may survive and re-infect you.

• To prevent abscesses:
  —Brush regularly with a toothbrush recommended by your dentist.
  —Floss daily and use a fluoride mouthwash, toothpaste, tablets, or supplements as instructed by your dentist or dental hygienist.
  —Reduce the amount of sugar in your diet.

Call Your Doctor If . . .
• You have a high temperature.
• Your pain becomes worse.
• You have any new symptoms or problems that may be due to the medicine you are taking.

Seek Care Immediately If . . .
• You have new or increased swelling in your face, jaw, cheek, eye, or neck.

Dermoid Cyst Removal

WHAT YOU SHOULD KNOW

A dermoid cyst is a sac filled with gas, liquid, or a jelly-like material that develops on the skin of the face, scalp, neck, or trunk. The cyst may remain small for years or slowly grow larger. Although such cysts are not dangerous, it may eventually need to be removed (excised) by a doctor.

WHAT YOU SHOULD DO

• After the removal, keep your bandage clean and dry. You may change it after 24 hours. If it sticks, use warm water to gently loosen it. Pat the area dry with a clean towel before putting on another bandage.
• If possible, keep the area where the cyst was removed raised. This will relieve soreness and swelling and promote healing.
• If you have stitches, keep them dry for 24 hours. After that time, you may clean them gently with a cotton swab dipped in a mixture of half water and half hydrogen peroxide.
• Do not go swimming or soak the area where the cyst was removed.
• Do not bump or overuse the area where the cyst was removed.

Call Your Doctor If . . .
- You develop a temperature of over 100.4 degrees F (38 degrees C).
- Blood continues to soak through the bandage.
- Pain in the area of the removal grows worse.
- You notice redness, swelling, pus, a bad smell, or red streaks leading from the stitches. These are signs of infection.

Diabetes

WHAT YOU SHOULD KNOW

To get energy from the starches and sugar we eat, everyone needs adequate supplies of a hormone called insulin. People with diabetes either do not make enough insulin or are unable to make efficient use of whatever insulin they do manage to produce. Without insulin, sugar builds up in the blood, eventually leading to a host of serious problems. Diabetes (referred to medically as diabetes mellitus) can start in childhood, but more often appears later in life. There is no cure for this disease, but it can be controlled. Left uncontrolled, it can result in damage to the heart, kidneys, eyes, blood vessels, and nerves.

Causes
In people with "Type I" diabetes—the kind that usually appears in childhood—the pancreas makes too little insulin or none at all. In those with "Type II" diabetes—which typically develops in adults— the pancreas continues to manufacture insulin, but the body fails to make use of it.

Signs/Symptoms
The tip-off that you have diabetes is a set of symptoms that includes fatigue, great thirst, weight loss, frequent urination, and increased vulnerability to infection. Wounds may heal slowly. You may also feel as though you are eating more than usual.

Care
People with Type I diabetes usually need regular injections of insulin. Type II diabetes can often be controlled with a special diet, exercise, and oral medicines, though temporary insulin injections may be necessary during periods of stress and times of illness. Since there is no cure, you will need treatment for the rest of your life.

WHAT YOU SHOULD DO

- The more closely you follow your doctor's instructions, the better your chances of preventing or delaying dangerous complications.
- It is very important to take the medication prescribed by your doctor exactly as directed. Never stop taking this medicine without talking to your doctor first.
- Be sure to test your urine or blood for sugar (glucose) as often as your doctor directs.
- Make a point of exercising regularly. Your doctor will suggest an exercise program you can follow.
- Eat wholesome, balanced meals at regular, fixed times. It is best to have 3 meals a day, plus 2 or 3 snacks. Your doctor or nutritionist will give you a special diet to guide your starch and sugar intake.
- Your doctor may advise you to lose weight. Losing as little as 10 to 15 pounds can improve your blood sugar levels.
- Always wear a medic-alert pendant or bracelet identifying you as a diabetic.
- Learn about your disease and about the signs of hypoglycemia and ketoacidosis (see below).

Call Your Doctor If . . .

- You have any questions about medicine, activity, or diet.
- You continue to have symptoms of diabetes (such as increased thirst and urination).

Seek Care Immediately If . . .

- You develop symptoms of low blood sugar (hypoglycemia). These symptoms include confusion, sweating, weakness, paleness, and a rapid heartbeat. In severe cases, hypoglycemia can progress to seizures and coma.
- You develop symptoms of ketoacidosis (a dangerous chemical imbalance in the body). These symptoms include a fruity odor on the breath, a speed-up or slow-down in breathing, and a very sleepy feeling.
- You develop vomiting or have diarrhea.
- You notice numbness, tingling, or pain in your feet or hands.
- You feel chest pain.
- Your symptoms get worse, even though you are following your doctor's orders.

Diabetic Foot Care

WHAT YOU SHOULD KNOW

Diabetes often causes poor blood supply to your legs and feet. As a result, your skin may become thinner, break more easily, heal more slowly, and become more vulnerable to infection. Diabetes can also lead to nerve damage, reducing the feeling in your feet. If this happens, you may not notice minor injuries that could cause an infection. Even a small cut or blister can lead to serious problems when you have diabetes. To prevent dangerous infections, you need to inspect and wash your feet daily.

Signs/Symptoms

If you have diminished blood supply to your feet, you may notice redness, warmth, or sores on your feet that heal slowly or not at all. If you have lost feeling in your feet, you may not feel any pain.

WHAT YOU SHOULD DO

- Do not go barefoot. Bare feet are easily injured.
- Check your feet daily for blisters, cuts, and redness.
- Wash your feet gently with warm (not hot) water and mild soap every day. Pat your feet and the area between your toes until completely dry.
- Apply moisturizing lotion to the dry skin on your feet and to dry, brittle toenails.
- Trim your toenails straight across. Do not dig under them or around the cuticle.
- Do not cut corns or calluses or try to remove them with medicine unless your doctor approves.
- Wear clean cotton socks or stockings every day. Make sure they are not too tight.
- Wear leather shoes that fit properly and have enough cushioning. To break in new shoes without injuring your feet, wear them just a few hours each day.
- If you find a minor scrape, cut, or break in the skin on your feet, keep it and the skin around it clean and dry.
- When you remove an adhesive bandage, be sure not to injure the skin around it.
- Check any wound several times a day to make sure it is healing.
- Follow your doctor's diet and exercise plan carefully, and take your medicines exactly as directed.

Call Your Doctor If . . .
• An injury is not healing or you notice redness, numbness, burning, or tingling.
• Your feet always feel cold.
• You develop pain or cramps in your legs and feet.

Diabetic Hypoglycemia

See Insulin Reaction

Diabetic Ketoacidosis

WHAT YOU SHOULD KNOW

Ketoacidosis (KEY-toe-ASS-ih-DOE-sis) is one of the many dangerous complications of diabetes. The problem develops when the body is unable to get enough energy from blood sugar and begins to use fat. As a byproduct of this process, chemicals called ketones flood the bloodstream. Together with excess sugar, the extra ketones can build up to dangerous, even life-threatening levels. This condition needs immediate care by your doctor.

Causes
The body needs insulin in order to process blood sugar efficiently and prevent excessive breakdown of fats; so diabetic ketoacidosis is often the result of a diabetic's failure to take enough insulin, or to take any insulin at all. The problem may also be triggered by infection, injury, and emotional stress. Often, doctors can find no immediate cause.

Signs/Symptoms
Early signs include excessive thirst, frequent urination, headache, nausea, and vomiting. The breath may begin to take on a fruity odor, and you may develop rapid deep breathing, sleepiness, and fatigue. Other symptoms include weight loss and a feeling of fullness or pain in the stomach.

Care
Call your doctor when you first notice early signs. You may need to be hospitalized for tests and treatment. If the condition is left untreated, it could lead to coma and death.

WHAT YOU SHOULD DO

• To keep from losing too much water from your body, drink 1 to 2 glasses of fluid (soda-can size) every hour, or sip 1 tablespoon of liquid every 10 to 15 minutes.

—If you can't eat, alternate between drinking fluids with sugar (soda, juices, flavored gelatin, or ice) and salty fluids (broth or bouillon).

—If you can eat, follow your usual diet and drink sugar-free liquids (water or diet drinks).

• Be sure to take your usual daily dosage of insulin, even if you can't eat.

• Continue to monitor your blood or urine glucose every 3 to 4 hours around the clock. Set your alarm clock or have someone awaken you. If you are too sick, have someone do the test for you.

• Your doctor will tell you the safe range for your blood or urine glucose levels. If either measures higher than that level, you will need to test for ketones.

• Rest and avoid exercise.

Call Your Doctor If . . .

• You have ketones in your urine or your blood sugar is over the level your doctor considers safe. You may need extra insulin.

• You cannot keep any liquids down.

• You have been vomiting for more than 1 hour.

• You develop any of the more advanced symptoms of ketoacidosis (fruity breath, rapid breathing, extreme sleepiness).

Seek Care Immediately If . . .

• You have signs of dehydration:

—Decreased urination.

—Increased thirst.

—Light-headed feeling.

• Your blood or urine glucose measurement remains higher than the level judged safe by your doctor even when you take 2 extra doses of insulin per 24 hours.

Diaper Rash

WHAT YOU SHOULD KNOW

Almost every child gets diaper rash, a skin irritation in the diaper area. The rash may get infected.

Causes

The rash usually starts when a wet diaper rubs your child's skin. Urine and stool sitting in the diaper for a long time also can cause a rash, as can diarrhea. Hot, humid weather can make the rash worse.

Allergies to soap, fabric softener, lotion, or powder are another possible cause. These chemicals can irritate the child's skin and cause diaper rash.

Diaper rash can develop from either cloth or disposable diapers.

Signs/Symptoms

Your child's diaper area may be red, raw, spotty-looking, cracked, painful, and itchy.

WHAT YOU SHOULD DO

• Most rashes improve in 3 days with proper care. Keep your child's diaper area clean and dry to help the area heal.
  —Check your child's diaper about once an hour. Wake the child up one time during the night to change the diaper until the rash improves. Change the diaper right away if it is wet or soiled from a bowel movement.
  —If the child has a bowel movement, use a mild soap with warm water to clean the diaper area. Gently rinse the area to remove any soap. Plain warm water and cotton balls or baby wipes also can be used.
  —Before closing the diaper, be sure the child's bottom is completely dry.
• Leave the child's bottom open to air as much as possible during naps or after bowel movements. To protect the bed, put a towel or diaper under the child.
• Diaper creams and ointments usually are not needed. However, an ointment such as zinc oxide can be helpful if the child's bottom is dry and cracked, or the child has diarrhea. Zinc oxide is available at drug stores. Make sure the child's bottom is clean and dry before applying any ointment.
• Do not use plastic pants until the rash improves.
• Punch small holes in disposable diapers to let air in. This will help the rash heal faster.
• After washing cloth diapers, rinse them twice to get rid of extra soap. Don't use fabric softeners if they make your baby's skin red or rashy.
• If the child's bottom stays bright red and raw-looking, or has small red dots, there may be an infection. Your doctor can give you a special ointment to treat the problem.

Call Your Doctor If . . .

• Additional redness, crusting, pus, or large blisters appear in the diaper area.
• The rash is not gone in 7 days.

• You see white spots in your child's mouth. This could indicate an infection called thrush. Your doctor can give you medicine to treat the problem.

Diarrhea, Traveler's

See Traveler's Diarrhea

Diarrhea and Vomiting

See Gastroenteritis

Diarrhea and Vomiting in Children

See Stomach Flu in Children

Dilatation and Curettage

WHAT YOU SHOULD KNOW

During dilatation (dill-uh-TA-shun) and curettage (CURE-eh-tazh)—also called a D & C—the lining of the uterus is scraped to remove tissue. The procedure is usually done to find out the cause of abnormal periods, to end a pregnancy, or to treat an incomplete abortion or miscarriage. After a D & C, you may have bleeding from the uterus for a few days, cramping, and some back or pelvic pain.

IF YOU'RE HEADING FOR THE HOSPITAL . . .

Remember These Pointers After You Leave
• Do not douche, use tampons, or have sex for 2 weeks or until your doctor gives you the okay.
• You may go back to work or resume normal activities in 2 to 4 days.
• You may begin eating or drinking as soon as you feel like it.

Call Your Doctor If . . .
• You have really bad pain that does not go away after taking medicine.
• You have a temperature greater than 99.6 degrees F (37.5 degrees C).
• You have heavy vaginal bleeding that gets worse instead of better.
• You have a vaginal discharge that smells bad.
• You get signs of infection such as headache, muscle aches, or dizziness, or you just feel sick.

Discectomy

See Lumbar Laminectomy

Disk, Slipped

See Slipped Disk

Dislocated Elbow

WHAT YOU SHOULD KNOW

An elbow dislocation occurs when the bones in the elbow are pulled apart, causing the ligaments that keep the bones together to stretch or tear. It may take from 2 to 8 weeks for the elbow to heal.

Causes
Most elbow dislocations are caused by falling on an outstretched hand.

Signs/Symptoms
Your elbow will probably swell, turn red, and be painful and difficult to move. It also may look misshapen.

Care
Your doctor will order an x-ray of the elbow. The bones may have to be put back into place, and, if you have a really bad dislocation, you may need surgery. After treatment, you will have to wear a splint or sling to keep your elbow from moving. If you scratched or tore some skin, you may also need a tetanus shot.

WHAT YOU SHOULD DO

• Apply ice to the injury for 15 to 20 minutes each hour for the first 1 to 2 days. Put the ice in a plastic bag and place a towel between the bag of ice and your skin.
• After the first 1 to 2 days, you may put heat on the injury to help ease the pain. Use a heating pad (set on low), a whirlpool bath, or warm, moist towels for 15 to 20 minutes every hour for 48 hours.
• For 48 hours, keep your arm lifted above the level of your heart whenever possible to reduce the pain and swelling.
• Wear your splint until your doctor says you may take it off or until your follow-up examination. If your fingers get numb or tingly, you may need to loosen the splint. Call your doctor for instructions if you don't know how.
• If the doctor prescribes pain medicine that makes you drowsy, don't

drive. You also may take over-the-counter medicines for pain. Take
all medications exactly as directed.

• If you have been given a tetanus shot, your arm may get swollen,
red, and warm to the touch at the shot site. This is a normal reaction
to the medicine in the shot.

Call Your Doctor If . . .
• The pain or swelling gets worse.
• You have trouble moving your elbow once the splint comes off.
• The bones in your elbow pop in and out of place more than once.

Seek Care Immediately If . . .
• Your arm feels numb or cold and looks pale.

Dislocated Elbow in Children

See Pulled Elbow

Dislocated Jaw

WHAT YOU SHOULD KNOW

When the jawbone becomes unseated at one or both joints, you have
a dislocated jaw. The condition is known medically as a dislocated
mandible.

Causes
The problem is usually the result of impact on the jaw. Dislocation
can also occur if you open your mouth too wide while yawning,
yelling, or biting large pieces of food.

Signs/Symptoms
Soon after the dislocation, the jaw muscles tighten, keeping the
mouth from closing normally. You'll have difficulty moving the jaw;
and swelling, pain, and redness will develop.

Care
Injection of a numbing medication near the joint and the jaw muscles
often allows the jawbone to pop back into place on its own. If this
doesn't work, however, the doctor may need to manually reseat the
bone in the joint.

WHAT YOU SHOULD DO

• Apply an ice pack to the jaw during the first 12 to 24 hours to relieve pain and swelling. Put ice in a plastic bag and place a towel between the ice pack and your skin. Keep the ice pack on your jaw for 15 to 20 minutes out of every hour.

- After 24 hours, you may use heat to ease the pain. Put the heat on your jaw for 15 minutes every 2 hours. Wait at least 24 hours after the injury before applying heat; it can increase swelling and bleeding if used any earlier.
- For one week, eat only soft foods, such as baby food, gelatin, cooked cereal, ice cream, applesauce, bananas, eggs, pasta, cottage cheese, soups, and yogurt. Your diet should be as well-balanced as possible.
- For about 6 weeks, do not open your mouth wide when you yawn, bite large pieces of food, scream or yell, sing, or call out loudly.
- If you need to yawn, put your fist under your chin to keep your mouth from opening up too wide.
- For the first few days, you may need to wear a bandage to hold the jaw in place.

Call Your Doctor If . . .
- You still have jaw pain after taking your pain medication.
- You think you have popped your jaw out of place again.

Seek Care Immediately If . . .
- You have trouble breathing.
- You get a rash, swelling, or redness after taking your medicine.

Dislocated Shoulder

WHAT YOU SHOULD DO

When the shoulder blade bone and the upper arm bone are pulled out of their normal position, the condition is called a dislocated shoulder. The injury takes anywhere from 2 to 8 weeks to heal. Each time it happens, the chances of a repetition increase.

Causes
Most shoulder dislocations result from an accident. Occasionally the cause is a diseased joint.

Signs/Symptoms
Sudden appearance of a bump in the front or back of the shoulder area may be a sign of dislocation. Other typical symptoms are swelling, pain, or redness in the injured area. The shoulder may feel weak, numb, or tingly; and you will have difficulty moving it.

Care

You'll probably get an x-ray of the shoulder. The doctor will need to tug on your arm or shoulder to pop the bones back into place. You may need to wear a splint or ace wrap to keep the shoulder from moving so it can heal. If the shoulder pulls apart easily and often, you may need surgery to prevent the problem from recurring. After the doctor puts the shoulder back in place, the pain may last for 24 to 48 hours.

WHAT YOU SHOULD DO

- Pack the injury with ice for 15 to 20 minutes each hour for the first 1 to 2 days. Put the ice in a plastic bag and place a towel between the bag of ice and your skin.
- After the first 1 to 2 days, you may put heat on the injury to help ease the pain. Use a heating pad (set on low), a whirlpool bath, or warm, moist towels for 15 to 20 minutes every hour for 48 hours.
- If you are wearing a sling, keep it on all the time. If you take the sling off to dress or bathe, be careful to avoid lifting or moving the arm.
- If you are wearing a special splint, keep it on until your doctor says you can remove it or until your follow-up visit. If your fingers get numb or tingly, you may need to loosen the splint. If you don't know how, ask your doctor for instructions.
- Take any medicine the doctor prescribes exactly as directed. Do not increase the dose or frequency. If the medicine makes you drowsy, avoid driving. Over-the-counter medications may be used for pain.
- If you are given a tetanus shot, your arm may get swollen, red, and warm to the touch at the injection site. This is a normal reaction to the medicine in the shot.

Call Your Doctor If . . .

- The pain or swelling gets worse.

Seek Care Immediately If . . .

- The arm on the same side as your injury becomes numb or tingly, or the skin looks pale or feels cold.

Diverticulitis

WHAT YOU SHOULD KNOW

Diverticulitis (di-ver-tik-u-LIE-tis) is an inflammation of small pouches called "diverticula" that often develop in the wall of the large bowel (colon). Waste from digested food can get trapped in the diverticula and cause swelling and pain.

Causes
Frequently no cause can be found. Having a family history of diverticulitis or eating a low-fiber diet may make you more likely to have this problem.

Signs/Symptoms
The main symptom is abdominal pain that either comes and goes or lasts all the time. You may also have a fever, feel like throwing up, or develop tenderness in the belly.

Care
Your doctor may order x-rays and tests. If the diverticula are infected, you may be given antibiotics. If you have a bad infection or if you need surgery to remove part of the colon, you may need a stay in the hospital.

Do's and Don'ts
To keep from having more attacks of diverticulitis, get plenty of rest, allow yourself plenty of time to move your bowels, eat foods with fiber in them, and drink plenty of water.

Risks
Without treatment, the problem could get worse, and the diverticula could bleed or burst, causing a life-threatening infection in the abdomen.

WHAT YOU SHOULD DO

- You may take over-the-counter medicines for constipation, but use them exactly as your doctor directs.
- If you feel a medication is not helping, call your doctor, but do not quit taking it on your own.
- You may also use stool softeners to make the stool easier to pass. Follow the directions on the label.
- If you have abdominal pain and a fever, take only clear liquids, such as ginger ale, juices, broth, or gelatin.
- Heat on the belly may help lessen the pain. Use an electric heating pad set on low.
- Stay in bed if you have pain and fever. When you feel better, you may begin your normal activities again.
- Don't strain while moving your bowels.

- To help prevent more attacks:
  —Eat foods that are high in fiber. Good choices are whole grain breads, oatmeal or bran cereals, and plenty of vegetables and fruits.
  —Drink lots of water.
  —Eat at regular hours.

Call Your Doctor If . . .
- You have a high temperature.
- You continue to have really bad abdominal pain even with treatment.
- Your stool is black or contains blood.
- You are throwing up or have swelling in your abdomen.

IF YOU'RE HEADING FOR THE HOSPITAL . . .

What to Expect While You're There
You may encounter the following procedures and equipment during your stay.

- **Colonoscopy** (co-lin-OS-ko-pee): A test that gives the doctor a view of the inside of the colon (large intestine). A soft tube with a light and camera lens on the end of it is inserted through the rectum and pushed into the colon.
- **Sigmoidoscopy** (sig-moid-OS-ko-pee): This test gives the doctor a view of only the lower end of the colon, called the sigmoid, and the rectum. A short, flexible tube with a light and camera lens is used for the test.
- **Barium Enema:** This is an x-ray of the bowel. You are given an enema with a chemical called barium in it. The barium blocks x-rays so that outline of bowel will appear on the film.
- **Activity:** You may need to rest in bed. Once you are feeling better, you will be allowed out of bed.
- **Medicines:**
  —**Antibiotics** will be prescribed to fight infection. They may be given in an IV, in a shot, or by mouth.
  —**Stool Softeners** will be given to make bowel movements easier. Some can be taken by mouth, others are placed in the rectum.
- **Taking Vital Signs:** These include your temperature, blood pressure, pulse (counting your heartbeats), and respirations (counting your breaths). A stethoscope is used to listen to your heart and lungs. Your blood pressure is taken by wrapping a cuff around your arm.
- **Pulse Oximeter:** You may be hooked up to a pulse oximeter (ox-IM-uh-ter). It is placed on your ear, finger, or toe and is connected to a machine that measures the oxygen in your blood.

- **Oxygen:** Your body may need extra oxygen at this time. It is given either by a mask or nasal prongs. Tell your doctor if the oxygen is drying out your nose or if the nasal prongs bother you.
- **Blood:** Usually taken from a vein in your hand or from the bend in your elbow. Tests will be done on the blood.
- **ECG:** Also called a heart monitor, an electrocardiograph (e-lek-tro-CAR-dee-o-graf), or EKG. The patches on your chest are hooked up to a TV-type screen or a small portable box (telemetry unit). This screen shows a tracing of each heartbeat. Your heart will be watched for signs of injury or damage that could be related to your illness.
- **Chest X-ray:** This picture of your lungs and heart shows how they are handling the illness.
- **IV:** A tube placed in your vein for giving medicine or liquids. It will be capped or have tubing connected to it.
- **Blood Transfusion:** If you are bleeding heavily, you may be given more blood.

After You Leave
Follow the directions listed under "What You Should Do."

Dizziness

WHAT YOU SHOULD KNOW

Dizziness, also called vertigo, is a common symptom. It can range from a sense of light-headedness or faintness to an intense feeling that the room is spinning. The problem may occur once in a while or may be present most of the time. It's usually not serious.

Causes
The problem can be brought on by an ear infection or disease, a head injury, or even a quick movement of your head. Sometimes no cause can be found.

Signs/Symptoms
The term "dizziness" covers a multitude of symptoms, including light-headedness; a sense of falling, losing your balance, or floating; a feeling that you are moving from one direction to another, or a conviction that you are going to faint. Your stomach may become upset. You may lose your balance and fall.

Care
If the problem persists, you may need medicine to relieve it.

WHAT YOU SHOULD DO

- If you are feeling dizzy, lie down until the feeling passes.
- To avoid an attack, rise slowly from a supine to a sitting position. Do the same when you go from a sitting to a standing position.
- Avoid driving a car or operating heavy machinery while dizzy.

Call Your Doctor If . . .
- You have prolonged, severe, or repeated attacks of dizziness.
- You notice some loss of hearing or hear strange noises in your ears.

Seek Care Immediately If . . .
- You have a severe headache, weakness in your arms or legs, numbness or tingling in any part of your body, blurred vision, or difficulty speaking or swallowing.
- You develop frequent morning headaches along with nausea and vomiting.
- You pass out, loose control of your bowels or bladder, bite your tongue, or sustain any injury from falling or unsteadiness.

Dog Bite

See Animal Bite

Domestic Violence

WHAT YOU SHOULD KNOW

Domestic violence (commonly called wife beating) is the use of strong, physical force by your spouse or another member of the household. It includes hitting, yelling, or touching when and where it is not wanted. Whether the abuser is angry or calm, it is important to remember that the violence is not your fault.

Physical abuse may be preceded or accompanied by emotional abuse. You are being emotionally abused if you are regularly insulted and made to feel worthless, or if you live in constant fear. Women are the most common targets of domestic violence (but men may be abused as well). At least 1 in every 6 women gets struck sometime during a relationship, and at least 1 million women each year are beaten repeatedly by their husbands or boyfriends.

If you are a victim of domestic violence, you should know that the abuse may get worse with time and may even end in death. It is important to remember that there are others like you, and help is available when you are ready. No one has the right to injure you; it is against the law.

Causes

While there are many reasons for domestic violence, is usually occurs because one partner's temper gets out of control. Excessive drinking often leads to a lack of control and then to physical force. The abusive partner may have been abused or witnessed abuse while growing up.

WHAT YOU SHOULD DO

- Leave if you feel that violence is going to occur. Warning signs of danger may include:
  —Your partner's use of alcohol
  —Your partner's threats to use a weapon or to harm the children, other family members, or pets
  —Forced sexual contact
  —Less frequent apologies by your partner after an attack.
- Domestic violence victims often fail to report their injuries out of fear or embarrassment. Nevertheless, you should report all attacks or beatings to the police so that the abuse is documented. The police can also protect you if you or the attacker is moving out. It is a good idea to get the officer's name and badge number and a copy of the report.
- Find somebody you can trust (your doctor, spiritual adviser, close friend, or family member, for example) and tell him or her what is happening to you. Talking about the abuse may make you feel better. Feeling ashamed is natural, but remember that no one deserves to be abused.
- It is important to have a safety plan in case you are being threatened:
  —Pack a suitcase or box with extra clothing for you and your children, medicines you may need, money, important phone numbers and papers, and an extra set of car and house keys. Keep it at a friend's or neighbor's house.
  —Tell a supportive friend or family member that you may show up at any time of day or night in case of an emergency.
  —If you do not have a close friend or family member you can trust, make a list of other safe places to go (shelters, hotels, or police or emergency departments).
- Many victims do not leave their homes because they do not have money or a job. Planning ahead may help you in the future. Try to save money and put it in a safe place. Keep your job or look for a job. If you cannot get a job, try to get the training you need to get ready for a job in the future.
- Look up the phone numbers of the following agencies and keep them close at hand in case you need them:
  —Social Services

—Local safe house or shelter
• The following organizations may also provide help in an emergency:
—**National Organization for Victim Assistance (NOVA):** 1-800-TRY-NOVA (1-800-879-6682).
—**National Coalition Against Domestic Violence:** (202) 638-6388 or (303) 839-1852.

Seek Care Immediately If . . .

• You fear you are about to be beaten or abused (**call 911 or 0 [operator] for help**).
• You are injured in a flare-up of violence.

Drug Allergy

WHAT YOU SHOULD KNOW

If you develop swelling, itching, or hives after taking a medication—even one you have had before—you have a drug allergy. When you stop taking the drug and the medication is completely out of your body, the reaction will disappear. Most allergic reactions are not a cause for alarm; but the severe reaction called anaphylaxis (AN-uh-fuh-LAX-is) is a life-threatening emergency that requires immediate medical care.

Causes

Just about any drug will trigger a reaction in a few individuals. However, most drug allergies are quite rare.

Signs/Symptoms

Mild Allergic Reaction: Skin rash, itching, and hives after taking a drug.
Anaphylaxis: Swollen mouth, trouble breathing, a pounding heart, fainting, chest tightness.

Care

You may be given medicine to stop the itching and swelling.

WHAT YOU SHOULD DO

• Stop taking the medicine that caused the reaction and call your doctor right away.
• If you are having trouble breathing, swelling in your throat or mouth, or other signs of anaphylaxis, **call 911 or 0 (operator)** right away for help.

- After you have determined what medicine caused your reaction, do not take it again and never take drugs in the same class. Whenever you are given a new prescription, make sure the doctor is aware of your allergy.
- Talk with your doctor before using any over-the-counter medications.
- After taking a new drug in your doctor's office, always stay there for at least 15 minutes.
- If you have hives or rash:
  —To relieve itching, apply cold compresses to the skin or take a cool bath or an oatmeal bath.
  —Do not take hot baths or showers. This will make the itching worse.
  —Wear loose fitting clothes and avoid tight underwear.
- If you have a severe allergic reaction:
  —Following a severe reaction, someone will need to stay with you for 24 hours in case the symptoms return.
  —You should wear a medic-alert bracelet or necklace that names the medication to which you are allergic.
  —Your doctor will suggest you buy an anaphylaxis kit and will teach you and your family when and how to give adrenaline shots.
  —If you have had a severe reaction before, always carry your anaphylaxis kit with you.
- You may return to your normal activities when the allergic symptoms are gone.

Call Your Doctor If . . .
- You suspect a drug allergy. Symptoms may occur as soon as 15 minutes after taking the medicine.
- Your rash, hives, or itching have not gone away in a few days.
- You develop a fever, upset stomach, or vomiting.
- You develop hives, swelling, or itching ALL OVER your body.

Seek Care Immediately If . . .
- You have trouble breathing, wheezing, tight feeling in your chest or throat, or a swelling in your mouth. **THIS IS AN EMERGENCY. Dial 911 or 0 (operator)** for help or have someone drive you to the nearest emergency room.

Drug Withdrawal, Barbiturates

See Barbiturate Abuse

Drug Withdrawal, Cocaine

See Cocaine Abuse

Drug Withdrawal, Narcotics

See Narcotic Abuse

Drug Withdrawal, Tranquilizers

See Benzodiazepine Abuse

DT Shot for Adults

See Tetanus and Diphtheria Vaccine for Adults

DVT

See Deep Vein Thrombophlebitis

Dysfunctional Uterine Bleeding

WHAT YOU SHOULD KNOW

Dysfunctional uterine (dis-FUNK-shun-ul U-ter-in) bleeding occurs in the uterus (and comes out the vagina) and is not part of the normal period. It mostly happens in women who are older than 45, and sometimes in young girls.

Causes

The bleeding results from a problem with estrogen, one of the body's reproductive hormones. If you do not manufacture the right amount of estrogen, there may be excessive growth in the lining of your uterus (womb), or you may not pass an egg (ovulate). As a result, you may see a change in the amount of bleeding during your period, as well as bleeding between periods.

Signs/Symptoms

The hallmark of this condition is bleeding between periods. The bleeding can be heavy, irregular ("spotting" at different times), or last longer than a normal period.

Care

Your doctor may need to examine you and take a small sample of the lining of your uterus. You may need a hormone medicine to help make your periods regular. If you have a lot of bleeding, you may lose too much iron, and your doctor may give you an iron supplement or ask you to eat foods that have lots of iron in them.

WHAT YOU SHOULD DO

- If your doctor prescribes medicine to make your periods regular, be sure to take it exactly as directed.
- If your bleeding is heavy and the doctor prescribes iron pills, take them regularly. They are an important part of therapy.
- Don't take aspirin or medicines that contain aspirin one week before or during your menstrual period. Aspirin may make the bleeding worse.
- If you need to change your sanitary pad or tampon more than once every 2 hours, stay in bed and rest as much as possible until the bleeding stops.
- Eat well-balanced meals with foods high in iron. Examples are leafy green vegetables, meat, liver, eggs, and whole-grain breads and cereals. Don't try to lose weight until the abnormal bleeding has stopped and your blood iron level is back to normal.
- Try not to get too stressed, or learn ways to control the tension. Stress may be making your problem worse.
- If you have pain or cramps, try a heating pad or hot bath.

Call Your Doctor If . . .
- You need to change your sanitary pad or tampon more than once an hour.
- You develop nausea and vomiting, dizziness, or diarrhea while you are taking your medicine.

Seek Care Immediately If . . .
- You have a high temperature or chills.

Dysmenorrhea

See Menstrual Cramps

Earache in Children

WHAT YOU SHOULD KNOW

Earaches are very common in children between the ages of 6 months and 2 years. They stem from an infection in the ear called otitis (o-TIE-tis) media (me-DEE-uh). Most children have at least one ear infection before their eighth birthday.

Causes

Ear infections often follow a cold, but cannot be spread from person to person. Some ear infections are caused by allergies.

Signs/Symptoms

Tugging of the ears and fever are signs of an ear infection. The child may cry more and seem fussier than normal. Simply touching the ears may cause pain.

Swallowing, chewing, and nose blowing can increase ear pain. The pain is caused by pressure changes inside the ear.

Older children may say their ears feel like they are under water. They may hear buzzing or ringing. Their speech may be unclear if they are just beginning to talk, because they can't hear clearly.

Ear infections can cause short-term hearing loss. The child may not hear far-away noises.

A child's eardrum can break if too much pressure builds up behind it. Signs of a broken eardrum are blood and pus draining from the ear. This drainage does not mean that the infection has gotten worse. The small break will heal on its own in a few days. However, the child could have a slight hearing loss until the infection is gone.

Hearing usually returns to normal after treatment. If it does not fully return, a hearing test may be needed.

If your child has frequent ear infections, your doctor may suggest putting tubes in the ears. The tubes let liquid drain from the ears and can help prevent additional infections.

Care

The doctor will use an otoscope (OH-toe-skope) to look in the ears for infection. A tympanogram (tim-PAN-uh-gram) is another test that may be done. It involves inserting an ear plug to see how the eardrum moves.

The doctor will prescribe an antibiotic. Use the entire prescription, even if the child feels better after the first few days.

You'll need to bring the child back to the doctor after finishing the medicine, usually in 2 to 3 weeks. The ears will be checked to see if the infection is gone. Sometimes more medicine is needed.

WHAT YOU SHOULD DO

- A heating pad set on low, or a warm water bottle placed on the ear, may ease the pain. You may also put a covered ice bag over the ear to relieve pain.
- Do not put anything in the child's ear unless suggested by your doctor.

- The child can swim if the eardrum is not broken. If there is no fever, the child can return to school.

Call Your Doctor If . . .
- The child does not feel better in a few hours.
- The child has a temperature.
- The child continues to cry, is fussy, and not as active as usual.
- The child starts vomiting or has diarrhea.
- The child has a skin rash.
- The child develops new problems that may be due to the medicine.

Seek Care Immediately If . . .
- The child has a high temperature.
- The child is crying, fussy, and tugging at the ears after taking the medicine for 48 hours.
- The child has swelling around the ear.
- The child seems to have pain or stiffness when moving the neck or complains of neck pain.
- The child is vomiting, less active, and more sleepy than usual.
- You feel the child is getting worse.

Ear Blockage

See Foreign Body in the Ear

Eardrum Perforation

See Perforated Eardrum

Ear Infection in Adults

See Otitis Media in Adults

Ear Infection in Children

See Earache in Children

Early Labor Signs

WHAT YOU SHOULD KNOW

Labor is a series of steps your uterus (womb) goes through to push out your baby. It may start at any time during pregnancy, but usually begins close to your due date.

Causes

It is not known for sure what causes labor to begin. Hormones made by you and your baby and changes in your uterus play a part in starting labor.

Signs

There are several signs that will tell you that labor is getting closer:

—**Lightening:** This is when your "baby drops." You may feel as if your baby has dropped lower into your abdomen. Your clothes may fit differently. You may find it easier to breathe, but may need to urinate more often. This can happen a few weeks to a few hours before labor starts.

—**Bloody Show:** This is also called "show" or "mucus plug." It is a thick plug of mucus that forms in your cervix (bottom part of your uterus) during pregnancy. As your cervix gets softer and starts to open, this mucus plug will come out. You will see clear, pink, or slightly bloody mucus coming from your vagina. This may happen up to 3 days before labor begins or at the start of labor.

—**Rupture of Membranes:** This is when your "water breaks." The bag of water is the water-like sack that surrounds your baby during pregnancy. When it leaks or breaks, you may feel a slow trickle from your vagina or a sudden gush of warm fluid. This may happen several hours before labor starts or any time during labor.

—**Braxton-Hicks Labor Pains:** These are called false-labor pains or contractions. You probably have had them during your pregnancy. As labor gets closer, these pains may get stronger and closer together. You will know they are not true labor pains because they go away when you walk around or rest. They often go away when you try to sleep. Braxton-Hicks pains are usually felt in your abdomen but not in your back.

—**Energy Burst:** You may have a burst of energy several days before labor begins.

Care

As labor gets closer, alert your doctor. Do **not** take medicines without talking to your doctor.

WHAT YOU SHOULD DO

Call Your Doctor If . . .

• Your bag of water breaks even though you are not having contractions or labor pains. Tell your doctor what color the fluid is when your bag of water breaks. Do not douche, take a bath (showering is fine), or have sex.

- You are bleeding from your vagina. You **do not** need to call if you have passed the mucus plug.
- Your labor pains (called contractions) are hard, regular, and going from your front to your back. Your doctor will tell you how frequently your contractions should be coming and how long they should be lasting before you call him or her.
- You have severe, constant pain rather than contractions that come and go.
- You do not feel your baby is moving as much as usual.

Ear Tubes

See Pressure-Equalizing Ear Tubes

Earwax Buildup

WHAT YOU SHOULD KNOW

The glands in your ear make wax, or cerumen (SIR-ooh-men), to protect the area between the eardrum and the outside of the ear. If you have too much wax, that passage will be blocked. Unless the blockage is removed, you risk developing an ear infection. Excess earwax can also cause damage to your eardrum.

Causes
Excess wax mixes with dust or water and collects in the ear.

Signs/Symptoms
Possible symptoms include hearing loss, ear pain, a ringing sound, or a feeling that something is plugging your ear.

Care
Your doctor can remove the excess wax with ear wash and special tools.

WHAT YOU SHOULD DO

- After removing the blockage, the doctor may advise you to remove earwax at home with wax-softening ear drops that you can buy without a prescription.
- To insert the ear drops:
  —Lie down with the affected ear pointed toward the ceiling.

—Put 2 or 3 drops into the ear, plug it with cotton, and wait 20 minutes.

—Using a soft rubber bulb syringe, squirt warm water gently into the ear canal several times to wash out the earwax.

• Do not try to remove earwax with a stick or cotton swab. This can damage the eardrum or cause an infection in the ear canal.

• If you work in a dusty area, wear earplugs to help keep your ear canals clean.

Call Your Doctor If . . .

• You continue to have pain in your ear.

• You develop a high temperature.

Ectopic Pregnancy

WHAT YOU SHOULD KNOW

An ectopic (ek-TOP-ik) pregnancy, also called a tubal pregnancy, is a pregnancy that grows outside the uterus (womb). Ectopic pregnancies often grow in one of the fallopian (fuh-LOW-pee-un) tubes. The pregnancy can also grow in the ovary, cervix (bottom part of uterus), or the abdomen.

A tubal pregnancy cannot grow like a normal pregnancy. As the fetus (baby) grows, the tube is stretched. If the tube bursts, there can be severe bleeding inside the abdomen. Your life could be in danger and emergency surgery must be done.

Causes

Some possible reasons for an ectopic pregnancy are IUD use, tubal infection, a growth pressing against the tube, past tubal surgery, past tubal pregnancy, or smoking. A condition called endometriosis (end-o-meet-ree-O-sis) can also cause an ectopic pregnancy.

Signs/Symptoms

Common symptoms are dull pain or sharp lower abdominal pain and spotty or heavy vaginal bleeding. You may have back and right shoulder pain. You could be nauseated, faint, weak; have vomiting or cold sweats; or feel as though your heart is racing.

Care

Surgery is usually needed to remove an ectopic pregnancy and repair or remove the damaged fallopian tube. It must be done even if the tube has not burst.

Risks
Women can die from an ectopic pregnancy. But the risks of serious illness or death are very small if the pregnancy is surgically removed.

WHAT YOU SHOULD DO

Call Your Doctor If . . .
• You have chills, headaches, dizziness, or muscle aches.
• You have a high temperature.
• You have pain or burning when you urinate. These are signs of an infection.

Seek Care Immediately If . . .
• You develop really bad abdominal pain or heavy vaginal bleeding.

IF YOU'RE HEADING FOR THE HOSPITAL . . .

What to Expect While You're There
You may encounter the following procedures and equipment during your stay.

• **Taking Vital Signs:** These include your temperature, blood pressure, pulse (counting your heartbeats), and respirations (counting your breaths). A stethoscope is used to listen to your heart and lungs. Your blood pressure is taken by wrapping a cuff around your arm.

• **Activity:** You will be asked to stay in bed before surgery. After surgery, you will be encouraged to get out of bed with help. You can walk more as you feel better.

• **IV:** A tube placed in your vein for giving medicine or liquids. It will be capped or have tubing connected to it.

• **Medicines:** You may need antibiotics to prevent infection. These may be given in your IV, in a shot, or by mouth.

• **Blood:** Usually taken from a vein in your hand or from the bend in your elbow. Tests will be done on the blood.

• **Chest X-ray:** This picture of your lungs and heart is usually taken before surgery. The doctors use it to see how your heart and lungs are handling the emergency.

• **Abdominal or Vaginal Ultrasound:** A painless test done while lying down. A dab of a jelly-like lotion is placed on your belly. The person doing the test will gently move a small handle through the lotion and across the skin. A TV-like screen is attached to the handle. To perform a vaginal ultrasound, a small tube is placed in your vagina. There is no pain.

• **Blood Transfusion:** A blood transfusion may be necessary if you lose too much blood.

• **After Surgery:**
—You will be returned to your hospital room when you are awake. Ask for medicine if you are having pain. You may want to have someone stay with you to give comfort and support.
—You will go home when you are eating, drinking, and able to care for yourself.

• **Grief:**
—You may feel scared, confused, and depressed because so much has happened in a short time. You may also feel sad or angry at the loss of your pregnancy.
—You may blame yourself and think you have done something wrong. These feelings are normal. Talk about them with your doctor or someone close to you.

After You Leave

• Take your medicine as directed by your doctor.
• Follow your doctor's suggestions about taking care of your stitches.
• Place a heating pad set on "low" or a hot water bottle on your abdomen if you experience pain.
• You can take warm baths to help sore muscles. Take them as often as needed.
• Rest and slowly get back to normal activity. Eating healthy foods and drinking liquids will help you return to your usual health.
• Talk to your doctor before you start exercising. He or she will tell you when you may begin.
• Your doctor will tell you when you may have sex.
• Schedule a check-up with your doctor.

Eczema

WHAT YOU SHOULD KNOW

Eczema, known medically as atopic (a-TOP-ik) dermatitis (DER-muh-TIE-tis), is a long-term skin irritation. It can come and go for months or even years, and often accompanies other allergic problems such as asthma or hay fever. There is no cure for the problem, but the symptoms can be managed. The disease will not spread from person to person.

Causes

The cause of eczema is unknown. It tends to affect people with a family history of atopic dermatitis or other allergic problems. It can be brought on by stress, food, or other irritants. Certain chemicals and fabrics may also trigger the problem.

Signs/Symptoms
In young children, the problem surfaces as a red, itchy, oozing, crusted rash on the face, scalp, diaper area, arms, and legs. In older children and adults the rashes may appear as dry, red, scaly patches on the eyelids, neck, and wrists, and in the folds of the elbows and knees, neck, hands, feet, genital area (between the legs), and around the rectum.

Care
Medicine may be used to relieve the itching.

WHAT YOU SHOULD DO

- To relieve itching and rash use the medication your doctor prescribed exactly as directed. Over-the-counter steroid creams may prove helpful, but check with your doctor before using any nonprescription medications.
- To relieve the problem in young children, take the following steps:
  —Give the child short baths or showers (10 minutes) in warm water. You may add nonperfumed bath oil to the bath water. It is best to avoid soap; if necessary, use a nondrying soap. Do not use any soap on the rash itself. NEVER use bubble bath.
  —Immediately after a bath or shower, when the skin is still damp, apply a moisturizing cream to the entire body. This will seal in moisture and help prevent dryness.
  —Keep your child's fingernails cut short. Wash the youngster's hands often. Because scratching makes the rash and itching worse, you may need to put soft gloves or mittens on the child at night.
  —Dress the child in clothes made of cotton or cotton blends. Avoid wool and synthetic fibers. Don't dress your child too warmly.
  —Avoid feeding the youngster cow's milk, peanut butter, eggs, wheat or other foods that may cause flare-ups.
  —Keep the child away from anyone that has fever blisters. The virus that produces fever blisters can cause a serious skin infection in children with eczema.

Call Your Doctor If . . .
- Itching interferes with sleep.
- The rash gets worse or is not better after 7 days of treatment.
- The rash develops pus or soft yellow scabs.
- A high temperature develops.
- The rash flares up after contact with someone who has fever blisters.

EEG

See Electroencephalography

Elbow Dislocation

See Dislocated Elbow

Elbow Dislocation in Children

See Pulled Elbow

Elbow Fracture

See Broken Elbow

Electrical Burns

WHAT YOU SHOULD KNOW

Electrical burns occur when current jumps from an electrical outlet, cord or appliance and passes through your body. The electricity can burn the skin—sometimes very deeply—and may also cause internal damage. How quickly you heal depends on the severity of the burns and injuries.

Signs/Symptoms

There are three degrees of severity, each with distinctive symptoms:
- First-degree burns are mild and injure only the outer layer of skin. The skin becomes red, but turns white when touched. The area may also be painful to the touch.
- Second-degree burns are deeper, more severe, and very painful. Blisters may form on the burned area. This type of burn takes about 2 weeks to heal.
- Third-degree burns are the deepest and most serious kind. The skin becomes white and leathery, but it does not feel very tender when touched.

There may be swelling in the burned area. Serious burns may be accompanied by headache, fever, and dizziness.

Causes

There are innumerable ways for anyone—particularly a child—to get an electrical burn. Among the leading causes are sticking a knife into a plugged-in toaster, dropping a plugged-in appliance into water, sucking or chewing on an electrical cord, and sticking something into an electrical outlet.

Care

Always call your doctor when you get an electrical burn. If the burn is small, you may be able to take care of it at home; but if the burn is large or you received a serious shock from the electricity, you should get to the hospital right away. Do not drive yourself.

WHAT YOU SHOULD DO

- Soak the burned skin in cold water for about 10 minutes.
- Gently wash the burn with warm, soapy water. Pat it dry with a clean towel, and cover it with a clean, dry bandage.
- You will need to clean the burn and put on a new bandage once a day. Be sure that everything that touches the burn is clean. Only use the burn medicine prescribed by your doctor. When changing bandages:
  —Wash your hands well with soap and water. Dry them with a clean towel.
  —Remove the outer bandage by cutting it off with a pair of scissors. Do not pull off the bandage if it is sticking to the burn. Instead, soak it in warm water for a few minutes and then remove it slowly.
  —Gently wash the burn with warm, soapy water. Use a clean, soft washcloth to help remove any old cream, blood, and loose skin. Do not break blisters. This may increase the pain.
  —Rinse the burn with clear warm water. Pat dry with a clean towel.
  —With a clean tongue depressor, apply a thin layer of the antibiotic cream prescribed by your doctor to a gauze pad. Throw the tongue depressor away when you're done. Do NOT put it back in the container of antibiotic cream.
  —Cover the burn with the gauze. Be careful not to touch the gauze that comes in contact with the burn. Carefully rewrap the burn with a clean bandage as directed by your doctor.
- Keep the bandage clean and dry. Change it if it gets wet.
- If the burn is on your arm or leg, keep it raised or propped up for the first 24 hours to help reduce swelling.
- You may use aspirin, acetaminophen, or ibuprofen for pain.
- Try to drink plenty of water or juice.
- Do not bump or overuse the burned area.
- For mouth burns (often suffered by children):
  —Feed the child bland, soft, cold foods such as baby foods, soft cooked eggs, cooked cereal, ice cream, and yogurt. Give lots of liquids such as water, milk, and fruit juices.
  —Brush the child's teeth 3 or 4 times a day. Use a soft toothbrush, with or without toothpaste.

—If the child is given a special device called a microstoma to help prevent scarring, use it exactly as directed.
• To prevent electrical burns:
  —Never stick foreign objects into an electrical plug. Cover unused electrical outlets with childproof plug covers, available in hardware stores and the baby section of department stores.
  —Do not use electrical appliances near standing or running water.
  —Do NOT stick forks or knives into toasters or other appliances when they are plugged in.
  —Repair or replace any frayed or worn electrical cords. Teach children to NEVER suck or chew on these cords.

Call Your Doctor If . . .
• You develop increasing pain and redness around the burn, or a bad-smelling drainage comes from the burn. These are signs of infection.
• You develop a high temperature.

Seek Care Immediately If . . .
• You have swelling, numbness, or tingling below a burn on your arm or leg.
• A child with a burn has trouble swallowing or breathing.

Electrocautery Wart Removal

See Wart Removal

Electroencephalography

WHAT YOU SHOULD KNOW

Electroencephalography (e-LEC-tro-en-SEF-uh-LAH-gruh-fee), also known as EEG, is a means of measuring the electrical activity of your brain. An electroencephalogram is helpful in determining whether you have epilepsy (seizures) or other brain diseases.

Risks
This test is painless and harmless.

IF YOU'RE HEADING FOR THE HOSPITAL. . . .

Before You Go
• Do not drink coffee, tea, or cola on the morning of your test. Do not smoke cigarettes the day of your test. You should eat your regular meals.

- Your doctor will tell you how many hours you should sleep the night before your test. Follow these directions exactly.
- Take any medicine prescribed by your doctor just as directed.
- Your hair should be clean and free from all oil or lotion. Before the test, you will need to remove everything made of metal (jewelry, for example) from your head and neck.

What to Expect While You're There

You may encounter the following procedures and equipment during your stay:

- **Taking Your Vital Signs:** These include your temperature, blood pressure, pulse (counting your heartbeats), and respirations (counting your breaths). A stethoscope is used to listen to your heart and lungs. Your blood pressure is taken by wrapping a cuff around your arm.
- **During Your EEG:**
  —The test will be done in a special room equipped with either a bed or a reclining chair.
  —About 20 sticky patches with wires will be placed on your head with paste. One patch may be put on each earlobe. You'll be asked to lie still and relax with your eyes closed. The test causes no pain.
  —You will be asked to breathe deeply 20 times a minute for 3 minutes. A bright light will be flashed over your face to see how it affects your brain waves. You may be asked to go to sleep.
  —The brain waves are recorded on a moving strip of paper for study by the doctor.
  —You may be given a short break so you can move around. After the test, the patches and wires will be taken off. The nurse may wash your hair to get rid of the paste.
  —The test takes between 45 minutes and 2 hours.

After You Leave

- You may return to your normal activities immediately.
- You will need to shampoo your hair to remove all the paste.

Electromyography

WHAT YOU SHOULD KNOW

Electromyography (e-LEC-tro-my-OG-ruf-ee) measures the electrical activity of muscles both at rest and contracted (flexed). It is performed when the doctor suspects a problem with your muscles or the nerves that control them.

Risks
There is a possibility that the muscles tested could be left temporarily sore or bruised. There is also a chance of skin infection.

IF YOU'RE HEADING FOR THE HOSPITAL . . .

Before You Go
• Tell your doctor if you:
  —Have a cardiac pacemaker.
  —Are taking an anticoagulant (blood thinner) or have a bleeding disease.
  —Have hepatitis, AIDS, or any other contagious disease.
• Do not take stimulants (drugs that make you nervous) or sedatives (drugs that make you sleepy) for 24 hours before the test.
• Do not drink coffee, tea, or cola on the morning of the test.

What to Expect While You're There
You may encounter the following procedures and equipment during your stay:
• **Taking Your Vital Signs:** These include your temperature, blood pressure, pulse (counting your heartbeats), and respirations (counting your breaths). A stethoscope is used to listen to your heart and lungs. Your blood pressure is taken by wrapping a cuff around your arm.
• **During the test:**
  —You will either lie in bed or sit in a chair that allows you to stay in a position that puts the muscle to be tested at rest.
  —A wire attached to a "hot box" will be placed on the nerve that controls the muscle. When the power is turned on to test the nerve, you may feel a very mild shock.
  —Thin needles will be put into the muscle to be tested. You may feel some pain when the needles are inserted and when you move the muscle during the test.
  —Electrical activity in the muscle will be recorded and displayed on a TV-like screen.
  —The test generally takes between 30 and 90 minutes.

After You Leave
• If the muscles that were tested feel sore, apply warm compresses and take a pain reliever such as acetaminophen.

EMG

See Electromyography

Emphysema

WHAT YOU SHOULD KNOW

Emphysema is one of the lung disorders classified as chronic obstructive pulmonary disease (COPD). In emphysema, damage to the air sacs in the lungs reduces their ability to pick up oxygen from the air we breathe.

Causes

Cigarette smoking is the leading cause. Others are air pollution, allergies, and infections. Dust or chemical-filled air at work can cause emphysema. The disease becomes more likely as we get older.

Signs/Symptoms

The most common symptom is gradually increasing difficulty in breathing that grows worse over a period of many years. Finally, breathing becomes difficult even when you're resting. You may also cough up small amounts of sputum or have swelling in your feet and hands. People with emphysema tend to have very pink skin, to be thin, and have a barrel-shaped chest.

Care

Treatment is aimed at helping you breathe more easily. If the problem is severe, you may need a stay in the hospital, where you can get oxygen, breathing treatments, and medicine.

Risks

If you don't follow your doctor's directions, this disease will get worse, ending in death. However, the illness can be controlled with medicine, exercise, and diet.

WHAT YOU SHOULD DO

- You will breathe easier if you take your medicine exactly as directed. If you feel it is not helping, call your doctor. Do not quit taking it on your own.
- If you are prescribed antibiotics, continue to take them until they are all gone—even if you feel well.
- If your medicine makes you drowsy, do not drive or use heavy equipment.
- Quit smoking. It's probably the cause of your emphysema, and will certainly make it worse. If you are having trouble quitting, ask your doctor for help.

- Try to avoid anything that makes your breathing harder, such as things that you're allergic to and polluted air.
- Try to avoid people who have colds or the flu. Get shots to prevent the flu and pneumonia.
- Eat foods that have plenty of protein, vitamins, and minerals in them. Your doctor can give you some suggestions.
- If you are coughing up sputum, do not eat or drink foods that contain milk. They can make sputum thicker.
- If you do not have to limit the amount of liquids you drink, drink 8 to 10 (soda-can size) glasses of water each day. This helps thin the sputum so it can be coughed up more easily.
- To help keep your lungs free of infection, take 2 or 3 deep breaths and then cough. Do this often during the day.
- A humidifier will help keep the air moist and your sputum thin, making it easier to cough up. Be sure to keep your humidifier free of fungus. Clean it every day.
- Stay inside during very cold or hot weather, or on days when the air pollution is high. If you work in a polluted area, you may need to change jobs.
- When you are active, you may feel short of breath. Here are some breathing exercises that may relieve the problem:
  —Breathe with pursed or puckered lips (as if you are playing the trumpet).
  —Breathe using your diaphragm. Put one hand on your abdomen and breathe in so that the hand moves outward or up. Breathing this way allows your lungs more room to expand and take in air.
- If you use medicine that you inhale, follow these steps:
  —First, shake the inhaler.
  —Breathe out slowly, all the way.
  —Put the mouthpiece of the inhaler in your mouth or 2 inches away (about half a finger's length), or use the spacer (a piece of plastic-like tubing that attaches to the inhaler).
  —Breathe in and push down on the inhaler at the same time (to create the mist).
  —Hold your breath for about 10 seconds.
  —Breathe out slowly through puckered lips or through your nose.
  —If you need to take 2 puffs, wait 2 to 5 seconds before taking the second one.
  —Gargling after using your inhaler may help relieve burning in your throat.

Call Your Doctor If . . .
• Your sputum gets thicker even though you're taking your medicine and drinking water as directed.
• You cough up sputum that is bloody, yellow, or green.
• Your nail beds stay gray or blue even after you are breathing easier.
• You have a high temperature.
• You have chest pain or trouble breathing during exercise that does not go away with rest.

Seek Care Immediately If . . .
• You are feeling confused, dizzy, or very drowsy, and have swollen hands and feet and blue or pale lips and nail beds.
• You have chest pain or trouble breathing even while resting.
• If you have these symptoms, **call 911 or 0 (operator)** to get to the nearest hospital or clinic. **Do not drive yourself!**

IF YOU'RE HEADING FOR THE HOSPITAL . . .

What to Expect While You're There
You may encounter the following procedures and equipment during your stay.
• **Activity:** At first you will need to rest in bed, with a few pillows to keep you sitting up a little. This will help your breathing. Do not lie flat. Once you are breathing more easily, you will be allowed to increase your exercise.
• **Oxygen:** You may need extra oxygen at this time. It is given either by a mask or nasal prongs. Tell your doctor if the oxygen is drying out your nose or if the nasal prongs bother you.
• **Pulse Oximeter:** While you are getting oxygen, you may be hooked up to a pulse oximeter (ox-IM-uh-ter). It is placed on your ear, finger, or toe and is connected to a machine. It measures the oxygen in your blood.
• **IV:** A tube placed in your vein for giving medicine or liquids. It will be capped or have tubing connected to it.
• **Medicines:** The drugs below will help you breathe easier. They can be taken by mouth or given in your IV.
  —**Antibiotics:** If you have an infection in the lungs, you'll be given antibiotics to clear it up.
  —**Bronchodilators** (bronk-o-DIE-lay-tors): The medicines may be needed to help open your lung's airways.
  —**Steroids** (STAIR-oids): You may be given one of these drugs to decrease the swelling and inflammation of the tissue in your lungs.
• **Breathing Treatments:** A machine will be used to help you inhale

medicine. A therapist will help with these treatments. They will help open your airways so you can breathe easier. At first you may need them frequently. As you get better, you may only need them when you are having trouble breathing.

- **Postural Drainage:** A nurse may tap your back briskly with his or her hands. This helps loosen the sputum in your lungs so you can cough it up more easily.
- **Taking Vital Signs:** These include your temperature, blood pressure, pulse (counting your heartbeats), and respirations (counting your breaths). A stethoscope is used to listen to your heart and lungs. Your blood pressure is taken by wrapping a cuff around your arm.
- **ECG:** Also called a heart monitor, an electrocardiograph (e-lec-tro-CAR-dee-o-graf), or EKG. The patches on your chest are hooked up to a TV-type screen or a small portable box (telemetry unit). This screen shows a tracing of each heartbeat. Your heart will be watched for signs of injury or damage.
- **12 Lead ECG:** This test makes tracings from different parts of your heart. It can help your doctor decide whether there is a heart problem.
- **Chest X-ray:** This picture of your lungs and heart is used to monitor your condition.
- **Blood Gases:** Blood taken from an artery in your wrist, elbow, or groin is tested for oxygen.
- **Blood:** Usually taken for testing from a vein in your hand or from the bend in your elbow.

Endometriosis

WHAT YOU SHOULD KNOW

The lining of the uterus (womb) is called the endometrium (end-o-MEET-ree-um). Endometriosis (end-o-meet-ree-O-sis) is a condition in which tissue from this lining grows in places other than the uterus. The tissue sometimes can be found in the ovaries, tubes, vagina, and abdomen. It can grow between these organs and cause them to stick together. The extra tissue gets red, swollen, and may cause pain.

The endometrium is shed each month during your period. When menstrual bleeding occurs, the extra tissue also bleeds. Bits of it float around and can find new places to grow.

You can get endometriosis only if you are having periods. It is most common in women ages 20 to 40. There is no complete cure. However, the disease goes away after menopause, when the ovaries stop making a hormone called estrogen. Estrogen stimulates growth of the endometrium. Without it, the extra tissue cannot thrive.

Causes
We do not know why one woman will develop this problem while another is spared. We do know that women who have relatives with the disease have a higher risk of getting it.

Signs/Symptoms
Belly pain related to your menstrual cycle is the main sign. The pain comes and goes as your estrogen level changes during your cycle.

Other possible symptoms are pain during sex, heavy bleeding during your period and at other times, problems getting pregnant, blood in your urine, and back pain. These signs can show up suddenly or develop over many years.

Care
Your care is determined by your age, your symptoms, your desire to get pregnant, and how much disease you have.

Your doctor will do a pelvic exam (an "internal") to check your female organs. He or she may want to check you between periods and again during your period to compare the changes that may have occurred between the two exams.

You may be given medicine to reduce the amount of estrogen your body makes. This medicine will slow down or stop your periods, and some of the tissue growing outside your uterus may get smaller or go away. The medicine can keep the disease from spreading, but is not a complete cure. You may also get other medicines to help your pain.

A test called a laparoscopy (lap-er-OS-ko-pee) may be done, in which your doctor examines your internal organs for signs of endometriosis. If the disease is severe, you may need a hysterectomy (his-toe-REC-toe-me) to keep the endometriosis from returning again and again. This is surgery to remove your uterus. However, no care, including surgery, guarantees a permanent cure.

WHAT YOU SHOULD DO

- Take your medicine as directed. You can also use over-the-counter medicines such as acetaminophen or ibuprofen for pain.
- Keep a record of your bleeding and other signs when you begin care. This will help your doctor when you go for another checkup.
- Use a heating pad set on "low" or a hot water bottle if you have belly or back pain. Hot baths also will relax your muscles and help the pain.
- Your doctor may suggest surgery to treat the endometriosis. Be sure all your questions have been answered before you decide to have surgery.

• Endometriosis can make it difficult to become pregnant. If you want children, you should consider having them before the disease does too much damage.

Call Your Doctor If . . .
• You have bad belly or back pain which does not go away.
• You have heavy or unusual vaginal bleeding.
• Your symptoms return after treatment.

Endoscopy, Colon

See Colonoscopy

Endoscopy, Sigmoid

See Sigmoidoscopy

Endoscopy, Upper GI

See Gastrointestinal Endoscopy

Endoscopy, Urinary Tract

See Cystoscopy

Enlarged Prostate

WHAT YOU SHOULD KNOW

The prostate is a small gland nestled around the duct that drains the bladder (the urethra). In many men over 45 years of age, the gland tends to gradually grow larger, a condition known medically as "benign prostatic hyperplasia," or BPH. If the gland grows too large, it can begin to squeeze the urethra, making urination increasingly difficult.

Causes
The cause is unknown. The condition may be a natural result of the aging process.

Signs/Symptoms
Men with BPH typically feel a frequent urge to urinate but are able to pass little or no urine. There may be dribbling or leaking during the day and while you're asleep, and you may need to urinate frequently during the night. You may find it difficult to begin urinating without pushing; the stream may seem weak; and you may notice flecks of

blood in the urine. After urination, your bladder may not feel empty. The condition can also affect sex.

Treatment

The doctor will have your urine tested to rule out an infection and may order a series of additional tests. If you are having severe difficulties, the doctor may thread a soft tube called a catheter (KATH-uh-ter) into the urethra to drain the bladder. For many men, a drug called Proscar will shrink the prostate and relieve symptoms, though it sometimes takes 6 months or longer for the drug to take effect. Surgery to cut incisions in the prostate can also relieve the pressure, allowing urine to flow.

WHAT YOU SHOULD DO

- Don't let your bladder get too full. Urinate as much as you can whenever you feel the urge.
- Sit on hard chairs instead of soft ones whenever possible.
- Avoid exposure to cold temperatures or dampness.
- Do not eat spicy foods: they often irritate the urinary tract.
- Frequent sex reduces the risk of a urinary blockage. However, you should avoid becoming sexually aroused without ejaculating.

Call Your Doctor If . . .

- Your symptoms don't clear up or they become more troublesome.
- You develop a high temperature. This may be a sign of an infection in your bladder or kidneys.

Seek Care Immediately If . . .

- You cannot urinate at all and your bladder is full and painful. If this happens, your bladder must be emptied with a catheter.

Enterobiasis

See Pinworms

Epididymitis

WHAT YOU SHOULD KNOW

Epididymitis (EP-ih-DID-ee-MY-tis) is an infection of the epididymis, a tube located behind the testicle. The infection is common in men 19 to 35 years old.

Causes
The problem may start with an infection of the bladder or prostate gland. The infection is sometimes contracted through sexual contact.

Signs/Symptoms
The usual symptoms are fever, pain, redness, and swelling of the scrotum and painful urination. You also may feel a lump in your scrotum.

Care
Your doctor will prescribe an antibiotic to fight the infection. Rest until you feel better, and follow the directions listed below.

WHAT YOU SHOULD DO

• Rest in bed until fever, pain, and swelling go down. The testicle may stay swollen and hard for several days or even a few weeks.
• If your doctor prescribes an antibiotic to fight the infection, take it exactly as directed and finish the entire prescription. If you stop taking the drug too soon, a few germs may survive and re-infect you.
• To help relieve pain and swelling, place a rolled-up towel between your legs under the scrotum. This helps support the weight of the scrotum and the tender testicles. Wearing briefs (jockey shorts) also provides support to the scrotum.
• Apply either cold or heat to the swollen area, whichever relieves the pain best. You may use warm or cold compresses, ice packs, an electric heating pad set on low, or a hot water bottle filled with warm water. Sitting in a warm bath for 15 minutes twice a day will help reduce the swelling more quickly.
• You may use acetaminophen, aspirin, or ibuprofen for the pain.
• Do not drink alcohol, tea, coffee, or carbonated beverages; they irritate the urinary system. Eat foods such as prunes, fresh fruit, whole-grain cereals, and nuts to prevent constipation.
• Wait at least 1 month after all symptoms disappear before having sex. Using a condom will help protect against sexually transmitted infections.
• Be careful not to injure the infected testicle for 2 or 3 months. When you resume normal activities, wear an athletic supporter (jock strap) or two pairs of briefs.

Call Your Doctor If . . .
• You have a high temperature.
• Your pain is not relieved by bed rest, applying heat or cold, or scrotal support.

- You become constipated.
- Your symptoms do not improve within 3 to 4 days after treatment starts.
- You have any problems that may be related to the medicine you are taking.

Epiglottitis

WHAT YOU SHOULD KNOW

Epiglottitis (ep-ee-glah-TIE-tis) is an infection that causes swelling of the area around the voice box. It affects children ages 2 to 12, and can be a very serious problem.

The infection is not common because most children get shots (Haemophilus Influenzae type B vaccine) to prevent the disease. The more children get the shots, the rarer the disease will become.

Causes

The infection is caused by a germ spread through the air. Children are usually not sick before getting epiglottitis. But some children may have a cold, cough, or sore throat.

Signs/Symptoms

The child may quickly get a high fever and sore throat. Breathing may be noisy and have a squeaky sound. There is no cough.

The child may want to sit or be held. The child will drool and may push his chin out, with his mouth open and tongue out.

The child may seem restless and anxious while trying to breathe.

Care

Hospitalization may be needed to watch for breathing problems, care for the infection, and administer medicine. Antibiotics are used for treatment.

Try to stay calm and reassure the child. Breathing problems will get worse if the child is afraid and crying.

Risks

Epiglottitis is dangerous, and can be fatal. But with proper treatment, the risks of serious illness or death are small.

WHAT YOU SHOULD DO

- Give your child medicine as directed by your doctor.
- Use a cool mist humidifier at night in the child's room. Place the

humidifier out of reach by the bed. Fill it with cool water. Use it for 2 to 3 weeks.

- Try to get your child to drink water, apple juice, tea, gelatin, broth, or ginger-ale. The liquids should be at room temperature. Do not worry about solid food until the child is better.
- Your child needs rest until the infection is gone. He or she can then go back to normal activity.
- Give acetaminophen if the child has a fever.

Call Your Doctor If . . .
- Your child has a high temperature.
- Your child is not drinking liquids.

Seek Care Immediately If . . .
- **Call 911 or 0 (operator)** for help if your child has any of the following signs: trouble breathing, the skin between the ribs is being sucked in with each breath, or lips or fingernails are turning blue or white.

IF YOU'RE HEADING FOR THE HOSPITAL . . .

What to Expect While You're There
- **Visiting:** You may stay with your child to give comfort and support. The child will feel safer with you nearby.
- **Room:** Your child will be kept from others to keep from spreading the disease. Hospital personnel will wear a face mask and gown around your child, which may seem scary.
- **Hand Washing:** Wash your hands after visiting to keep from spreading the infection.
- **Oxygen:** Your child may be placed in a clear plastic mist tent or a high humidity room to help make breathing easier. Oxygen also can be given with a face mask that goes over the mouth and nose.
- **Breathing Tube:** Your child may need a tube in the nose or throat to help him or her breathe. Oxygen will be given through the tube. It will be left in for about 36 hours and taken out when breathing is easier.
- **Pulse Oximeter:** Your child may be hooked up to a pulse oximeter (ox-IM-uh-ter). It is placed on the ear, finger, or toe and is connected to a machine that measures the oxygen in your child's blood.
- **Taking Vital Signs:** These include temperature, blood pressure, pulse (counting heartbeats), and respirations (counting breaths). A stethoscope is used to listen to the heart and lungs. Blood pressure is taken by wrapping a cuff around the arm.
- **ECG:** Also called a heart monitor, an electrocardiograph (e-lec-tro-

CAR-dee-o-graf), or EKG. The patches on your child's chest are hooked up to a TV-type screen. This screen shows a tracing of each heartbeat. Your child's heart will be watched for signs of injury or damage that could be related to the illness.

- **Neck X-Ray:** This picture of your child's neck will show the swollen area around the vocal cords. It will help your doctor decide on treatment.
- **Laryngoscopy:** Your child may have a test called a laryngoscopy (lair-in-GOS-ko-pee). It is done to check on the breathing problems. Before the test, your child will either be put to sleep or be given medicine to make him or her sleepy.
- **IV:** A tube placed in your child's veins for giving medicine or liquids. It will be capped or have tubing connected to it.
- **Medicines:** Your child will get antibiotics to treat the infection. They can be put in the IV or taken by mouth.
- **Blood:** Usually taken from a vein in your child's hand or from the bend in the elbow. Tests will be done on the blood.
- **Blood Gases:** Blood is taken from an artery in your child's wrist, elbow, or groin. It is tested for the amount of oxygen in it.

Epistaxis

See Nosebleeds

Erythema Infectiosum

WHAT YOU SHOULD KNOW

Erythema (air-uh-THEE-ma) infectiosum (in-fek-tee-OH-sum), also called Fifth disease, is an infection that mostly occurs in children. It usually starts with a rash on the face that spreads to other parts of the body. In most cases, it is mild and lasts for 5 to 10 days, although it can sometimes come and go for up to 5 weeks. It goes away by itself without care.

Causes

The problem is caused by a virus. It occurs most often during the spring. A pregnant woman who gets this infection can pass it on to her unborn child.

Signs/Symptoms

The first sign of the infection is a rash on the face that looks like the child has been slapped. After 1 or 2 days, the rash spreads to other parts of the body. The child may also have flu or cold symptoms such as a low fever, headache, runny nose, pain in the joints, sore throat, and cough. Some children get an upset stomach or may throw up. The rash may get brighter and itch after the child has been out in the sun and following exercise or a warm bath.

Care

There is no cure, and the symptoms usually go away on their own after about a week.

WHAT YOU SHOULD DO

- No treatment is needed for the infection. Medicine such as acetaminophen to reduce fever or ease pain may be given if needed.
- This disease is not very contagious, and it is usually not necessary to keep your child away from other children. Once the rash appears, the infection usually no longer will spread.
- Pregnant women should stay away from places where children have this infection.
- The rash may get brighter and itch after the child has been out in the sun or after exercise. Try to have your child avoid these things for a week.

Call Your Doctor If . . .

- Your child develops a high temperature or seems to be getting worse.
- The rash becomes itchy.

Eyelid Infection

See Blepharitis

Facial Fracture

WHAT YOU SHOULD KNOW

A facial fracture may involve one of several facial bones: the orbit (bones around the eye), the cheek bones, or the bones in the upper jaw. An x-ray will show when the broken bone is healed; it may take weeks or months.

Causes

Facial fractures are usually the result of an accident.

Signs/Symptoms

You'll have swelling, pain, bruising, or bleeding. The face may feel numb or tingly. Because of swelling or the break itself, your face may not look normal. You may also have double vision or numbness in your cheek.

Care
Although the fracture won't be put in a cast, the break must be carefully protected until it has healed. If you have a bad fracture, surgery may be necessary.

WHAT YOU SHOULD DO

• Apply ice to the injury for 15 to 20 minutes each hour for the first 1 to 2 days. Put the ice in a plastic bag and place a towel between the bag of ice and your skin.
• After the first 1 to 2 days, you may put heat on the injury to help ease the pain. Use a heating pad (set on low), a whirlpool bath, or warm, moist towels for 15 to 20 minutes every hour for 48 hours.
• Do not play any contact sports or indulge in other dangerous activities until your doctor says it's all right.
• You may gently wash and dry your face.
• If the doctor prescribes pain medicine that makes you drowsy, don't drive. You also may take over-the-counter medicines for pain. Take all medications exactly as directed.
• If you have been given a tetanus shot, your arm may get swollen, red, and warm to the touch at the shot site. This is a normal reaction to the medicine in the shot.

Call Your Doctor If . . .
• You develop a high temperature.
• You have really bad headaches or your vision becomes worse.
• You have new numbness or tingling in your face.

Seek Care Immediately If . . .
• You have even worse trouble seeing.
• You become dizzy or pass out.
• You have trouble speaking, breathing, or swallowing.

Fainting

WHAT YOU SHOULD DO

Fainting, known medically as syncope (SIN-coe-pea), strikes quickly and passes just as fast—typically within a few seconds to 1 or 2 minutes. It usually occurs while you are standing.

Causes

Fainting episodes usually occur when the brain fails to get enough blood. This can be the result of various heart conditions, a change in your heart rate, low blood pressure, or a sudden change in position. The problem is sometimes an allergic reaction to a drug. In addition, low blood sugar can lead to a fainting spell, as can hyperventilation. Sometimes, no cause can be found.

Signs/Symptoms

Warning signs of an impending attack typically include lightheadedness and a sudden feeling that you are going to pass out. These are often accompanied by sweating, weakness, dizziness, or nausea. You may also develop rapid breathing and a fast heartbeat.

WHAT YOU SHOULD DO

- When you feel faint, lie down or sit down and bend over. If possible, keep your legs higher than your head. This will send blood back to your heart and help blood flow to your brain.
- You may resume your normal activities when you are feeling better.
- Make an appointment with your doctor to find out what caused the problem.
- If you have low blood sugar, eat 5 or 6 small meals a day. Make sure they are high in protein (meat, chicken, fish, cheese) and complex carbohydrates (grains and cereals). Avoid sugar and simple carbohydrates (candy and other sweets).

Call Your Doctor If . . .

- You have another fainting spell.

Seek Care Immediately If . . .

- You develop chest pain. **THIS IS AN EMERGENCY.** Get medical help at once. **Call 911 or 0 (operator). Do NOT** drive yourself to the hospital.
- You have trouble breathing, get a really bad headache, feel dizzy, or develop a rapid heartbeat.
- You have pain in your back; severe pain in your abdomen; or pain, numbness, burning, or tingling in your arms or legs.
- You have a seizure.
- You notice any signs of bleeding, including bloody vomit and bloody or black stools.

Febrile Seizure

WHAT YOU SHOULD KNOW

A febrile (FEB-rile) seizure (SEE-zhur) is a type of convulsion. It causes your child's face or body to tighten up and jerk or twist. It is the most common type of seizure, and may last from 1 to 10 minutes. Children between 6 months and 2 years are more likely to have a febrile seizure. The seizures do not cause brain damage. Most children will not have another one.

Causes
A temperature of about 104 degrees F (40 degrees C) or more. The fever may be the result of an infection.

Signs/Symptoms
Jerking or twitching of the arms, legs or face. When a seizure starts, the child may pass out. He or she may not be aware of the jerking. The child may urinate or have a bowel movement without knowing it, or may throw up. After the seizure, the child may seem irritable, confused, or sleepy.

WHAT YOU SHOULD DO

- If your child develops a fever, give a sponge bath to try to reduce the fever. The bath should be done in a warm room with warm water. Using a damp washcloth, gently rub the entire body. The child should be damp but not dripping wet. Do not use a fan or ice or cold water, and do not chill the child.
- During a convulsion, protect the child from injury by moving dangerous objects away. Do not try to hold the child down. Do not put anything in his or her mouth.
- When the seizure has passed, give the child acetaminophen for fever control. **Do not give your child aspirin.** Your doctor will tell you whether you need other medicines to prevent more seizures.
- If the child has another febrile seizure, write down details for the doctor, including when it began, whether both sides of the body were jerking, how long the convulsion lasted, the length of time between the rise in temperature and the start of the seizure, and whether the child slept afterward.

Call Your Doctor If . . .
- The child still has a fever 3 days after the febrile seizure, or has an uncontrolled fever of any duration.

Seek Care Immediately If . . .
• Your child has another convulsion.
• Your child is injured during a convulsion.
• Your child develops vomiting, headache, or a stiff neck.

Fever Blister

See Cold Sores

Fever in Adults

WHAT YOU SHOULD KNOW

You have a fever if your body temperature, taken by mouth, is over 99.5 degrees F (37.5 degrees C). Running a fever is a sign that your body is fighting an infection. In most cases, it is not a sign of a life-threatening illness.

Causes
Fever is typically associated with a viral infection such as a cold or flu. Certain other infections and diseases also cause fever.

Signs/Symptoms
Typical symptoms include a reddened face, warm forehead, body chills, and sweating. You may feel hot and may be tired.

WHAT YOU SHOULD DO

• To reduce your fever:
  —You may use aspirin, acetaminophen, or ibuprofen.
  —Place a cold compress under your arm or on the back of your neck, or sponge off with lukewarm water.
• You may feel better if you decrease your activity or rest in bed.
• Drink an 8-ounce glass of water every hour while you are awake.

Call Your Doctor If . . .
• Your fever lasts more than 3 or 4 days.
• You notice any new symptoms.

Seek Care Immediately If . . .
• You develop a very high temperature.

Fever in Children

WHAT YOU SHOULD KNOW

Fever is a symptom, not a disease. It is the body's normal reaction to an infection. The fever helps fight the infection.

A fever does not cause long-term problems until it reaches 107 degrees F (41.7 degrees C). A high fever may sometimes cause convulsions (seizures).

Your child has a fever if:

- The mouth temperature is higher than 99.5 degrees F (38 degrees C).
- The rectal temperature is higher than 100.4 degrees F (38 degrees C).
- The armpit temperature is higher than 98.6 degrees F (37 degrees C).

Exercise, a hot bath, too much clothing, and hot weather can raise a child's temperature. Drinking or eating warm foods can also cause the temperature to rise. Wait 30 minutes and take the child's temperature again.

WHAT YOU SHOULD DO

- If the child's temperature is higher than 101 degrees F (38.3 degrees C), restrict activity or put the child to bed.
- Encourage the child to drink extra fluids.
- Give acetaminophen for the fever. **Do not give your child aspirin.**
- If the child's temperature remains higher than 104 degrees F (40 degrees C), it may be helpful to give the child a sponge bath. This should be done in a warm room with warm water. Using a damp wash cloth, gently rub the entire body. The child should be damp but not dripping wet. Do not use a fan or ice or cold water, and do not chill the child.
- Take the child's temperature in the morning, at bedtime, and every 4 hours during the day, or more often if he or she looks ill.

Call Your Doctor If . . .

- The child develops a temperature higher than 103 degrees F (39.4 degrees C).
- The child's temperature is higher than 101 degrees F (37 degrees C) for more than 24 hours.
- The child develops new symptoms.
- The child has a marked change in behavior, level of consciousness, or level of activity.

Seek Care Immediately If . . .
• The child develops a rectal temperature higher than 105 degrees F (40.6 degrees C).
• Your child has a seizure, develops abnormal movements of the face, arms, or legs, or has difficulty breathing.

Fifth Disease

See Erythema Infectiosum

Finger Fracture

See Broken Finger

Fingernail Removal

See Nail Removal

Flu in Adults

WHAT YOU SHOULD KNOW

Flu (influenza) is a common infection of the lungs, airways, and throat. It can spread easily, most often during the winter. Most people start to feel better after a few days, and feel normal again after 1 to 2 weeks.

Causes
The infection can come from any of a large variety of influenza viruses. A flu shot will protect you from some of the worst kinds of flu viruses—but not every kind. Even with the shot you may still get the flu, but it may not last as long as it would otherwise.

Signs/Symptoms
Typical symptoms are chills, fever, an achy feeling, cough, sore throat, and headache. You also may feel very tired.

Care
Antibiotics are no help against the flu. There are virus medicines your doctor can prescribe if the flu gets very bad, but they won't provide a cure. The best strategy is plenty of rest, lots of liquids, and acetaminophen for pain and fever. Your doctor can also prescribe medicine to help you stop coughing.

WHAT YOU SHOULD DO

- You may use acetaminophen or ibuprofen for fever and body aches. Do NOT take aspirin if you have a fever.
- Use a cool-mist humidifier to increase air moisture. This will make it easier for you to breathe and will help relieve your cough.
- Gargling may help relieve your sore throat. Use warm salt water (1 teaspoon of salt in a cup of water) or warm or cold double-strength tea.
- Wash your hands often to avoid spreading germs. This is especially important after blowing your nose and before touching food. Cover your mouth and nose when you cough or sneeze.
- Rest until your temperature is normal (98.6 degrees F or 37 degrees C). This usually takes 3 to 4 days. Get plenty of sleep.
- Drink as much water or other liquid as you comfortably can. Drink 8 to 10 (soda-can size) glasses a day, if possible.
- You may want to get a flu shot in the fall to keep from getting the flu again next year, particularly if you are over 65 or have a medical condition.

Call Your Doctor If . . .
- Your fever lasts more than 3 or 4 days or you have a high temperature.
- You have trouble breathing while resting, a deep cough with lots of mucus, or chest pain.
- You have nausea, vomiting, or diarrhea.

Seek Care Immediately If . . .
- You are very breathless or have dark or bluish fingernails, toenails, or skin.
- You get really bad neck pain or stiffness.
- You feel confused, start acting strangely, or have a seizure.

Flu in Children

WHAT YOU SHOULD KNOW

Flu, known medically as influenza (in-flew-EN-zuh) is an infection of the nose, throat, windpipe, and airways in the lung.

Causes
Influenza is caused by a virus. The germ is quickly spread from an infected person to others by coughing and sneezing.

Signs/Symptoms

Typical symptoms include chills, fever, headache, body aches, sore throat, cough, swollen glands, vomiting and diarrhea. The child also may have a runny nose; earache; and red, watery, sore eyes.

The disease is worst during the first 1 to 2 days. Cough and tiredness may last another week or more.

Care

There is no cure for the flu. Antibiotic medicine will not work. The best remedy is plenty of rest and liquids.

WHAT YOU SHOULD DO

- DO NOT GIVE ASPIRIN if a child with influenza is under 18 years of age. This could lead to brain and liver damage (Reye's syndrome). Carefully check for aspirin on the label on any over-the-counter medicines.
- Acetaminophen will help relieve fever and body aches.
- Use a cool-mist humidifier to increase moisture in the child's room. This will make breathing easier.
- The child should rest until his or her temperature is normal (98.6 degrees F or 37 degrees C). This usually takes 3 to 4 days.
- Give plenty of liquids such as juice, water, broth, gelatin, or lemonade. Do not worry about giving solid food until the child is better.
- Wash the child's hands often to prevent spread of germs. This is especially important after blowing the nose and before touching food. Be sure the child covers his or her mouth when coughing or sneezing.
- Keep your child home from daycare or school until the fever is gone (usually 2 or 3 days).

Call Your Doctor If . . .
- The fever lasts more than 36 hours.
- The child has shortness of breath while resting, a deep cough with lots of mucus, or chest pain.
- The child has nausea, vomiting, or diarrhea.

Seek Care Immediately If . . .
- Your child is not drinking enough fluids and has signs of water loss such as listlessness, dry mouth, little or no urination, wrinkled skin, no tears, dizziness, or, in babies, a sunken soft spot on the top of the head.
- The child has trouble breathing or the skin or nails turn bluish.

• The child develops severe neck pain or stiffness.
• The child acts confused or too sleepy, has changes in behavior, or has seizures.
• The child has a very high fever.

Foley Catheter

WHAT YOU SHOULD KNOW

A Foley catheter (KATH-uh-ter)—a soft, thin rubber tube with a balloon on the end—is used to drain urine from the bladder. It can remain in place for a short or long period of time. The catheter is threaded through the urinary duct (urethra) and into the bladder.

A Foley catheter is needed when normal urination is disrupted by an infection, a swollen prostate gland, bladder stones, or, sometimes, an injury. In very sick people, a catheter may be used to keep track of urine production.

Risks
Your bladder or urethra could be injured when the Foley catheter is inserted. You could also develop an infection. But, if you follow your doctor's directions, you should not have problems.

IF YOU'RE HEADING FOR THE HOSPITAL . . .

What to Expect While You're There
You may encounter the following procedures and equipment during your stay:

• **Taking Your Vital Signs:** These include your temperature, blood pressure, pulse (counting your heartbeats), and respirations (counting your breaths). A stethoscope is used to listen to your heart and lungs. Your blood pressure is taken by wrapping a cuff around your arm.
• **Inserting the Foley Catheter:**
   —You will lie on your back covered by a sheet. Using sterile gloves, your doctor will carefully clean the area around your urethra.
   —The catheter will be gently inserted in your urethra and passed up to your bladder.
   —When the tube reaches your bladder, the balloon at the tip will be filled with sterile water by your doctor. This will hold the catheter in place.
   —The balloon presses against the wall of your bladder. This may make you feel the need to urinate. However, the urine will drain out the catheter, instead.

—To keep it secure, the catheter will be taped to your belly or leg.

—The insertion will take about 10 minutes.

After You Leave

- Do NOT pull on the catheter or try to remove it. Keep the catheter tube taped or tied to your leg to prevent accidental pulling.
- Always keep the urine drainage bag below the level of your bladder. This prevents urine from running back into your bladder and reduces your chances of getting a bladder infection.
- Do not puncture, cut, or clamp the catheter.
- To help keep the catheter from clogging, drink 8 glasses of water a day. Your urine should be clear or pale yellow.
- Empty the drainage bag frequently. Do not allow the urine to sit in the bag for more than 2 or 3 hours. This helps prevent infection and also reduces odor and the chance of leakage. Measure and write down the amount of urine you empty from the bag.
- If crusty deposits form on the catheter, they should be washed off gently with warm water and mild soap. Rinse the area well after washing. Do not put creams or ointments on the catheter unless prescribed by your doctor.
- You may shower with the catheter in place, but do not take tub baths.
- The catheter will need to be changed regularly. Be sure to keep your appointments.

Call Your Doctor If . . .

- The catheter's point of entry is painful.
- You feel pain or burning in your bladder.
- You begin to see blood in your urine.
- Bloody or pus-like discharge appears around the catheter.
- You have a high temperature.
- The catheter slips out.
- No urine is draining into the urine bag.

Seek Care Immediately If . . .

- Your symptoms get worse.
- Your temperature gets very high.
- You notice blood specks in your urine, or the urine becomes red or smelly.

Food Allergy

WHAT YOU SHOULD KNOW

An allergic reaction to food is a mistaken attack by the body's immune system against a substance that other people find harmless. Food allergies are more common in children than adults.

Causes
Just about any food can be the source of an allergic reaction. However, the most common culprits are cow's milk, eggs, wheat, soybeans, peanuts, fish, chocolate, shellfish and tree nuts such as walnuts or pecans. You are at higher risk if you have a family history of food allergies.

Signs/Symptoms
A mild reaction may produce diarrhea, stomach pain, gas, or a full feeling in your stomach. You may develop a skin rash with hives and itching. There may be nausea and vomiting, a bad headache, or fainting. Swelling around the mouth is common. In a severe reaction (known medically as anaphylaxis [AN-uh-fuh-LAX-is]), you may become congested, lose your breath, and be in danger of suffocating.

WHAT YOU SHOULD DO

- If you are not sure what caused the reaction, keep a diary of the foods you have eaten and any symptoms that followed. Don't eat any of the foods that cause reactions.
- If you develop hives or a rash:
  - —Take the medicine prescribed for your hives exactly as your doctor directs.
  - —You may use a nonprescription antihistamine. Take it until the hives have been completely gone for 24 hours.
  - —Apply cold compresses to the skin or take baths in cool water. Don't take hot baths or showers; the warmth will make the itching worse.
  - —Wear loose fitting clothes and avoid tight underwear.
- If you are severely allergic:
  - —Following a severe reaction, someone will need to stay with you for 24 hours in case the symptoms return.
  - —You should wear a medic-alert bracelet or necklace stating the nature of your allergy.
  - —Your doctor will suggest you buy an anaphylaxis kit and will teach you and your family when and how to give adrenaline shots.
  - —If you have had a severe reaction before, always carry your anaphylaxis kit with you.

Call Your Doctor If . . .

- You suspect a food allergy. Symptoms usually occur within 30 minutes of eating, but sometimes take up to 2 hours to appear.
- The symptoms have not gone away within 2 weeks.
- You develop new symptoms.
- You want to retest a child with a food you think causes an allergic reaction.

Seek Care Immediately If . . .

- You develop wheezing, a tight feeling in your chest or throat, a swollen mouth, and difficulty breathing. **THIS IS AN EMERGENCY. Call 911 or 0 (operator)** for medical help or have someone drive you to the nearest emergency room.
- You develop hives, swelling, or itching ALL OVER your body.

Food Poisoning

See Salmonella Food Poisoning

Foot Fracture

See Broken Foot

Foreign Body in the Ear

WHAT YOU SHOULD KNOW

Children often put beans, peas, beads, or small pieces of toys into their ears. Insects can also crawl inside. If the object gets stuck, the situation is not dangerous, but does require professional attention.

Signs/Symptoms

Likely complaints include ear pain, discharge, or loss of hearing. Smaller children may be very fussy and try to scratch the ear to get the foreign body out.

Care

Do not try to remove the object with tweezers or your finger. This can push the object further into the ear canal and possibly damage the eardrum. Instead, see your doctor.

WHAT YOU SHOULD DO

- Once the doctor removes the object from the ear, there usually is no further problem.
- Keep small objects out of reach of young children and tell them not

to put anything in their ears. Tell the child to inform you or another
adult immediately if it happens again.

Call Your Doctor If . . .
• Bleeding from the ear develops.
• Pain and discharge from the ear continue. This may be a sign of in-
fection or may indicate that the object was not completely removed.
• Another small object gets stuck in the ear canal.

Foreign Body in the Eye

WHAT YOU SHOULD KNOW

In windy weather, or when you're working with power tools without
wearing safety glasses, it's easy to get something in your eye. This
foreign body can scratch or irritate your cornea (the transparent area
of the eyeball over the iris and pupil).

Signs/Symptoms
Symptoms range from redness, a scratchy feeling, or frequent
blinking to severe eye pain.

Care
Do not rub the eye or try to remove the object yourself; let your doctor
get it out. You will probably have to use medication and wear an eye
patch after the foreign body is removed.

WHAT YOU SHOULD DO

• If you are wearing an eye patch:
  —Do NOT loosen or remove the patch until your doctor gives the
    go-ahead. If the tape comes loose, retape it just as it was before.
  —Do not drive or operate machinery while your eye is patched;
    your ability to judge distances will be impaired. In some states,
    driving with one eye patched is against the law.
• If you are not wearing an eye patch:
  —Keep your eye closed as much as possible. Do not rub the eye.
  —Wear dark glasses for a few days to protect your eye from bright
    light.
• Do not wear contact lenses until your doctor says it's okay.
• To avoid future problems, wear protective eye covering if your job
  or hobby involves the risk of eye injury. This is especially important
  when you are working with high-speed tools or power saws.

Call Your Doctor If . . .
• Pain increases in your eye or your vision changes.
• You have any problems with your eye patch.
• You develop a high temperature.

Foreign Body in the Nose

WHAT YOU SHOULD KNOW

Children sometimes put small objects such as beans, peas, candy, beads, or small pieces of toys into their nose. These foreign bodies often get stuck or cannot be found.

Signs/Symptoms
The nose may have a watery discharge that later turns thick, yellow, and foul-smelling. The child may have trouble breathing through the nose, and may complain of pain in the nose. The object may or may not be visible.

Care
Blowing the nose may push the object out. If that doesn't work, see the child's doctor. If you try to get the object out by yourself, you could injure the nose.

WHAT YOU SHOULD DO

• Once the doctor removes the object, there usually are no more problems.
• Keep small objects out of reach of young children and tell them not to put anything in their noses. Tell the child to inform you or another adult immediately if it happens again.

Call Your Doctor If . . .
• The nose begins to bleed.
• The nose continues to drain (the object may still be inside).
• If the child develops a fever, earache, headache, pain in the cheeks or around the eyes, or yellow-green nasal discharge. These are signs of a possible sinus or ear infection.

Foreskin Removal

See Circumcision

Fractured Ankle

See Broken Ankle

Fractured Arm

See Broken Arm

Fractured Collarbone

See Broken Collarbone

Fractured Elbow

See Broken Elbow

Fractured Face

See Facial Fracture

Fractured Finger

See Broken Finger

Fractured Foot

See Broken Foot

Fractured Hand

See Broken Hand

Fractured Jaw

See Broken Jaw

Fractured Leg

See Broken Leg

Fractured Nose

See Broken Nose

Fractured Rib

See Rib Fracture

Fractured Shoulder Blade

See Broken Shoulder Blade

Fractured Toe

See Broken Toe

Frostbite

WHAT YOU SHOULD KNOW

Frostbite (frozen skin) usually affects bare skin on the hands, fingers, feet, toes, nose, and ears during cold and windy weather.

People who have drunk alcohol or smoked before going outside are most likely to get frostbite. Those who have medical problems, such as diabetes or blood vessel diseases, are also highly susceptible.

Causes

Frostbite occurs when ice forms in the skin and blood vessels during extended exposure to subfreezing temperatures.

Signs/Symptoms

You'll first notice numbness and pain. The skin will be hard and look white. After the skin warms up, its color will change from white to red or purple and you may feel pain, tingling, burning. The skin may swell and sometimes develops blisters.

Care

You may need medicine to relieve the pain or to fight infection.

WHAT YOU SHOULD DO

- If you get frostbite:
  —Get out of the wind.
  —Do NOT walk on frostbitten feet. Do NOT use snow or direct heat, and do NOT rub the area.
  —Immediately cover the frozen area with extra clothing or blankets, or warm it against your body.
  —When out of the cold, remove clothes from the frostbitten skin and soak it in warm water.
  —Drink warm fluids.
- To prevent getting frostbite again:
  —If you must go out in freezing weather, wear several layers of warm clothes under a windproof and waterproof coat.
  —Be sure to protect your hands, ears, and feet.
  —Once outside, try to stay dry.
  —Do not drink alcohol before you go out in the cold.

Seek Care Immediately If . . .

- You have increased pain, swelling, redness, or discharge in the area that was frostbitten.
- You have a high temperature or feel achy, dizzy, or generally ill.
- You get any new, unexplained symptoms.

Fungal Meningitis

WHAT YOU SHOULD KNOW

Fungal (FUN-gul) meningitis (MEN-in-JIE-tis) is an infection that causes swelling and irritation of the tissue around the brain and spinal cord. It usually strikes people whose weakened immune systems can't fight off infection. The disease is not common, but it can be very serious.

Causes

This type of meningitis is caused by a fungus. It usually results from an infection that spreads to your brain from another part of your body. The infection does not pass easily from person to person.

Signs/Symptoms

Typical symptoms are headache, blurred vision, confusion, tiredness, irritability, vomiting, and a stiff neck. You may also have a fever.

Care

Medicines that fight the fungus are used to treat the disease. You may be put in the hospital for tests and care.

Risks

Left untreated, this disease can be fatal. If you don't get treatment soon enough, you could end up with brain damage (hearing loss, learning problems, difficulty talking, seizures, or paralysis).

IF YOU'RE HEADING FOR THE HOSPITAL . . .

What to Expect While You're There

You may encounter the following procedures and equipment during your stay.

- **Activity:** You will rest in bed in a darkened room. You may not be allowed to have certain visitors if it is felt that you could catch a cold from them or they could catch your infection.
- **Taking Vital Signs:** These include your temperature, blood pressure, pulse (counting your heartbeats), and respirations (counting

your breaths). A stethoscope is used to listen to your heart and lungs. Your blood pressure is taken by wrapping a cuff around your arm.

- **Pulse Oximeter:** If you need to take oxygen, you may also be hooked up to a pulse oximeter (ox-IM-uh-ter). It is placed on your ear, finger, or toe and is connected to a machine that measures the oxygen in your blood.
- **Neuro Signs:** The doctor will check your memory and your eyes, and see how easily you awaken. These are important signs that show how well your brain is handling the infection.
- **Blood:** Usually taken from a vein in your hand or from the bend in your elbow. Tests will be done on the blood.
- **Blood Gases:** Blood is taken from an artery in your wrist, elbow, or groin. It is tested for its oxygen content.
- **Chest X-ray:** This picture of your lungs and heart shows how well they are handling the illness.
- **Lumbar** (LUM-bar) **Puncture:** (Also called a spinal tap.) Fluid is taken from your spine and is sent for tests.
- **Body fluid cultures:** Blood, urine, throat, and nose fluids may be tested to help your doctor decide which medicine to give you.
- **CT Scan:** (Also called a "CAT" scan.) This computerized x-ray may be used to take pictures of your brain.
- **IV:** A tube placed in your vein for giving medicine or liquids. It will be capped or have tubing connected to it.
- **ECG:** Also called a heart monitor, an electrocardiograph (e-LEK-tro-CAR-dee-o-graf), or EKG. Patches on your chest are hooked up to a TV-type screen or a small portable box (telemetry unit). This screen shows a tracing of each heartbeat.
- **Medicines:**
  —**Anti-Fungal medicine** to kill the infection may be given in your IV or by mouth.
  —**Pain medicine** may be given in your IV, as a shot, or by mouth. If the pain does not go away or comes back, tell a doctor right away.
  —**Fever medicine** such as acetaminophen will be given by mouth or in your rectum to bring your temperature down.
  —**Anti-nausea medicine** may be given to get rid of your nausea and control your vomiting so that you don't lose too much body fluid (become dehydrated).

After You Leave

- If you are still taking anti-fungal medicine, continue to take it until it is all gone, even if you feel well. If you stop treatment too soon,

some of the fungus may survive and give you a second bout of the illness.
- If you are taking medicine that makes you drowsy, do not drive or use heavy equipment.
- If you feel a medication is not helping, call your doctor. Do not quit taking it on your own.
- No special diet is needed. Just drink about 6 to 8 glasses (soda-can size) of water a day, even if you don't feel like it. Do not drink alcohol.
- Eat healthy foods and get lots of rest.
- If you still have headaches, rest in a dark, quiet room.
- When you feel better, you may start your normal activities again.
- For protection against other likely infections, get shots for flu and pneumonia. Stay away from anyone who has an infection.
- Wash your hands after going to the bathroom and before eating to keep from spreading germs.

Call Your Doctor If . . .
- You have new symptoms, such as a rash, itching, swelling, or trouble breathing, that started after you began taking a medicine. You may be allergic to the drug.
- You develop a high temperature while you are taking medicine.

Seek Care Immediately If . . .
- Your symptoms come back or someone else in the family develops them.
- You or someone in your family becomes confused or difficult to wake up, or has a high temperature.
- You or someone in your family has seizures.

Furuncle

See Boils

Gallstones

WHAT YOU SHOULD KNOW

The gallbladder is a small pouch near the liver where bile is stored. Bile helps to break down food, especially fats. The gallbladder can become irritated and swollen. A common cause of gallbladder disease is gallstones. Pain from gallstones is also called "biliary (BILL-ee-air-ee) colic."

Many people have gallstones but do not know it. Often, gallstones stay in the gallbladder or pass through it without causing problems. However, if one gets stuck on its way out of the gallbladder, intense pain can result.

Causes

You are more likely to have gallstones if your parents had them. Your chances of developing gallstones also increase if you weigh too much, have many children, take birth control pills, drink too much alcohol, and have a high-fat diet.

Whenever the gallbladder cannot completely empty, gallstones may develop. For instance, infection and swelling of the tubes that carry bile out of the liver can produce gallstones.

Signs/Symptoms

You may not have any symptoms, or you may have stomach pain, nausea, vomiting, fever, or jaundice (yellow skin or eyes). You may also feel bloated, not be able to eat fatty food, and burp more than usual.

Care

Your doctor may suggest aspirin, acetaminophen, or ibuprofen for pain. Rest until you feel better. You may need to go into the hospital for more tests and treatment.

If your gallstones or other gallbladder disease causes problems such as infection, you may need to have the gallstones broken apart or removed. Surgery may be needed to remove your gallbladder.

Risks

The disease is not life-threatening, but could get worse if you do not get treatment.

WHAT YOU SHOULD DO

- You may take aspirin, acetaminophen, or ibuprofen for pain.
- Rest in bed until you are feeling better.
- During an attack, drink clear fluids if you are able. Don't eat anything.
- To prevent further attacks, don't eat foods that give you indigestion. Make sure everything you eat is low in fat.

Seek Care Immediately If . . .

- You have a high temperature.
- You have severe pain in the upper right side of your abdomen or between your shoulder blades.

- You start to vomit.
- You have shortness of breath.
- Your skin or eyes turn yellow, or your urine is dark brown.

IF YOU'RE HEADING FOR THE HOSPITAL . . .

What to Expect While You're There

You may encounter the following procedures and equipment during your stay.

- **Abdominal Ultrasound:** This painless test to look at your gallbladder is done while you're lying down. A dab of a jelly-like lotion is placed on your stomach. The person doing the test will gently move a small handle through the lotion and across the skin. A TV-like screen is attached to the handle.
- **Lithotripsy** (lith-uh-TRIP-see): Your gallstones may be broken apart with medicine, shock waves, or both.
- **Surgery:** You may need to have surgery to remove your gallbladder.
- **Antibiotic Medicines:** You may be given these drugs by IV, shot, or mouth. They fight infection.
- **Pain Medicine:** This medicine may be given in your IV, as a shot, or by mouth. If your pain is not better after you take the medication, tell your nurse at once.
- **Taking Vital Signs:** These include your temperature, blood pressure, pulse (counting your heartbeats), and respirations (counting your breaths). A stethoscope is used to listen to your heart and lungs. Your blood pressure is taken by wrapping a cuff around your arm.
- **Pulse Oximeter:** If you are getting oxygen, you may be hooked up to a pulse oximeter (ox-IM-uh-ter). It is placed on your ear, finger, or toe, and is connected to a machine that measures the oxygen in your blood.
- **IV:** A tube placed in your vein for giving medicine or liquids. It will be capped or have tubing connected to it.
- **Blood:** Usually taken from a vein in your hand or from the bend in your elbow. Tests will be done on the blood.
- **Chest X-ray:** This picture of your lungs and heart shows how they are handling the illness.

Ganglion Cysts

WHAT YOU SHOULD KNOW

A ganglion (GANG-lee-un) cyst is a swelling under the skin that is filled with a thick, jelly-like substance. It occurs most often at the wrist. Sometimes the problem goes away without treatment.

Causes

These cysts are usually the result of an injury or trauma that you may not recall.

Signs/Symptoms

Typically, you'll notice a dull ache or wrist tenderness. You may or may not have a lump. Other signs are numbness, weakness, or swelling of your hand or wrist. Often there are no symptoms.

Care

If the cyst is very painful, you may need to have minor surgery.

WHAT YOU SHOULD DO

• Do not try to break the cyst yourself by pressing on it, poking it with a needle, or hitting it with a heavy object.

Call Your Doctor If . . .

• The cyst becomes larger or more painful.
• You develop weakness or numbness in your hand or wrist.
• You notice sudden increased redness or swelling.

Gardnerella Vaginosis

See Bacterial Vaginosis

Gastritis

WHAT YOU SHOULD KNOW

Gastritis (gas-TRY-tis) is inflammation of the stomach. Most of the time it goes away in a few days if you avoid things that upset your stomach.

Causes

Common causes of gastritis are drinking alcohol, smoking, overeating, and eating spicy foods. The condition may also be caused by pain medicines, such as aspirin and ibuprofen. Sometimes an infection is to blame.

Signs/Symptoms

Common symptoms include loss of appetite, an upset stomach, or stomach cramping. Gastritis can also cause vomiting, diarrhea, burping, a bad taste in your mouth, weakness, fever, stomach bloating, and chest pain.

Care
Treatment consists of antacids and rest.

WHAT YOU SHOULD DO

- You may take over-the-counter antacids to keep stomach acid in check.
- Ask your doctor before taking any other medications. Don't take aspirin or ibuprofen. They will make your gastritis worse. If you need a painkiller, use acetaminophen.
- Don't eat solid foods on the first day of the attack. Drink plenty of liquids such as milk or water—about 8 glasses a day.
- Resume a normal diet slowly. Eat bland foods or those that you know agree with you. Eat only a little at a time.
- Start normal activities when you feel better.
- To avoid another attack:
  —Eat and drink moderately. Avoid hot and spicy foods or those that you find hard to digest. Don't skip meals.
  —If you smoke or use alcohol, quit or cut down as much as possible.

Call Your Doctor If . . .
- You have pain or vomiting that lasts for more than a few hours.

Seek Care Immediately If . . .
- You vomit blood.
- You have blood in your stool or black bowel movements.
- You become weak and dizzy.
- You have severe pain.
- You develop a high temperature.

Gastroenteritis

WHAT YOU SHOULD KNOW

Gastroenteritis (gas-tro-ent-er-I-tis) is an inflammation of the stomach and bowel that is often wrongly called the "flu." It should only last 1 or 2 days.

Causes
The problem can be caused by infections with either viruses or bacteria. Food poisoning also can cause gastroenteritis.

Signs/Symptoms
Common symptoms are diarrhea and vomiting, Others include fever, stomach cramps, nausea, headache, tiredness, and muscle aches.

Care

Gastroenteritis can be treated at home.

WHAT YOU SHOULD DO

- Decrease activity until you feel better or the diarrhea and vomiting are gone.
- Take clear liquids, such as ginger ale, cola, water, tea, broth, and gelatin, for the first 24 hours or until the diarrhea and vomiting stops. During the next 24 hours, you may eat bland foods such as cooked cereals, rice, soup, bread, crackers, baked potatoes, eggs, or applesauce. Do not eat fruits, vegetables, fried or spicy foods, bran, candy, dairy products such as milk or ice cream, or alcoholic beverages. You may resume your normal diet after 2 to 3 days.
- Drink 8 to 12 glasses of liquid a day. Most problems are caused by loss of water through vomiting and diarrhea.
- You may take ibuprofen or acetaminophen for fever and muscle aches.

Seek Care Immediately If . . .

- Your symptoms last for more than 3 days.
- You have severe pain in the abdomen (area around the stomach) or rectum.
- You have a high temperature.
- You find blood, mucus, or worms in your stool.
- You have signs of water loss, including dry mouth, excessive thirst, crinkled skin, little or no urination, dizziness, or light-headedness.

Gastroenteritis in Children

See Stomach Flu in Children

Gastroesophageal Reflux

See Heartburn

Gastroesophageal Reflux in Babies

See Spitting Up in Infants

Gastrointestinal Bleeding

WHAT YOU SHOULD KNOW

Gastrointestinal (gas-tro-in-TES-tin-ul) bleeding can occur anywhere within the gastrointestinal (GI) tract. This includes the mouth, the esophagus (ih-SOF-uh-gus) leading to the stomach, the stomach it-self, and the intestines.

Causes
Infections, some medicines, and alcohol can damage tissue in the GI tract and produce bleeding. So can growths or the swollen pockets that sometimes form in the walls of the intestines. Blood vessels that are not formed correctly also can bleed.

Signs/Symptoms
Symptoms depend on the cause and place of the bleeding, and how fast the blood is flowing. Among the common signs of gastro-intestinal bleeding are vomit that contains dark specks or blood, and bloody or black, sticky stools. Other signs include dry mouth, thirst, urinating less than usual—or not urinating at all.

In some cases, additional symptoms may result from other ill-nesses or medicines. For example, someone with heart disease could have chest pain as a result of blood loss from GI bleeding.

If you experience dizziness; confusion; low blood pressure; and fast heart rate and breathing, you may be going into shock from ex-cessive blood loss.

Care
Treatment depends on where the blood is coming from and how fast and how much you are bleeding. Your doctor will do tests to find the answers. Medications may be prescribed. In the hospital, you will be watched carefully and given IV fluids. Most GI bleeding stops on its own. But you may need to be given blood, have surgery, or both.

Risks
Without treatment, it's possible that you could bleed to death.

WHAT YOU SHOULD DO

Call Your Doctor If . . .
• You have bad stomach or abdominal pain, even if you have taken your medicine.
• You have a rash, swelling, or trouble breathing. Your medicine may cause these symptoms.
• You feel weak or light-headed, or look pale.

Seek Care Immediately If . . .
• You throw up what looks like coffee grounds (black specks) or blood, or you have bloody or black, sticky stools.

• You have a fast heart rate and breathing, or you feel confused or dizzy. These are signs of shock. **THIS IS AN EMERGENCY. Call 911 or 0 (operator)** to get to the nearest hospital or clinic. **Do not drive yourself!**

IF YOU'RE HEADING FOR THE HOSPITAL . . .

What to Expect While You're There

You may encounter the following procedures and equipment during your stay.

• **Endoscopy** (end-OS-ko-pee): Your doctor will run a tube through your mouth and down into your stomach. A light and camera at the end allows the doctor to inspect the upper GI tract.

• **Nasogastric Tube:** This tube may be threaded through your nose or mouth and down into your stomach. The tube is then attached to suction that will keep the stomach empty. This can help your doctor see if you have bleeding in the upper part of your GI tract.

• **Blood Transfusion:** If the bleeding is heavy, you may need a transfusion to replace the lost blood.

• **Activity:** You may need to rest in bed. Once you are feeling better, you will be allowed to move around.

• **Taking Vital Signs:** These include your temperature, blood pressure, pulse (counting your heartbeats), and respirations (counting your breaths). A stethoscope is used to listen to your heart and lungs. Your blood pressure is taken by wrapping a cuff around your arm.

• **Oxygen:** Your body may need extra oxygen at this time. It is given either by a mask or nasal prongs. Tell your doctor if the oxygen is drying out your nose or if the nasal prongs bother you.

• **Pulse Oximeter:** While you are getting oxygen, you may be hooked up to a pulse oximeter (ox-IM-uh-ter). It is placed on your ear, finger, or toe and is connected to a machine that measures the oxygen in your blood.

• **IV:** A tube placed in your vein for giving medicine or liquids. It will be capped or have tubing connected to it.

• **Blood:** Usually taken from a vein in your hand or from the bend in your elbow. Tests will be done on the blood.

• **ECG:** Also called a heart monitor, an electrocardiograph (e-LEK-tro-CAR-dee-o-graf) or EKG. The patches on your chest are hooked up to a TV-type screen or a small portable box (telemetry unit). This screen shows a tracing of each heartbeat. Your heart will be watched for signs of injury or damage that could be related to your illness.

After You Leave
- Always take your medicine as directed. If you feel it is not helping, call your doctor, but do not quit taking it on your own.
- Do not eat things that upset your stomach, such as alcohol, coffee or certain medicines. Your doctor can suggest foods that will not irritate your GI tract.
- Get lots of rest and eat a healthy diet.

Gastrointestinal Endoscopy

WHAT YOU SHOULD KNOW

Upper gastrointestinal (GAS-troh-in-TES-tin-uhl) endoscopy (en-DOS-co-pee) is a visual examination of your esophagus, stomach, and first part of the intestine with a fiberoptic instrument. Tissue may be taken for tests.

Risks
There is a small chance of injury to your esophagus, stomach, or intestine during the test. Liquid or other matter could get into your lungs.

IF YOU'RE HEADING FOR THE HOSPITAL . . .

Before You Go
- Your doctor will tell you when you must stop eating. DO NOT eat or drink after that time.
- If your doctor says you need to empty your bowel, you may have to take a laxative or other medicine to clear it out.

What to Expect While You're There
You may encounter the following procedures and equipment during your stay:
- **Taking Your Vital Signs:** These include your temperature, blood pressure, pulse (counting your heartbeats), and respirations (counting your breaths). A stethoscope is used to listen to your heart and lungs. Your blood pressure is taken by wrapping a cuff around your arm.
- **Pulse Oximeter:** You may be hooked up to a pulse oximeter (ox-IM-uh-ter). It is placed on your ear, finger, or toe and is connected to a machine. It measures the oxygen in your blood.
- **IV:** A tube placed in your vein for giving medicine or liquids. It will be capped or have tubing connected to it.
- **Medicine:** You may be given medicine to help prevent pain during the test.

• During the Endoscopy:

—You will be asked to lie on your left side with one knee bent. You may have to wear a mouthpiece to keep your mouth in the right position. A suction tube may be used to drain saliva out of your mouth.

—A soft tube will be put into your mouth. As you swallow, the tube will go down your throat. The tip of the tube contains a light and camera lenses. The camera will display pictures on a TV-like screen as the tube advances down your throat.

—Air may be pumped into your stomach to give the camera an un-obstructed view. This may result in a feeling of pressure or bloating.

—A sample of tissue from inside your throat, stomach, or intestine may be taken for tests.

—The procedure will take about 30 minutes.

After You Leave

• If medicine has made you drowsy, do not drive.
• You may resume normal activities and begin eating and drinking as soon as you feel up to it.

Call Your Doctor If . . .

• You have a generally ill feeling, headache, chills, and muscle aches.
• You develop a temperature over 101 degrees F (38.3 degrees C).

Seek Care Immediately If . . .

• You begin to vomit blood or have black stools.
• You feel dizzy, short of breath, or faint.
• You have problems swallowing.
• You develop nausea, vomiting, and sharp pain in your stomach.

Genital Herpes

WHAT YOU SHOULD KNOW

Genital herpes is an infection of the sex organs caused by the herpes (HER-peez) simplex virus (HSV). Painful sores develop on or around the sex organs when you first get the virus. Once the virus is no longer active, the sores should begin to heal. However, the virus remains in the body permanently, and can cause renewed symptoms at any time.

Cause

The virus is acquired through sexual contact with someone who has an active case of the disease. Although genital herpes is usually

caused by the herpes simplex 2 virus (HSV-2), sometimes it is caused
by the herpes simplex 1 virus (HSV-1), which produces cold sores in
and around the mouth. Both viruses can be found in either place.

Signs/Symptoms
Typically, the symptoms are itching, burning or pain on or around the
sex organs, followed by painful blisters; difficulty or pain when trying
to urinate; swollen lymph glands; fever and feeling sick.

Care
There is no cure, but there is medicine that works against the virus to
help you feel better and heal more quickly. Acetaminophen can help
with the pain. Try to get plenty of rest, too.

Risks
Without treatment, you have a greater risk of inflammation of the
brain, spinal cord, or bone marrow, as well as nerve pain.

WHAT YOU SHOULD DO

- If your doctor prescribes medicine to help the sores heal, take it exactly as directed. You may use acetaminophen to help relieve pain.
- Tell partners with whom you had sex before you were treated that
you have herpes. They also may be infected and need treatment.
- Don't have sex until all the sores clear up (about 1 month). Also
avoid sex when either partner has blisters or sores. Don't have oral
sex with a partner who has cold sores around the mouth.
- When it is safe to have sex, use a latex condom. Using a condom or
spermicide that contains nonoxynol-9 increases protection against
herpes and also helps prevent the spread of gonorrhea and other
infections.
- Warm baths can help relieve pain and inflammation. Add a tablespoon of salt to the water. Applying wet tea bags or petroleum jelly
to the sores may also be soothing.
- Urinating in the shower or through a tube (toilet paper roll) can help
women relieve pain. Pouring a cup of warm water between the legs
while urinating also helps.
- Women should wear cotton panties or pantyhose with a cotton crotch. Douching is not recommended unless the doctor has
ordered it.
- Try to avoid stress, fatigue, and illness. They increase the chances
that your symptoms will return.
- Pregnant women should be sure to tell the doctor that they have
genital herpes. They are at greater risk for miscarriage or early labor.

Herpes also can be passed on to the baby during birth and cause serious problems.

Call Your Doctor If . . .
• There is any unusual bleeding from the vagina.
• You get a high temperature during treatment or you feel generally ill.
• You get a headache or start throwing up.
• Your symptoms become worse or do not improve one week after starting treatment.
• Your symptoms return after you have been treated. Your herpes may have come back, and you may need to be treated again.
• You have any problems that may be related to the medicine you are taking.

IF YOU'RE HEADING FOR THE HOSPITAL . . .

What to Expect While You're There
You may encounter the following procedures and equipment during your stay.
• **Taking Vital Signs:** These include your temperature, blood pressure, pulse (counting your heartbeats), and respirations (counting your breaths). A stethoscope is used to listen to your heart and lungs. Your blood pressure is taken by wrapping a cuff around your arm.
• **Pulse Oximeter:** You may be hooked up to a pulse oximeter (ox-IM-uh-ter). It is placed on your ear, finger, or toe and is connected to a machine. It measures the oxygen in your blood.
• **IV:** A tube placed in your vein for giving medicine or liquids. It will be capped or have tubing connected to it.
• **Blood:** Usually taken from a vein in your hand or from the bend in your elbow. Tests will be done to measure certain chemicals normally found in the blood.
• **CT Scan:** Also called a "CAT" scan, and similar to an x-ray, this machine will be used to check for inflammation in the brain.
• **ECG:** Also called a heart monitor, an electrocardiograph (e-LEK-tro-CAR-dee-o-graf), or EKG. The patches on your chest are hooked up to a TV-type screen or a small portable box (telemetry unit). The TV-type screen shows a tracing of each heartbeat. Your heart will be watched for signs of injury or damage that could be related to the virus.
• **Lumbar Puncture:** In this procedure, fluid is taken out of an area near your spine, then tested for blood and signs of infection.

Genital Warts

WHAT YOU SHOULD KNOW

Genital warts grow on or around your sex organs. They are seen most often in young adults. In the United States, warts are one of the most common sexually transmitted diseases.

Causes
The warts are caused by the human papilloma (PAP-ih-LOW-muh) virus (HPV). This virus is spread by vaginal, anal, and oral sex.

Signs/Symptoms
You'll notice one or more warts—small, soft bumps that can be pink, red, white, or brown. In men, they appear in or around the opening of the penis or around the rectum. Women may develop them inside the vagina, rectum, or the urinary canal. They may also appear in the genital area (between the legs). Left untreated, the warts may spread and grow.

Care
The doctor may give you a medicine to remove the warts. They can also be removed by freezing, burning, or cutting. Since HPV can cause cancer, it's important to get rid of the infection completely. If you are pregnant (or think you might be), tell the doctor.

WHAT YOU SHOULD DO

- It is important that you follow your doctor's instructions carefully. The warts will not go away without repeated treatment.
- Do NOT try to treat the warts with medicine used for hand warts. This type of medicine is very strong and can burn the skin in the genital area.
- Tell all sexual partners with whom you had sex before treatment that you have genital warts. They also may be infected and need treatment.
- Do not have sex while you are being treated for warts. After that, use of a latex condom during sex will help protect both of you from possible re-infection.
- Do not touch or scratch the warts; you could spread them to other parts of your body.
- Women with genital warts should have a cervical cancer check (Pap smear) at least once a year. This type of cancer is slow-growing and can be cured if found early.

Call Your Doctor If . . .
• The treated skin becomes red, swollen, or painful.
• You have a high temperature.
• You feel generally ill.

German Measles

WHAT YOU SHOULD KNOW

German measles is a mild infection that is also called rubella (ru-BELL-uh) or three-day measles. The infection is no longer common because nowadays most children get a rubella shot (immunization) to prevent the disease.

Causes
Rubella is caused by a virus. It is spread in the air by the coughing and sneezing of an infected person.

Signs/Symptoms
The hallmark of this infection is a skin rash of tiny, flat or slightly raised, pink-red spots all over the body. Other symptoms are fever, headache, sore eyes, runny nose, cough, sore throat, and swollen glands. The child also may have muscle aches and not want to eat.

Rubella can be spread to others from 7 days before the rash starts until 5 days after it first appears. The rash is gone in 3 to 4 days.

Care
There is no cure for rubella, but acetaminophen will help relieve fever and aches. Keep your child at home and **away from pregnant women.**

WHAT YOU SHOULD DO

• Do NOT give aspirin if a child with rubella is under 18 years of age. This could lead to brain and liver damage (Reye's syndrome). Be sure to check for aspirin on the label on any over-the-counter medicines you buy.
• Put calamine lotion on the skin to help itching.
• Give acetaminophen for fever.
• Keep your child away from other people, ESPECIALLY PREGNANT WOMEN, until the fever has been gone for 12 hours. Rubella can cause birth defects in unborn babies. If your child has been in contact with a pregnant woman, be sure to warn her so that she can tell her doctor.

• Have the child rest as much as possible until the fever is gone. This usually takes about 4 days. He or she does not need to stay in bed.
• The child may return to school or daycare when the fever has been gone for 12 hours.

Call Your Doctor If . . .
• The fever lasts more than 3 days.
• The rash starts to itch.

Seek Care Immediately If . . .
• The child's temperature becomes very high.
• The rash turns purple.
• The child acts very sick.

Giardiasis

WHAT YOU SHOULD KNOW

Giardiasis (jee-are-DIE-uh-sis) is an infection of the bowel (intestines). Without medicine, it may take as long as 1 month to get better.

Causes
The infection is caused by a parasite called Giardia (jee-ARE-dee-uh) lamblia (LAM-blee-uh) found in dirty water. You can get the infection from drinking the water itself or eating uncooked food that has been rinsed in it. The disease spreads easily from one person to another.

Signs/Symptoms
Symptoms usually start about 1 to 3 weeks after the parasite gets into your body. They include sudden diarrhea and stomach cramps; loose, bulky, and bad smelling stools; an upset stomach that comes and goes; fever (not common); and weight loss. There are often no signs or symptoms at all.

Care
Your doctor will need one or more stool samples in order to pinpoint the cause of the problem. You will need medicine to kill the parasite. You also will need to drink plenty of liquids. If you lose too much body water with your diarrhea, you may need a stay in the hospital to get IV fluids.

Risks

Without treatment, persistent diarrhea can rob the body of the vitamins and minerals you need to stay healthy. You may lose too much weight. There is also a danger of losing too much body water and salts. If this dehydration becomes too severe, it can lead to dangerous complications.

WHAT YOU SHOULD DO

- Take the medicine prescribed to get rid of the Giardia exactly as directed.
- Do NOT use any over-the-counter drugs for diarrhea unless your doctor recommends them.
- Drink at least 6 to 8 glasses (soda-can size) of water or other liquid each day.
- Wash your hands well with soap and water every time you go to the bathroom and before you touch food. If you have a child in diapers, wash your hands after each diaper change.
- To avoid getting giardiasis again:
  —Don't drink water from streams, even if it looks clear and clean. Boil any water that is not safe or treat it with a chemical purifier.
  —Wash or peel fruits and vegetables before eating.
  —Stay away from crowded or unclean living conditions.
- Everyone in contact (household and sexual) with an infected person should be seen by a doctor.

Call Your Doctor If . . .

- Your diarrhea lasts more than 24 hours after starting treatment.
- You have a high temperature.
- You lose a lot of weight during treatment.

Seek Care Immediately If . . .

- You have blood in your stools.
- You have severe pain or bloating in your abdomen or rectum.
- You begin showing signs of water loss (dehydration), such as dry mouth, increased thirst, little or no urine, and feelings of dizziness or light-headedness.

IF YOU'RE HEADING FOR THE HOSPITAL . . .

What to Expect While You're There

You may encounter the following procedures and equipment during your stay.

- **Taking Vital Signs:** These include your temperature, blood pressure, pulse (counting your heartbeats), and respirations (counting your breaths). A stethoscope is used to listen to your heart and lungs. Your blood pressure is taken by wrapping a cuff around your arm.

- **Pulse Oximeter:** You may be hooked up to a pulse oximeter (ox-IM-uh-ter). It is placed on your ear, finger, or toe and is connected to a machine that measures the oxygen in your blood.
- **Blood:** Usually taken from a vein in your hand or from the bend in your elbow. Tests will be done on the blood.
- **Stool Sample:** Your doctor may need to send a sample of your stool to the lab. The sample can confirm the cause of the illness and determine which medicine you need.
- **IV:** A tube placed in your vein for giving medicine or liquids. It will be capped or have tubing connected to it.
- **Strict Intake/Output:** Nurses will carefully watch how much liquid you are drinking or getting in your IV. They will also measure how much you are urinating.
- **Daily Weight:** You will be weighed daily.
- **Activity:** You may need to rest in bed. Once you are feeling better, you will be allowed to get up.
- **Medications:** Drugs will be prescribed to fight the infection. They may be given by IV, in a shot, or by mouth.

GI Bleeding

See Gastrointestinal Bleeding

Gingivitis

WHAT YOU SHOULD KNOW

Gingivitis (JIN-ji-VIE-tis)—swelling and redness of the gums—is an early sign of gum disease. It's also a sign that you need to take better care of your teeth.

Causes

The disease is usually caused by a sticky film called plaque that forms on the teeth. Plaque is a buildup of food, germs, and mucus at the bottom of your teeth. Certain medicines may encourage it.

Signs/Symptoms

Symptoms include red and swollen gums, bad breath, and separation of the gums from the teeth. The gums may look bumpy and may bleed easily. The swelling may come and go. Usually there is no pain.

Care

Gingivitis that isn't treated can lead to serious gum disease or tooth loss. Daily brushing and flossing will help remove plaque before it builds up. Once it has hardened, however, it must be removed at the dentist's office. You should have your teeth checked and cleaned by a dentist every 6 months.

WHAT YOU SHOULD DO

• Make an appointment with a dentist as soon as possible.
• Brush your teeth twice a day and after meals (if possible) with a soft toothbrush and a fluoride toothpaste that contains a plaque fighter. Floss them with dental floss at least once a day. Be sure to clean between your teeth. Your dentist can give you instructions on the correct way to brush and floss.
• Do not smoke or use alcoholic beverages while your gums are inflamed.
• Eat a well-balanced diet. Cut back on foods and beverages that contain sugar.

Call Your Dentist If . . .

• The bleeding in your gums gets worse.
• Your gums become painful.
• You develop a high temperature.
• You have swelling in your face or neck.

Seek Care Immediately If . . .

• You have trouble swallowing.
• You have trouble breathing.

Gonococcal Urethritis

See Gonorrhea

Gonorrhea

WHAT YOU SHOULD KNOW

Gonorrhea (GON-o-REE-uh) is an infection that affects the sex organs and sometimes the throat and rectum. It is most common among adults of either sex who are between 15 and 29 years old. If not treated, gonorrhea can spread throughout the body and can cause sterility.

Causes

The disease is caused by a bacteria. You catch the disease by having sex with an infected partner. The throat or rectum can become infected from having oral or anal sex.

Signs/Symptoms

Typical symptoms include a discharge of thick yellow-green fluid from the penis or vagina; fever, pain or burning when urinating; and the need to urinate frequently. The sex organs may become red, swollen, and itchy. Some women who have gonorrhea may show no signs; others may develop a smelly vaginal discharge or have pain during intercourse.

Care

The doctor will prescribe antibiotics to cure the infection. Be sure to take them exactly as prescribed. Even if you think you are well, use the entire prescription. If you stop taking the antibiotics too soon, some bacteria may remain to re-infect you.

WHAT YOU SHOULD DO

- It is important to follow your doctor's instructions carefully. Gonorrhea can be cured. However, if you don't follow through with treatment, serious problems may develop. The infection can spread to the internal sex organs, joints, skin, eyes, and heart. Gonorrhea can cause damage to the uterus and fallopian tubes, and can make it difficult to get pregnant.
- Don't have sex until you have taken all your medicine. After that, use of a condom can help protect both partners from catching or spreading gonorrhea and other infections.
- Tell all partners with whom you had sex before treatment that you have gonorrhea. They may have contracted the infection, and may need treatment.
- Wash your hands often, especially after urination or bowel movements. Do not touch your eyes with your hands.
- If you find out you are pregnant, be sure to tell your doctor that you have gonorrhea. The disease can be passed on to an infant during birth.

Call Your Doctor If . . .

- You have abdominal pain, swelling of the testicles, chills, joint pain, rash, or a high temperature.

Seek Care Immediately If . . .
• Your temperature becomes extremely high.

Guillain-Barré Syndrome

WHAT YOU SHOULD KNOW

Guillain-Barré (GEE-yan Bar-A) syndrome is a disorder of the nervous system that leads to increasing muscular weakness. The problem is marked by the unexplained loss of sections of the protective sheath that surrounds the nerves in the body. The nerves then become swollen and inflamed. The disease takes between a couple of weeks and a few months to clear up. It is also known as infectious polyneuropathy (POL-ee-noor-AH-path-ee) or acute idiopathic polyneuritis (ID-e-o-PATH-ic POL-ee-noor-EYE-tis).

Causes
Doctors do not know the precise cause. One theory is that your body attacks its own tissues. The disease most often develops between 5 days and 3 weeks after a shot, an infection, or surgery.

Signs/Symptoms
The disease is marked by weakness and mild loss of sensation in the body. Weakness usually starts in the legs and moves up into the arms over a period of about 72 hours. It may affect the belly and chest muscles, making it hard to breathe. You may go into shock (symptoms include weakness or faintness, cold hands and feet, fast heart rate, and sweating). Later, paralysis may occur.

Care
Initially, you will have to be hospitalized for close observation and testing. Other care will depend on how weak you are.

Risks
Without treatment, Guillain-Barré can get worse and cause serious, even life-threatening, complications. For more information, call the Guillain-Barré Foundation at (215) 667-0131.

IF YOU'RE HEADING FOR THE HOSPITAL . . .

What to Expect While You're There
• **Activity:** You may need to rest in bed. Once you are feeling better, you can get up.
• **Taking Your Vital Signs:** These include taking your temperature, blood pressure, pulse (counting your heartbeats), and respirations

(counting your breaths). A stethoscope is used to listen to your heart and lungs. Your blood pressure is taken by wrapping a cuff around your arm.

- **Oxygen:** Your body may need extra oxygen at this time. It is given either by a mask or through nasal prongs. Tell your doctor if the oxygen is drying out your nose or if the nasal prongs bother you.
- **Pulse Oximeter:** You may be hooked up to a pulse oximeter (ox-IM-uh-ter). It is placed on your ear, finger, or toe and is connected to a machine that measures the oxygen in your blood.
- **Blood:** Usually taken from a vein in your hand or from the bend in your elbow and sent to a laboratory for testing.
- **Blood Gases:** For this test, blood is taken from an artery in your wrist, elbow, or groin and tested to see how much oxygen and carbon dioxide it contains.
- **ECG:** Also called a heart monitor, an electrocardiograph (e-LEK-tro-CAR-dee-o-graf), or EKG. The patches on your chest are hooked up to a TV-type screen or a small portable box (telemetry unit) that shows a tracing of each heartbeat. Your heart will be watched for signs of injury or damage stemming from your illness.
- **IV:** A tube placed in your vein for giving medicine or liquids. It will be capped or have tubing connected to it.
- **Lumbar Puncture:** Also called spinal tap. Fluid is taken from your spine and sent to a laboratory for testing.
- **Electromyography** (e-LEK-tro-mi-AH-gruh-fee): This test is used to measure the activity of muscles and nerves.
- **Coughing and Deep Breathing:** Doing this frequently will help prevent lung infections.
- **Incentive Spirometer** (in-SEN-tive spir-OM-ih-ter): A small plastic device used to encourage you to take deep breaths.
- **Chest X-ray:** A picture of your lungs and heart that helps your doctor determine how these organs are handling the illness.
- **ET Tube:** This tube is inserted through the mouth or nose and threaded into the windpipe. It is often hooked up to a breathing machine. While the tube is in place, you will be unable to talk.
- **Ventilator:** A special machine used to help with breathing.
- **Postural Drainage:** In this procedure, a nurse will tap briskly on your back with his or her hands. This helps loosen the sputum in your lungs so you can cough it up more easily.
- **Foley Catheter:** A tube inserted in the bladder to empty urine when you cannot urinate on your own.
- **Pressure Stockings:** You may need to wear these special stockings to prevent blood from sitting in your legs and causing clots.

- **Cold/Heat:** A cool towel or a heating pad (set on low) may be used to relieve pain.
- **Medicine:**
  —**Heparin** may be given to keep the blood thin and prevent clots from forming. It is given in an IV. Later, blood thinners may be taken by mouth.
  —**Laxatives** may be needed to keep you from getting constipated.
- **Plasmapheresis** (PLAZ-muh-fer-E-sis): In this treatment, plasma is taken from the blood and processed to remove the antibodies that may be attacking the nerves. The plasma is then returned to the bloodstream.

After You Leave

- If you are going to a special hospital or "skilled nursing facility" before going home, the caregivers there will help you dress and feed yourself until you are stronger.
- If you are going home:
  —You may need to install special ramps and side rails to help you get around the house safely.
  —You may need to have physical and occupational therapy when you get home. Your therapy sessions should take place during the time of day when you are least tired.
  —Work closely with the therapists. It is important to do the exercises they teach you.
- Stay as active as your muscle strength allows. Daily exercise helps to keep your muscles in shape, strengthens the heart, lowers blood pressure, and keeps you healthy.
- Do not keep to yourself; try to see your friends and family as much as you can without getting too tired.
- Always take your medicine exactly as directed. If you feel it is not helping, you may call your doctor, but do not stop taking it on your own.
- For a while, you may not have much sensitivity to heat or cold. To keep from burning yourself, test the water carefully before bathing or washing.
- Keep coughing to keep your lungs free of mucus and infection so you can breathe more easily.
- Drink at least 8 glasses (soda-can size) of liquid every day to prevent constipation.
- Use a heating pad set on low or warm wet towels to ease pain.
- Check with your doctor before you get flu or pneumonia shots.

Call Your Doctor If . . .
- You develop a high temperature.
- You have trouble breathing, develop sores on your skin, experience vision problems, have swollen or tender calves, or become constipated.
- You develop redness, a rash, or swelling of your skin. This may be caused by the medicine you are taking.

Haemophilus Vaginalis

See Bacterial Vaginosis

Hand Fracture

See Broken Hand

Hay Fever

WHAT YOU SHOULD KNOW

If you have hay fever—known medically as allergic rhinitis (rine-I-tis)—the inside of your nose will become red and swollen when you breathe in particles to which you are sensitive. Seasonal allergic rhinitis occurs only at certain times of the year (for example, the spring or fall), while nonseasonal allergic rhinitis can affect susceptible people during any season. Treatment can relieve the symptoms but will not cure the problem.

Causes
Seasonal allergic rhinitis is caused by pollen from ragweed, grasses, and trees, depending on the time of year. House dust, feathers, mold, and animals cause the nonseasonal variety. Tobacco smoke, air pollution, and sudden changes in temperature may make the condition worse.

Signs/Symptoms
The most familiar symptoms are sneezing and an itchy, runny, or stuffy nose. In addition, the eyes may be itchy, red, swollen, burning, or watery. Other possible symptoms include an itchy throat, coughing, and headache.

Care
Your doctor may give you skin tests to see what's causing the reaction. Medications may relieve or prevent symptoms.

WHAT YOU SHOULD DO

- If your doctor prescribes a medication, take it only as directed.
- You may use nonprescription medicines to relieve your symptoms. Antihistamines are the best drugs for hay fever; eyedrops will help itchy, watery eyes. Do not use decongestants, nose drops, or nasal sprays. They usually aren't helpful and may make your symptoms worse.
- Blow your nose as often as needed. Be careful not to blow too hard or you can have a nosebleed. To prevent injury to your ears, do not plug one side of your nose while blowing your nose.
- Do not rub your eyes; it will make them feel worse. Contact lenses also may bother your eyes.
- Keep your house as clean as possible. Get an air cleaning filter for your house and have all the vents and ducts cleaned. Wear a face mask if you do the cleaning. Do not touch things that are covered with dust.
- If you find out that you are allergic to your pets, you will have to give them away.
- If you have seasonal allergic rhinitis, stay inside with the windows and doors closed on days when the air pollution is bad or the pollen count is high; drive an air-conditioned car, and have someone else mow the lawn.
- Don't smoke.

Call Your Doctor If . . .

- Your symptoms get worse or keep you from doing your normal activities.
- You feel pain or pressure in your sinuses.
- You have any problems with a medicine you are taking.
- You develop a high temperature, headache, muscle aches, face or ear pain, severe headache, or thick, greenish-yellow drainage from your nose. These are signs of infection.

Headache, Cluster

See Cluster Headache

Headache, Migraine

See Migraine Headache

Headache, Tension

See Tension Headache

Head Injury

See Concussion

Head Lice

WHAT YOU SHOULD KNOW

Head lice favor the hairy areas of the body and bite the skin for food. You can catch them by using a hat, comb, or headphones belonging to an infested person. The problem is known medically as pediculosis (peh-DIK-u-LO-sus). With treatment, it should clear up in 5 days.

Causes

These tiny, gray bugs lay white eggs (called nits) in hair near the skin. The eggs hatch in about 7 days. The lice themselves move quickly, and are hard to see.

Signs/Symptoms

You'll notice itchy, red bite marks in hair-covered areas of the body. The problem is most common in hair that grows on the head.

Care

Medication will kill the lice. Follow the measures listed below to get rid of the eggs.

WHAT YOU SHOULD DO

- If your doctor prescribes medicine, use it exactly as directed. A medication that kills lice does not always kill all the nits. You must remove them from your hair with a special fine-toothed comb. If this kind of comb does not come with your medicine, you can buy one at a drugstore.
- Removing the nits will be easier if you first soak your hair in a solution of 1/2 vinegar and 1/2 water. Comb the lice-infested hair completely—from the skin outward—once a day until treatment is complete. You do not have to shave or cut the hair in the affected area.
- Avoid close contact with anyone until your doctor tells you the lice are all gone.
- All clothing, bedding, and towels that have been worn or used either three days before or during treatment should be machine washed in hot water and dried in a hot dryer for at least 20 minutes. Items that cannot be washed should be dry cleaned, hung outside for 2 days, or sealed in a plastic bag for 10 days.

- Soak combs, brushes, barrettes, and curlers in an antiseptic solution, rubbing alcohol, or lice-killing shampoo for 1 or 2 hours. Or boil them for 5 to 10 minutes. Vacuum all rugs, mattresses, and furniture carefully.
- If a child develops the problem, be sure to tell the school or daycare center that the youngster has head lice. They will tell you when the child may return to school.

Call Your Doctor If . . .

- The bites become pus-filled or crusty, and the hair becomes matted and foul-smelling. These are signs of infection.
- Itching or rash return to the scalp after treatment.
- The medication causes any kind of reaction.

Heart Attack

WHAT YOU SHOULD KNOW

A heart attack is also called a myocardial (my-o-CARD-e-ul) infarction (in-FARK-shun), or MI for short. It is the leading cause of death in America.

A heart attack occurs when an artery in the heart is blocked or has spasms. As a result, that part of the heart does not get enough blood or oxygen. It then becomes injured or dies.

Signs/Symptoms

The most common one is chest pain. It may feel crushing, tight, or heavy. It may spread to the neck, jaw, shoulders, back, or left arm. The pain may also feel like indigestion or burning, occurring under the breastbone.

Other common signs are trouble breathing; sweating; nausea and vomiting; having pale, cool skin; and feeling light-headed or weak.

Some people have no symptoms at all. This is called a "silent" MI or heart attack.

Hospital Care

You will be given pain medicine, hooked up to a TV-type monitor (ECG), and given oxygen. Other tests also will be done to find out why you had a heart attack.

If you arrive within 12 hours of your first pain, you may be given medicine to help break up the clots that are blocking the arteries in your heart. If the arteries are cleared of clots, there will be no more damage to your heart. This is why it is important to go to the nearest hospital if you think you are having a heart attack.

Do's and Don'ts

To keep from having more attacks, eat foods low in fat, salt, and cholesterol; stop smoking; exercise; take your medicines; and avoid situations that cause you anxiety.

Risks

Heart attacks are the leading cause of death in America. If you are not treated, you may have another heart attack or even die. The sooner you get care, the less damage you may have to your heart.

WHAT YOU SHOULD DO

- Always take your medicine as directed by your doctor. If you feel it is not helping, call your doctor, but do not quit taking it on your own.
- Aspirin helps thin the blood so blood clots don't form. Do not take acetaminophen or ibuprofen instead.
- If you have other illnesses like diabetes or high blood pressure, you need to control them. Take medicines as directed. Because of these illnesses, you have a higher chance of getting a heart attack.
- Cardiac Rehabilitation: This is a special exercise program for persons who have had an MI. Ask your doctor for details.
- Exercise daily. It helps make the heart stronger, lowers blood pressure, and keeps you healthy. If your exercise plan is too hard or too easy, talk to your doctor.
- Get at least 7 hours of rest each night. Take a nap during the day if you are tired.
- Since it is hard to avoid stress, learn to control it. Learn new ways to relax (deep breathing, relaxing muscles, meditation, or biofeedback). Talk to someone about things that upset you.
- Quit smoking. It harms the heart and lungs. If you are having trouble quitting, ask your doctor for help.
- Weighing too much can make the heart work harder. If you need to lose weight, ask your doctor about the best way of doing it.
- A diet low in fat, salt, and cholesterol is very important. It keeps your heart healthy and strong. Ask your doctor what you should and should not eat.
- It may take time getting used to a new diet. Special cookbooks may help you and the cook in your family find new recipes.
- Ask your doctor how often you may have sex and whether you may drive.
- Do not lift or push or pull anything heavy or work with your arms above shoulder level until your doctor says you may.
- For more information, contact the **American Heart Association** at

1-800-AHA-USA1 (1-800-242-8721) or call your local **Red Cross**.

Call Your Doctor If . . .
• You have chest pain anytime that does not go away with rest.
• You have chest pain that does not go away after using your medicine as directed by your doctor.
• You are light-headed or dizzy, sweaty, or nauseated after taking your medicine.
• Your blood pressure or pulse is higher or lower than usual.
• You have trouble breathing while resting, you have swelling in your feet or ankles, or you are more tired than usual.
• You are bleeding from your gums or nose, or have blood in your urine or stools. This may be due to your blood thinners.

Seek Care Immediately If . . .
• You have chest pain that spreads to your arms, jaw, or back, and find that you are sweating, sick to your stomach (nauseated), and are having trouble breathing. These are signs of a heart attack. **THIS IS AN EMERGENCY. Call 911 or 0 (operator)** to get to the nearest hospital or clinic. **Do not drive yourself!**

IF YOU'RE HEADING FOR THE HOSPITAL . . .

What to Expect While You're There
You may encounter the following procedures and equipment during your stay.
• **Taking Vital Signs:** These include your temperature, blood pressure, pulse (counting your heartbeats), and respirations (counting your breaths). A stethoscope is used to listen to your heart and lungs. Your blood pressure is taken by wrapping a cuff around your arm.
• **Pulse Oximeter:** While you are getting oxygen, you may be hooked up to a pulse oximeter (ox-IM-uh-ter). It is placed on your ear, finger, or toe and is connected to a machine that measures the oxygen in your blood.
• **ECG:** Also called a heart monitor, an electrocardiograph (e-LEK-tro-CAR-dee-o-graf), or EKG. The patches on your chest are hooked up to a TV-type screen or a small portable box (telemetry unit). This screen shows a tracing of each heartbeat. Your heart will be watched for signs of injury or damage that could be related to your illness.
• **12 Lead ECG:** This test makes tracings from different parts of your heart. It can help your doctor gauge the seriousness of the problem.
• **Oxygen:** Your body may need extra oxygen at this time. It is given

either by a mask or nasal prongs. Tell your doctor if the oxygen is drying out your nose or if the nasal prongs bother you.

- **IV:** A tube placed in your vein for giving medicine or liquids. It will be capped or have tubing connected to it.
- **Blood:** Usually taken from a vein in your hand or from the bend in your elbow. Tests will be done on the blood.
- **Blood Gases:** Blood is taken from an artery in your wrist, elbow, or groin. It is tested for the amount of oxygen in your blood.
- **Chest X-ray:** This is a picture of your lungs and heart. The caregivers use it to see how your heart and lungs are handling the illness.
- **Medicine:**
  —**Heparin:** Keeps the blood thin so no other clots form. It is given in an IV.
  —**Other Blood Thinners:** These include aspirin and warfarin. They are given by mouth as a replacement for heparin. Like heparin, they keep the blood from forming clots.
  —**Clot Busters:** Break clots apart. They are given in your IV, usually at the same time as heparin. This medicine can make you bleed or bruise easily.
  —**Blood Pressure Medicine:** Given for constant high blood pressure. At first it can be given in an IV, and later taken by mouth.
  —**Pain Medicine:** May be given in your IV, as a shot, or by mouth. If the pain does not go away or comes back, tell a doctor right away.
- **Heart Tubes/Wires:** You may be attached to many different tubes and wires. Some may enter your body under your collarbone or in your groin. They will then be threaded into your heart. They are attached to monitors that measure your heart while it's working. These readings help your doctor guide your treatment.
- **Other Tests:** May be needed to find out what is causing your chest pain.
  —**Stress Test:** Used to watch your heart during exercise.
  —**ECHO:** Also called an echocardiogram (ek-oh-CAR-dee-o-gram). This uses sound waves to view your heart while it is beating. It can help caregivers decide what is causing your heart failure.
  —**Cardiac Catheterization** (cath-uh-ter-i-ZAY-shun): A test used to study the arteries sending blood to your heart.
- **Angioplasty:** A procedure that may be needed to open up a blocked artery to your heart.
- **Surgery:** May be needed if the arteries to your heart are severely blocked.

Heartburn

WHAT YOU SHOULD KNOW

Heartburn, known medically as reflux esophagitis (e-sof-uh-JIE-tis), occurs when stomach acid flows back into the esophagus (e-SOF-uh-gus), the tube connecting the mouth to the stomach. With time, the stomach acid can irritate your esophagus and cause problems, such as ulcers.

Causes

In most patients, no specific cause is discovered. A hiatal hernia is one possible cause. Others are taking certain medicines, coughing too hard, or a stomach that empties too slowly. Esophagitis may also occur when you are pregnant.

Signs/Symptoms

You may feel burning in your chest, especially at night. Other signs of esophagitis may be burping, trouble swallowing, a sour or acid taste in your mouth, or a sore throat.

WHAT YOU SHOULD DO

- You may use an over-the-counter antacid. Follow the directions on the label. Check with your doctor first if you are pregnant.
- Eat 6 small meals instead of 3 big ones. This keeps your stomach from getting too full. Eat slowly. Don't lie down for 2 or 3 hours after eating. Don't eat or drink anything 1 to 2 hours before going to bed.
- Avoid alcohol, caffeine beverages (colas, coffee, cocoa, tea), fatty foods, citrus fruits, and other foods and drinks that seem to increase heartburn.
- To help prevent heartburn at night, place 4- to 6-inch blocks under the head of your bed. This will keep your head and esophagus higher than your stomach. If you can't use blocks, sleep with several pillows under your head and shoulders.
- Avoid bending over, especially after eating. Also avoid straining during bowel movements, or when you're urinating or lifting things.
- Don't wear clothing that constricts your chest or stomach.
- Don't smoke. Smoking often causes the stomach to make more acid.
- If you are overweight, lose weight. Ask your doctor for a weight loss plan.

Call Your Doctor If . . .
• Your symptoms don't improve in a few days or they get worse.
• You develop a high temperature.

Seek Care Immediately If . . .
• You vomit blood or have recurrent vomiting.
• You develop severe chest pain along with nausea, sweating, or shortness of breath.

Heart Failure

See Congestive Heart Failure

Heat Cramps

WHAT YOU SHOULD KNOW

Heat cramps are usually provoked by hard work or exercise during hot weather. The cramps are most severe in the muscles that get the most use. Among those most likely to develop the cramps are people who don't routinely exercise in hot weather, older people, and small children, whose bodies cannot easily adapt to high temperatures.

Causes
Heavy sweating causes the body to lose salt and water, disrupting muscle activity.

Signs/Symptoms
The cramping pain may be accompanied by hard knots in the muscles.

WHAT YOU SHOULD DO

• Drink plenty of sports drinks and similar beverages. You can make your own by stirring 1/4 teaspoon of salt into 1 quart (about 4 glasses) of water. One glassful will replace the water and salt you have lost from sweating. Do NOT take salt tablets; they may upset your stomach and cause you to throw up.
• Drink until your urine looks light or pale yellow or clear. If it is dark yellow, keep drinking.
• Rest in a cool place until you are feeling better.
• To keep from getting heat cramps again:
  —Do not exercise heavily during the hottest part of the day, especially in direct sunlight.

—Start exercising slowly, and gradually increase the amount of exercise you do over several weeks.

—Drink liquids before and during exercise, or eat foods containing salt.

—Wear loose, lightweight clothes that keep sunlight off of your body.

Call Your Doctor If . . .

• You have been out in the heat and feel confused, tired, and dizzy; have a headache or upset stomach; feel like throwing up, and have cold, wet skin. These are signs of heat exhaustion, a potentially dangerous condition.

Heat Exhaustion

WHAT YOU SHOULD KNOW

Heat exhaustion, also called heat prostration, is always a danger when you work or exercise for a long time in very hot weather. Older people and children are most likely to get heat exhaustion, but it can happen to anyone.

Causes

The condition results when the body loses too much salt and water through heavy sweating. It is more common in the young and old because their systems are not quick to adjust to temperature changes.

Signs/Symptoms

You're likely to experience fatigue, confusion, nervousness, weakness, dizziness, or faintness. You may also have muscle cramps, a headache, an upset stomach, and cold, clammy skin.

Care

You can recover from a moderate attack by resting in a cool place until you are feeling better. However, a severe attack may require a brief stay in the hospital, where your body fluids can be restored with IV liquids containing salt.

WHAT YOU SHOULD DO

• Drink plenty of sports drinks and similar liquids. You can make your own by mixing 1/4 teaspoon of salt with 1 quart (about 4 glasses) of water. These liquids will replace the water and salt you have lost from sweating. Do NOT take salt tablets.

- Keep drinking cool, salty liquids until your urine is a light or pale yellow or clear.
- If you are throwing up and can't keep fluids down, try sucking on ice chips or taking sips of liquids.
- Get out of the heat, remove your outer clothing, lie down with your feet up, rest, and cool off.
- Taking a bath in cold water may help.
- To keep heat exhaustion from happening again:
  —Try not to exercise heavily during the hottest part of the day, especially in direct sunlight.
  —Start exercising slowly, and gradually increase the amount of exercise you do over several weeks.
  —Drink liquids, such as water or sports drinks, before and during exercise.
  —Wear loose fitting, lightweight, light-colored clothing. Protect your head and neck with a hat or umbrella when you are outdoors.

Seek Care Immediately If . . .
- You feel very hot, confused, and light-headed. These are signs of a severe attack that may require hospitalization. Go to the emergency room or **call 911 or 0 (operator)**. If you cannot get to the hospital right away, take off your clothes, and put cold wet cloths next to your skin. You can also use ice packs if you put a thin cloth between your skin and the ice.

Hematoma

See Bruises

Hematoma, Periorbital

See Black Eye

Hematuria

See Blood in the Urine

Hemorrhoids

WHAT YOU SHOULD KNOW

Hemorrhoids (HEM-uh-roids)—also called "piles"—are swollen veins in the rectum or anus. You can have hemorrhoids for years before they cause pain or bleeding.

Causes

Hemorrhoids tend to develop during pregnancy, and in people who are overweight. They may also result from excessive straining during bowel movements and from sitting too long on hard chairs. They are also associated with liver problems.

Signs/Symptoms

The primary symptom is a swelling or a soft lump at the anus, sometimes accompanied by pain and itching. You may pass some mucus after a bowel movement. You may also feel that you need to pass more stool. There may be streaks of bright-red blood on the toilet paper or on the stool. The water in the toilet may also be reddish from blood.

Care

Your doctor may need to examine your rectal area using a short tube. Usually, medications, warm baths, and ice packs will relieve the problem. Surgery may be necessary if the hemorrhoids cause you problems for a long time.

WHAT YOU SHOULD DO

- To reduce pain and swelling, apply an over-the-counter hemorrhoid medicine. Follow the directions on the label.
- Sit in a tub of comfortably hot water for 20 minutes, 3 times a day.
- If a hemorrhoid is very painful and swollen, apply an ice pack to the anal area.
- Clean the anal area gently with soft, moist toilet paper after each bowel movement.
- You may do normal activities if you are not in pain. Avoid sitting or standing for long periods of time. If the hemorrhoid is painful, lie down as much as possible.
- You may use a stool softener to make your bowel movements easier to pass. Don't try to hurry bowel movements and don't strain.
- Lose weight if you are overweight.
- Eat a high-fiber diet. Good choices are fruits and vegetables, oat and bran cereal, whole-grain bread, and brown rice. Drink plenty of liquids, at least 6 to 8 glasses (soda-can size) every day.
- Exercise regularly.

Call Your Doctor If . . .

- Your hemorrhoids cause severe pain that is not relieved by the above steps.

- You have rectal bleeding that is more than a trace or streak on the toilet paper or in the stool.
- You notice a hard lump in the location of the hemorrhoid.

Hepatitis A

WHAT YOU SHOULD KNOW

Hepatitis A (hep-uh-TIE-tis A) is a viral infection that causes the liver to become irritated and swollen. There are many different types of viral hepatitis, including A, B, C, D, and E. There is no cure or special medicine for hepatitis A; and it may be weeks or even months before you feel better. This disease spreads quickly from person to person. However, a shot is available to prevent the disease.

Causes

The hepatitis A virus spreads through infected food and water. The virus appears in the stool of infected persons, and can be passed on to others through poor hand washing, especially by restaurant workers and food handlers. Day care workers who do not wash their hands after changing a diaper can also spread the virus. The disease can also be picked up from eating infected raw shellfish.

Signs/Symptoms

Early signs are fever, nausea, vomiting, diarrhea, loss of appetite, and tiredness. Later you may have jaundice (yellow eyes and skin). Your urine may be darker in color and your stools may be lighter in color. You may, however, have no symptoms at all.

Care

There is no effective treatment. Your best strategy is keep up your strength as much as possible. Maintain a healthy diet and get plenty of rest. If complications set in, you may need a stay in the hospital.

Risks

Serious problems such as brain swelling and damage, or long-term damage to your liver can occur, but they are rare.

WHAT YOU SHOULD DO

- To prevent spreading the infection to others:
  —Don't share dishes and eating utensils. Wash dishes and utensils in boiling water or an automatic dishwasher, or use disposable ones.
  —Avoid close contact with other people, including kissing.

  —Wash your hands well before eating and after using the toilet. Be careful not to touch your bowel movements.

  —Wash clothing and bedding at the hottest water setting.

  —Clean toilets with a product that kills germs.

- You will feel tired and tire easily for quite a while. Get plenty of rest. You don't need to stay in bed. When you are feeling better, slowly return to your normal activity.

- Even if your appetite is poor, try to eat a balanced diet. Eating several small meals a day may be helpful. Drink at least 8 glasses (soda-can size) of water each day.

- Until you recover, do not take medicines that contain acetaminophen. These will cause your liver to work harder. Be sure to check the label of all medicines that you buy.

- Don't drink any alcohol (including beer and wine) for a few weeks. Alcohol also makes your liver work harder.

- Your friends and family can get a shot to keep them from catching the disease.

Call Your Doctor If . . .

- You can't drink fluids or keep food down.
- You develop a rash, itching, or swelling of your abdomen or legs.

Seek Care Immediately If . . .

- You feel confused or unusually sleepy.
- You have vomiting or diarrhea that lasts longer than a few days, or severe abdominal pain.
- You have signs of water loss, such as dry mouth, excessive thirst, wrinkled skin, little or no urination, or dizziness or light-headedness.
- You notice that you bruise easily.

IF YOU'RE HEADING FOR THE HOSPITAL . . .

What to Expect While You're There

You may encounter the following procedures and equipment during your stay.

- **Liver biopsy:** In this test, a special needle is pushed through the wall of the abdomen and into the liver. A small sample of liver tissue is then removed for study.

- **CT Scan:** This computerized x-ray will be used to take pictures of your liver so that the doctor can check for problems.

- **Neuro Signs:** The doctor will examine your eyes, see how easily you awaken, and check your memory. These are important signs that can detect any problems the infection may be causing in the brain.

- **Taking Vital Signs:** These include your temperature, blood pressure, pulse (counting your heartbeats), and respirations (counting your breaths). A stethoscope is used to listen to your heart and lungs. Your blood pressure is taken by wrapping a cuff around your arm.
- **Pulse Oximeter:** You may be hooked up to a pulse oximeter (ox-IM-uh-ter). It is placed on your ear, finger, or toe and is connected to a machine that measures the oxygen in your blood.
- **IV:** A tube placed in your vein for giving medicine or liquids. It will be capped or have tubing connected to it.
- **Blood:** Usually taken from a vein in your hand or from the bend in your elbow. Tests will be done on the blood.

Hepatitis B and C

WHAT YOU SHOULD KNOW

Hepatitis (hep-uh-TIE-tis) is an inflammation and swelling of the liver, often due to viral infection. There are many types of viral hepatitis, including A, B, C, D, and E. There is no cure or special medicine for any of them, and it may take weeks or months to recover. The disease can leave lasting effects.

Causes
The hepatitis viruses that cause these diseases travel easily from person to person. You can get hepatitis B by having sex with an infected person. A pregnant woman with hepatitis B can pass the disease to her baby.

Hepatitis C, on the other hand, is usually picked up by using dirty needles to inject drugs or by getting a blood transfusion from an infected person. Sometimes the source of the infection can't be determined.

Signs/Symptoms
Early signs are fever, nausea, vomiting, diarrhea, loss of appetite, and tiredness. Later you may have jaundice (yellow eyes and skin). Your urine may be darker in color and your stools may be lighter in color. You may, however, have no symptoms at all.

Care
Medicine is available to reduce liver swelling and irritation, and to relieve other problems these diseases can cause. If your condition becomes serious, you may need to go to the hospital.

Risks

With or without treatment, there is a possibility of damage to the liver, liver failure, or liver cancer. Fatalities can result.

WHAT YOU SHOULD DO

- To keep from spreading the infection to others:
  —Don't share dishes and eating utensils. Wash dishes and utensils in boiling water or an automatic dishwasher, or use disposable ones.
  —Avoid close contact with other people, including kissing. Don't have any sexual contact, including oral and anal sex, until your doctor tells you it is okay.
  —When having sex, use a latex condom to help prevent the spread of hepatitis B and other infections.
  —Wash your hands well before eating and after using the toilet. Be careful not to touch your bowel movements.
  —Wash clothing and bedding at the hottest water setting.
  —Clean toilets with a product that kills germs.
- You will feel tired and tire easily for quite a while. Get plenty of rest. You don't need to stay in bed. When you are feeling better, slowly return to your normal activity.
- Even if your appetite is poor, try to eat a balanced diet. Eating several small meals a day may be helpful. Drink at least 8 glasses (soda-can size) of water each day.
- Until you recover, do not take medicines that contain acetaminophen. These will make your liver work harder. Be sure to check the label of all medicines that you buy.
- Don't drink any alcohol (including beer and wine) for several weeks. Alcohol also makes your liver work harder.

Call Your Doctor If . . .

- You can't drink fluids or you vomit after you eat.
- You develop a rash, itching, or swelling of your abdomen or legs.

Seek Care Immediately If . . .

- You feel confused or unusually sleepy.
- You have vomiting or diarrhea that lasts longer than a few days, or you develop severe abdominal pain.
- You have signs of water loss, such as dry mouth, excessive thirst, wrinkled skin, little or no urination, or dizziness or light-headedness.
- You find that you bruise easily.

IF YOU'RE HEADING FOR THE HOSPITAL . . .

What to Expect While You're There
You may encounter the following procedures and equipment during
your stay.
- **CT Scan:** This computerized x-ray will be used to take pictures of
  your liver so that the doctor can check for problems.
- **Liver biopsy:** In this test, a special needle is pushed through the
  wall of the abdomen and into the liver. A small sample of liver tissue
  is then removed for study.
- **Taking Vital Signs:** These include your temperature, blood pressure, pulse (counting your heartbeats), and respirations (counting
  your breaths). A stethoscope is used to listen to your heart and lungs.
  Your blood pressure is taken by wrapping a cuff around your arm.
- **Pulse Oximeter:** You may be hooked up to a pulse oximeter (ox-
  IM-uh-ter). It is placed on your ear, finger, or toe and is connected to
  a machine. It measures the oxygen in your blood.
- **IV:** A tube placed in your vein for giving medicine or liquids. It will
  be capped or have tubing connected to it.
- **Blood:** Usually taken from a vein in your hand or from the bend in
  your elbow. Tests will be done on your blood.

Hernia

WHAT YOU SHOULD KNOW

A hernia (HER-nee-uh) develops when a part of your inner organs
pushes through a hole or a weak part of a nearby muscle. There is
swelling or a lump at the place where this occurs. Most hernias are in
the belly or groin.

Causes
The weak area or hole in the muscle wall may have been present since
birth. The weakness can also develop in later life as a result of
surgery, straining at bowel movements, or just getting older. Pregnancy, coughing hard, or excess weight can also lead to a hernia.

Signs/Symptoms
Typically, there is a swelling or lump in the abdomen or groin that
sometimes hurts. The lump usually disappears when you lie down or
gently push on it. There may be painful swelling in the area of the testicles. You may have a hard time moving your bowels. Vomiting is a
rare—but dangerous—sign.

Care

You may be given something to wear to keep the lump from pushing out, or you may need surgery to fix the problem. You can use over-the-counter pain-killers for minor pain.

Risks

Without treatment, the hernia could become strangulated (lose its blood supply). This can cause a blockage in the intestines that produces fever and vomiting, and may even prove fatal.

WHAT YOU SHOULD DO

- You do not need to rest in bed. You may continue your normal activities; but avoid heavy lifting or straining. Cough gently.
- Don't wear anything tight over the hernia. Don't try to keep it in with an outside bandage or truss unless your doctor recommends it.
- You may eat a normal diet. Try to get plenty of fiber (fruits, vegetables, and grains). This will promote easier bowel movements.
- Check with your doctor before taking any new medicine.

Call Your Doctor If . . .

- You have a high temperature.
- You have bad pain in the area of the hernia.

Seek Care Immediately If . . .

- You have symptoms of a strangulated (trapped) hernia:
  —A high temperature.
  —Increasing abdominal pain.
  —Nausea and throwing up.
  —The hernia becomes stuck outside the belly, looks gray, and feels hard.

IF YOU'RE HEADING FOR THE HOSPITAL . . .

What to Expect While You're There

You may encounter the following procedures and equipment during your stay.

- **Taking Vital Signs:** These include your temperature, blood pressure, pulse (counting your heartbeats), and respirations (counting your breaths). A stethoscope is used to listen to your heart and lungs. Your blood pressure is taken by wrapping a cuff around your arm.
- **Pulse Oximeter:** While you are getting oxygen, you may be hooked up to a pulse oximeter (ox-IM-uh-ter). It is placed on your ear,

finger, or toe and is connected to a machine that measures the oxygen in your blood.

- **Blood:** Usually taken from a vein in your hand or from the bend in your elbow. Tests will be done on the blood.
- **IV:** A tube placed in your vein for giving medicine or liquids. It will be capped or have tubing connected to it.
- **ECG:** Also called a heart monitor, an electrocardiograph (e-lec-tro-CAR-dee-o-graf), or EKG. The patches on your chest are hooked up to a TV-type screen or a small portable box (telemetry unit). This screen shows a tracing of each heartbeat. Your heart will be watched for signs of injury or damage that could be related to your illness.
- **Oxygen:** Your body may need extra oxygen at this time. It is given either by a mask or nasal prongs. Tell your doctor if the oxygen is drying out your nose or if the nasal prongs bother you.
- **Activity:** You may need to rest in bed. Once you are feeling better, you will be allowed to get up.
- **Pain Medicine:** May be given in your IV, as a shot, or by mouth. If the pain does not go away or comes back, tell a doctor right away.

Herniated Disk

See Slipped Disk

Herpes, Genital

See Genital Herpes

Herpes, Oral

See Cold Sores

Herpes Stomatitis in Children

WHAT YOU SHOULD KNOW

Herpes (HER-pees) stomatitis (sto-ma-TIE-tis) is an infection in the mouth caused by the herpes virus. The condition is also called herpetic stomatitis and herpes gingivostomatitis. For the most part, it occurs in young children who have never had the virus before. There are usually many small open blisters inside the mouth, on the tongue and gums. The blisters usually heal in 1 to 2 weeks.

Causes

This infection comes from the same herpes virus that causes cold sores, but not the one that is spread by having sex.

Signs/Symptoms

The chief symptoms are sore, open blisters and swelling of the lips, mouth, and tongue. Your child may have a high fever and feel tired. Because the mouth hurts, it will be hard to eat and swallow. The child may also have a sore throat.

Care

Your child may need medicine for pain and fever. You may also be given pain medicine that can be put on the sores. In very bad cases, medicine that helps to control the virus may be prescribed.

WHAT YOU SHOULD DO

- You may give acetaminophen for pain or fever, but do NOT give aspirin.
- Give the child cool liquids. This may be soothing to the mouth and help numb the pain. Good choices are milk, milkshakes, and clear liquids. Don't give citrus or carbonated drinks such as orange or grapefruit juice, lemonade, or soda. These will make the sores hurt more. Use a straw if there are blisters on the lips or end of the tongue.
- Feed the child soft foods to make chewing and swallowing easier. Good choices are strained baby foods, soft fruits, mashed potatoes, applesauce, yogurt, and pudding. Avoid salty, spicy, and hard foods.
- After each meal, rinse the child's mouth with warm water. You may be asked to have the child rinse or gargle with salt water.
- Wash your hands and the child's hands often, and especially before eating.
- Wash any toys that find their way into the child's mouth before and after the child plays with them.
- To keep from spreading the virus, tell your child not to share drinks or food with others.

Call Your Doctor If . . .

- Your child will not drink and cannot swallow.
- Your child has a high temperature.
- Your child becomes more fussy or won't stop crying.
- Your child isn't better in a few days.

Seek Care Immediately If . . .

- Your child has a very high temperature.
- Your child becomes dehydrated from not getting enough fluids. Signs of dehydration include no urination in 8 hours, dry and

cracked lips, no tears when crying, and, in babies, sinking of the soft
spot on the top of the head.
• Your child is weak or more sleepy than usual and is hard to wake up.

Herpes Zoster

See Shingles

Hiatal Hernia

WHAT YOU SHOULD KNOW

A hiatal (hi-A-tul) hernia occurs when a part of the stomach slides
above the diaphragm (DIE-uh-fram), the thin muscle separating the
stomach from the chest. This is a common problem and most people
are not bothered by it.

Your hernia may allow stomach acid to flow back into your
esophagus (ee-sof-uh-gus), the tube that connects the mouth to the
stomach. With time, the stomach acid may irritate your esophagus
and cause problems. If this happens, you may need surgery to repair
the hernia.

Causes

You can be born with a hiatal hernia or develop one when you are
older. A trauma or surgery can cause the problem too.

Signs/Symptoms

The most common symptom is burning in your chest (heartburn), especially at night when you are lying down. Other possible signs include burping and trouble swallowing.

Care

Usually, treatment at home is all that's needed. Surgery is required
only if your symptoms get worse.

WHAT YOU SHOULD DO

• You may use an over-the-counter antacid. Follow the directions on
the label.
• Eat 6 small meals instead of 3 big meals. This keeps your stomach
from getting too full. Eat slowly. Don't lie down for 2 or 3 hours
after eating. Don't eat or drink anything 1 to 2 hours before going
to bed.
• Avoid alcohol, caffeine beverages (colas, coffee, cocoa, tea), fatty

foods, citrus fruits and other foods and drinks that seem to increase heartburn.

- To help prevent heartburn at night, place 4- to 6-inch blocks under the head of your bed. This will keep your head and esophagus higher than your stomach. If you can't use blocks, sleep with several pillows under your head and shoulders.
- Avoid bending over, especially after eating. Also avoid straining during bowel movements or when urinating or lifting things.
- Don't wear clothing that constricts the chest or stomach.
- Don't smoke. Smoking often causes the stomach to make more acid.
- If you are overweight, lose weight. Ask your doctor for a weight loss plan.

Call Your Doctor If . . .
- Your symptoms don't improve in a few days, or they get worse.
- You develop a high temperature.

Seek Care Immediately If . . .
- You vomit blood or have recurrent vomiting.
- You develop severe chest pain along with nausea, sweating, or shortness of breath.

Hiccups

WHAT YOU SHOULD KNOW

Hiccups, also called hiccoughs, are repeated spasms of the diaphragm, the large, flat muscle that divides your chest from your stomach. In most cases, hiccups are mild and last less than an hour, although they can persist for hours or days or return repeatedly.

Causes
Hiccups occur when overeating, eating too rapidly, drinking carbonated beverages, or illness irritates the phrenic nerve in the diaphragm.

Signs/Symptoms
Hiccup spasms close the muscles in the back of the throat when you exhale, resulting in the typical hiccup sound.

Care
Try one of the home remedies listed below. If the problem won't subside, medication may be necessary.

WHAT YOU SHOULD DO

- There are many home remedies for hiccups. Some that might help include:
  —Swallow dry bread crumbs, crushed ice, or 1 teaspoon of dry sugar.
  —Hold your breath and count silently to 10 (or higher, if possible).
  —Drink a glass of water very quickly, sip ice water, or gargle with water.
  —Pull gently on your tongue or push down the back of your tongue with your finger or a spoon handle.
  —Press the end of a finger into each ear for 20 seconds.
  —Close your eyes and push lightly and gently on your eyeballs.

Call Your Doctor If . . .
- Hiccups last longer than 3 hours in children or 8 hours in adults.

High Altitude Sickness

See Mountain Sickness

High Blood Pressure

See Hypertension

Hip Joint Replacement

See Total Hip Replacement

Hives

WHAT YOU SHOULD KNOW

Hives, known medically as urticaria (UR-tih-KARE-e-uh), is an allergic reaction appearing on the skin. The problem may disappear quickly or last for months or years.

Causes
The reaction can be caused by medicines, pets, foods, insect bites, or infections. Cold, heat, sunlight, exercise, and water may also produce hives in susceptible individuals. Hives tend to run in families.

Signs/Symptoms
The reaction produces red, itchy, swollen bumps called wheals that quickly change in size, shape, and location. The wheals may come

and go in minutes or last for hours. In some people, they are accompanied by more serious allergic symptoms. Hives cannot be spread from person to person.

Care

Medicine may relieve the itch and irritation and prevent more hives from developing. If you suffer violent allergic reactions, you may need to keep an emergency medicine kit with you at all times.

WHAT YOU SHOULD DO

- If you know what causes the hives, avoid whatever brought on the attack. Your doctor may suggest that you see an allergy specialist.
- If your doctor prescribes medication to relieve itching and rash, take it exactly as directed. You may use an over-the-counter antihistamine until the hives are completely gone for 24 hours. Do not take any medications, including aspirin, laxatives, vitamins, antacids, pain killers, or cough syrups, without first checking with your doctor.
- Apply cold compresses to the skin or take baths in cool water. Don't take hot baths or showers; the warmth will make the itching worse.
- Wear loose fitting clothing; avoid tight underwear. Any skin irritation may trigger another attack.

Call Your Doctor If . . .

- You still have a lot of itching after taking medicine for 24 hours.
- You develop a high temperature.
- You have any pain or swelling in your joints.
- The condition lasts more than 1 week.
- You develop new, unexplained symptoms.

Seek Care Immediately If . . .

- You have the following symptoms during an attack of hives: swollen lips or tongue, difficulty breathing or swallowing, or abdominal pain. These may be the first signs of a life-threatening allergic reaction. **THIS IS AN EMERGENCY. Call 0 (operator) or 911** for medical help.

HIV Testing

WHAT YOU SHOULD KNOW

HIV, the human immunodeficiency virus, is the infection that leads to AIDS (acquired immunodeficiency syndrome). The virus attacks the body's disease-fighting immune system, eventually weakening it so much that it can no longer fend off disease. The infection may take many years to do its work. When someone first contracts HIV, there may be no symptoms at all. Later, AIDS-like symptoms will begin to develop. Finally, AIDS itself will take hold.

If you have an HIV infection, your body will make antibodies in an attempt to fight it off. A blood test for HIV searches for evidence of these antibodies. A positive test means that you have the virus and may need treatment. It doesn't mean you have AIDS.

If you know that you were exposed to HIV or if you are at high risk of getting HIV (you are a gay or bisexual man, or an IV drug user), and your test results are negative, the test should be done again in 6 months. If you have the virus, your body can take from 2 weeks to 6 months to make antibodies.

You may have to wait for up to 2 weeks to get the test results. In some states, only you will be given the results. In others, results must also be reported to the Health Department. Before having the test, ask about this.

Although there is no cure for HIV infection, there are medicines that may slow down the development of AIDS. Other medicines can fight the infections that AIDS allows to take hold.

Causes
You can get an HIV infection from contact with blood or other body fluids, like semen or vaginal discharge. Most people get the virus from having sex with an infected partner or from using dirty needles. You can get HIV from having sex with ANYONE, not just someone who is gay. Infected blood transfusions are another source of the virus, and a pregnant woman with HIV can pass the virus to her baby.

Signs/Symptoms
At first, there are usually no symptoms. Later, people with an HIV infection may feel tired, lose weight, have a fever, contract skin or lung infections, or develop cancer. They can also have diarrhea that lasts for a long time, swollen glands, mouth sores, or night sweats.

Care
There is no cure, but your doctor can give you medicine to try to slow down the HIV infection. You may develop AIDS months or years later. If this happens, additional medicines can be prescribed to fight the new infections.

WHAT YOU SHOULD DO

- If you test positive for the virus, see a doctor right away. Early treatment may help.
- Get tested if you even suspect that a sexual partner has HIV or AIDS. You also should be tested if you have had sex with several people. It doesn't matter whether you are gay or straight.
- If you have used a needle that might have been used by someone else, you should be tested.
- If the test is negative, but you think you might have had contact with HIV, get tested again in 6 months.
- If you have the virus, tell all of the people you have had sex with so they can get tested. Always tell a new partner BEFORE you have sex. There are ways to have sex and be safe.
- Use a condom when you have sex whether you have the HIV virus or not.
- If you have the virus, do not give blood or donate organs, and tell any health care workers you come in contact with, so they can take steps to avoid infection.

HIV Transmission

WHAT YOU SHOULD KNOW

HIV (human immunodeficiency virus) is the infection that leads to AIDS. The virus may not cause any symptoms at first, but it will eventually weaken the immune system to the point that it can no longer fight off disease

The virus is spread by contact with blood or body fluids. It may be in all body fluids; but only blood, semen, discharge from the vagina, and possibly breast milk have enough of the virus to infect other people. It can be spread from male to male, male to female, female to male, or female to female. It can be passed from a mother to her unborn child or a nursing baby. Most people get the virus from having sex or using dirty needles.

Causes

If you have sex with someone who has HIV, or use the same needle as someone with HIV, you can get the virus. It doesn't matter whether you are gay or straight; and your sexual partner may not be sick or even know that he or she has the virus. You can also get HIV from an infected blood transfusion. A pregnant woman with HIV can pass the virus to her baby.

Signs/Symptoms

There are usually no symptoms at first. Months or years later, when the virus has broken down the immune system, you may feel tired, lose weight, have a fever, get skin or lung infections, or develop cancer. You can also have diarrhea that lasts for a long time, swollen glands, mouth sores, or night sweats.

Care

There is no cure, but there are medicines that may slow down the development of AIDS. Other medicines can be prescribed to fight the infections that AIDS allows to take hold.

WHAT YOU SHOULD DO

- Keep your risk to a minimum. Having multiple sexual partners and using IV drugs put you at greatest risk.
- Don't have sex without a condom. Use a condom every time you have oral, vaginal, or anal sex. Always use a latex condom. Condoms made from animal skin (lamb skin) will not protect you from the virus.
- Use water-based lotions such as K-Y Jelly, Foreplay, and Wet with a condom. NEVER use oils such as Vaseline, Crisco, baby oil, or hand lotion. They could cause the condom to break.
- Safer forms of sex include massage, hugging, masturbation, dry kissing, or oral sex with a condom.
- If you and your partner both have HIV, you should still have safe sex. You might have slightly different strains of the virus, and you could infect each other.
- Drug users should always use clean needles and syringes. They can be cleaned with bleach for 30 seconds and rinsed with clean water.
- Ear piercing and tattooing should always be done with a clean needle.
- Working or living in the same house with someone who is infected with HIV is safe. Sneezing, talking, touching, handshaking, and sharing dishes or glasses, toilets, and air space does not spread AIDS. You cannot get AIDS from mosquito bites, from donating blood, or from touching a doorknob, table top, telephone or something else that a person with AIDS may have used.
- Since April 1985, all donated blood has been tested for HIV. Only blood that has tested negative and has been specially treated to kill the virus is used for transfusions. There is still a small risk of HIV infection from blood, however. Donors may give blood before they know they're infected. Some people store their own blood if they

know in advance that they are going to have surgery. This procedure is called autotransfusion.

• If you even suspect you've had contact with HIV, get tested. If you have HIV, see a doctor right away. Early treatment may help you. Do not donate blood or organs. Do not have sex without telling your partner that you may have HIV.

Human Bite

WHAT YOU SHOULD KNOW

A bite from another human can be every bit as worrisome as one from an animal. Human bites often break the skin, and sometimes go very deep. Because the human mouth carries plenty of germs, the wound is likely to become infected if it is not cleaned right away. Healing may take days or weeks, depending on the severity of the bite.

Signs/Symptoms

You may have bleeding, pain, bruising, or swelling in the area of the bite.

Care

Clean the wound thoroughly right away. If it is large or deep, it may require stitches. Otherwise, soak the wound 3 to 4 times a day, keeping it clean and dry between soakings. If you have not had a tetanus shot recently, you may need one. Your doctor also may prescribe antibiotic medicine to keep an infection from developing.

WHAT YOU SHOULD DO

• If you have stitches, keep them clean and dry for several days. Then you can clean the wound. Make an appointment with your doctor to have your stitches taken out.

• Keep the area of the bite clean. Wash the wound with soap and water 3 to 4 times a day.

• If you have a bandage, keep it clean and dry. Change it whenever it gets dirty. To loosen the bandage if it sticks to the wound, put a little water on it, then gently pull it off the wound.

• If possible, raise the site of the bite above the level of your heart to keep the swelling down.

• If you have been given a tetanus shot, your arm may get swollen, red, and warm to the touch at the site of the shot. This is a normal re-action to the medicine.

• If you are taking antibiotics, continue to take them until they are all gone, even if you feel well. If you feel they are not helping, call your doctor. Do not quit taking them on your own.

Call Your Doctor If . . .

• You have numbness or tingling in the area of the bite.
• You have any signs of infection (redness, red streaking or pus coming from the wound, or warmth or swelling in the area of the bite).
• You have a high temperature.
• You have pain or trouble moving the injured part.
• Tender lumps appear in your groin or under your arm.
• You develop a rash, itching, or swelling after taking your medicine

Hyperemesis Gravidarum

WHAT YOU SHOULD KNOW

When nausea and vomiting in pregnancy become really severe, the condition is called hyperemesis (hi-per-EM-uh-sis) gravidarum (grav-uh-DARE-um). It is more serious than morning sickness, and can be unsafe for both you and your baby. Without food the baby cannot grow, and your own health can get worse if the condition is not treated.

Causes

The cause of this problem is unknown. Emotional changes may be a factor. A multiple pregnancy can encourage it. Changes in your hormones may have a role.

Signs/Symptoms

Typical signs of this condition include vomiting more than 3 or 4 times a day, not keeping any food down, losing weight, feeling tired and dizzy, and urinating less than usual.

Your heart may seem to race; you may suffer headaches and confusion; and your skin may become pale-looking and dry. These are signs of dehydration that can harm both you and your baby.

Care

Your doctor will weigh you, talk to you, and examine you. Your blood will be tested for certain chemicals called electrolytes (ee-LECK-trow-lights). Too much vomiting can cause the balance of these chemicals to change in your blood. Your urine also will be tested for signs that the vomiting is too severe.

If your condition is serious, you may need to go into the hospital for treatment.

Risks

You can die from serious untreated hyperemesis gravidarum. But the risks of serious illness are very small if you follow your doctor's suggestions.

WHAT YOU SHOULD DO

- Take your medicine as directed. Call the doctor if you feel it is not helping. Do not quit taking it on your own.
- Do not take over-the-counter medicine without talking to your doctor. Rest often. Exercise and work without getting too tired. Your body will tell you when to rest.
- If your stomach is upset in the morning, eat dry toast or saltine crackers before getting out of bed.
- Eat small, frequent meals. Avoid fried or spicy foods that can upset your stomach. After eating, sit up for 45 minutes.

Call Your Doctor If . . .

- Your nausea and vomiting get worse.
- You are losing weight.

IF YOU'RE HEADING FOR THE HOSPITAL . . .

What to Expect While You're There

You may encounter the following procedures and equipment during your stay.

- **Taking Vital Signs:** These include your temperature, blood pressure, pulse (counting your heartbeats), and respirations (counting your breaths). A stethoscope is used to listen to your heart and lungs. Your blood pressure is taken by wrapping a cuff around your arm.
- **IV:** A tube placed in your vein for giving medicine or liquids. It will be capped or have tubing connected to it.
- **ECG:** Also called a heart monitor, an electrocardiograph (e-lec-tro-CAR-dee-o-graf), or EKG. The patches on your chest are hooked up to a TV-type screen or a small portable box (telemetry unit). This screen shows a tracing of each heartbeat. Your heart will be watched for signs of injury or damage resulting from your illness.
- **Blood:** Usually taken from a vein in your hand or from the bend in your elbow. Tests will be done on your blood.
- **Medicines:** You may get medicines by shot, in your IV, or in your rectum as a suppository.

• **Monitoring the Baby's Heartbeat:**
   —If it is late in your pregnancy, you will have a loose-fitting belt strapped around your abdomen. The belt secures a patch which is attached to a machine with a TV-type screen. This screen shows a tracing of your baby's heartbeat.
   —Your baby's heartbeat may be monitored all the time during the early part of your hospital stay. As you improve, a tracing may be taken several times a day.

• **Urine Tests:** You will be asked to urinate in a container. Hospital personnel will measure and test your urine to make sure you are getting enough liquids. Do not throw away your urine unless your nurses have given the okay.

• **Other Tests:** You may have tests of your liver, kidney, pancreas, and bowels to find reasons for the vomiting.

• **Weight:** You will be weighed daily to see if there have been any changes.

• **Food:** Until your vomiting stops, you will not be given any meals. Instead, you will receive food and vitamins through your IV. You can slowly begin to drink and eat small amounts of food when your vomiting has stopped.

• **Emotions:** Try to relax and avoid stress. Talking to your doctor or someone close to you may be helpful.

Hypertension

WHAT YOU SHOULD KNOW

Hypertension (hi-per-TEN-shun) is another name for high blood pressure. Blood pressure is a measure of the force the blood puts on the walls of veins, arteries, and the heart.

There are 2 parts to a blood pressure reading. One is called systolic (sis-TAHL-ic). It is the first number in a blood pressure reading. The other is called diastolic (DI-as-tahl-ic). It is the second number in the reading. For example: in the reading of 120/80, 120 is the systolic number, and 80 is the diastolic number.

The systolic (first) number tells you how hard the blood is pushing against the walls of the arteries, veins, and heart when the heart is pumping blood (during a heartbeat).

The diastolic (second) number gives the pressure when the heart is resting between beats.

A good systolic number is between 100 and 140 millimeters of mercury (mm Hg). For some people, a number between 80 and 100 is normal. A good diastolic number is usually lower than 90 mm Hg. Your doctor can tell you what is normal for you.

If the systolic number is higher than 140 or the diastolic number is higher than 90, you are said to have high blood pressure. Only one of the numbers needs to be high. For example, you have high blood pressure if your reading is 120/98, because even though the first number (systolic) is normal, the second (diastolic) number is high. Likewise, you have a problem if your reading is 180/88, where the first number is high even though the second is not.

Causes
Often there is no specific cause. Some illnesses that can cause high blood pressure are kidney or other organ problems, pregnancy, or taking drugs.

Do's and Don'ts
To bring your blood pressure down, you need to quit smoking, lose weight, exercise, eat a diet low in salt and fat, avoid alcohol and caffeine, and avoid or learn to control stress. Talk to your doctor about how to make these changes.

Risk Factors
Your risk of high blood pressure is greater if someone in your family has it, if you are over 50, male, or black, and if you smoke or are overweight.

Care
You may need to take medicine to lower your blood pressure. If so, take it as directed and do not stop taking it unless you are told to by your doctor. If there is another illness causing your high blood pressure, that illness will be treated also.

Risks
Millions of Americans have high blood pressure and don't know it. High blood pressure is often called "the silent killer" because often it has no symptoms. Without treatment, however, it can lead to heart disease, a stroke, kidney failure, or a heart attack. With treatment to keep your blood pressure under control, there is less chance of having these problems.

WHAT YOU SHOULD DO

- Always take your medicine as directed by your doctor. If you feel it is not helping, call your doctor. Do not quit taking it on your own.
- If you take aspirin regularly, continue to take it. Aspirin helps thin

the blood so blood clots don't form. Do not take acetaminophen or ibuprofen instead.

- If you are taking more than one medicine, make a list of what you are taking and when you take it. You can buy a plastic pill holder that has 7 sections, one for each day of the week.
- If you are on blood pressure medicine:
  —You may get dizzy when you change from a lying to a sitting position. Get up slowly. If you feel faint lie down right away.
  —Your medicine may make your nose stuffy or make you feel weak. It can also diminish your appetite.
  —You may need to have your medicine or the dose changed many times before finding the right treatment.
  —Take your blood pressure and pulse regularly. Ask your doctor to teach you or a family member how.
  —Vomiting, diarrhea, or heavy sweating can lower your blood pressure and make you dizzy. Hot baths, hot weather, fever, or drinking alcohol can also lower your blood pressure. If this happens, call your doctor so your medicine or its dose can be changed.
- A diet low in fat, salt, and cholesterol is very important. It keeps your heart healthy and strong. Ask your doctor what you should and should not eat.
- It may take time getting used to a new diet. Special cookbooks may help you and the cook in your family find new recipes.
- Quit smoking. It harms the heart and lungs. If you are having trouble stopping, ask your doctor for help.
- Exercise daily. It helps make the heart stronger, lowers blood pressure, and keeps you healthy. If your exercise plan seems too hard or too easy, speak with your doctor.
- Excess weight can raise your blood pressure. If you need to lose weight, talk to your doctor about a plan.
- Since it is hard to avoid stress, learn to control it. Ways to relax include deep breathing, relaxing the muscles, and imagery. Also, don't hesitate to talk to someone about things that upset you.
- If you have other illnesses like diabetes or high blood pressure, you need to control them. Take medicines as directed. Because of these illnesses, you have a higher chance of getting a heart attack.
- For more information about the heart, call the **American Heart Association at 1-800-AHA-USA1 (1-800-242-8721)** or call your local **Red Cross**.

Call Your Doctor If . . .
• You are dizzy and the feeling does not go away.
• You have chest pain during exercise that doesn't go away with rest.
• You have a fever, vomiting, or diarrhea that makes you dizzy.

Seek Care Immediately If . . .
• Your blood pressure is higher than usual.
• You pass out or have a seizure.
• You have chest pain that does not go away with rest or medicine.
• You have a headache; are sleepy, confused, or have numbness and tingling in your hands and feet; are coughing blood; have nosebleeds; or have a lot of trouble breathing. These are signs of very high blood pressure. **Call 911 or 0 (operator)** to get to the nearest hospital or clinic. **Do not drive yourself!**

IF YOU'RE HEADING FOR THE HOSPITAL . . .

What to Expect While You're There
You may encounter the following procedures and equipment during your stay.
• **Taking Vital Signs:** These include your temperature, blood pressure, pulse (counting your heartbeats), and respirations (counting your breaths). A stethoscope is used to listen to your heart and lungs. Your blood pressure is taken by wrapping a cuff around your arm.
• **Oxygen:** Your body may need extra oxygen at this time. It is given either by a mask or nasal prongs. Tell your doctor if the oxygen is drying out your nose or if the nasal prongs bother you.
• **Pulse Oximeter:** While you are getting oxygen, you may be hooked up to a pulse oximeter (ox-IM-uh-ter). It is placed on your ear, finger, or toe and is connected to a machine that measures the oxygen in your blood.
• **IV:** A tube placed in your vein for giving medicine or liquids. It will be capped or have tubing connected to it.
• **ECG:** Also called a heart monitor, an electrocardiograph (e-lec-tro-CAR-dee-o-graf), or EKG. The patches on your chest are hooked up to a TV-type screen or a small portable box (telemetry unit). This screen shows a tracing of each heartbeat. Your heart will be watched for signs of injury or damage that could be related to your illness.
• **12 Lead ECG:** This test makes tracings from different parts of your heart. It can help your doctor decide whether there is any problem with your heart.
• **Medicine:**
  —**Blood Pressure Medicine:** Given for constant high blood pressure. It may be given in an IV at first, and later taken by mouth.

—**Diuretics** (di-your-ET-ics): Also called "water pills," these medicines make you pass urine more often and thus get rid of any extra fluid your body or lungs may have collected. It can be given as a pill or in your IV.

- **Activity:** It is important to rest and relax until your blood pressure is lower. If you are anxious, call a doctor. Keeping the head of your bed up slightly may help lower your blood pressure.
- **Blood:** Usually taken from a vein in your hand or from the bend in your elbow. Tests will be done on the blood.
- **Other tests:** Chest and kidney x-rays may need to be done to help find the cause of your high blood pressure.

Hyperventilation

WHAT YOU SHOULD KNOW

In hyperventilation (hi-per-ven-tuh-LAY-shun), your breathing is so rapid that it upsets the balance of gases in your blood. One of these gases is carbon dioxide. Hyperventilation reduces the carbon dioxide level in the blood, causing symptoms that resemble a heart attack.

Causes

Hyperventilation is usually brought on by anxiety, stress, or hysteria.

Signs/Symptoms

Common symptoms are shortness of breath; fast breathing; chest pain; weakness; dizziness; and numbness and tingling around the mouth, hands, and feet. You may have blurred vision, feel like your heart is racing, have muscle tightness in your hands and feet, or feel faint.

Care

Since it is hard to avoid stress, try to control it. Learn new ways to relax (deep breathing, relaxing muscles, meditation, or biofeedback). Talk to someone about things that upset you.

WHAT YOU SHOULD DO

- During an attack, try to slow your breathing. Take 1 breath every 10 seconds.
- Do **not** breathe into a paper bag. This can be dangerous because you may not get enough oxygen.
- You may need help to deal with the stress or anxiety that may be causing you to hyperventilate. Family, friends, clergy, your doctor, or a mental health center may be able to help.

Call Your Doctor If . . .
• Your symptoms do not go away.
• You have a sudden fever.

Seek Care Immediately If . . .
• You have a seizure.
• You have fainting spells or chest pain.

Hyphema

WHAT YOU SHOULD KNOW

Hyphema (hi-FEE-muh) is bleeding in the space between the cornea and the iris of your eye. A mild hyphema usually disappears in 1 week. If the injury is serious, you may develop long-term eye problems.

Causes
Injury to the eye, especially in sports.

Signs/Symptoms
Typical symptoms include eye pain, blurring or loss of vision, and blood in the white of the eye.

Care
The doctor will probably prescribe an eye shield. Resting the eye is very important. Surgery may be needed if other treatment does not work.

WHAT YOU SHOULD DO

• Follow your doctor's directions carefully. Otherwise, the injury may start to bleed again and you might experience a permanent loss of vision.
• Rest in bed as much as possible until the doctor says you may resume your normal activities. Lie on your back and use two pillows to keep your head elevated. You may get up to go to the bathroom, eat, and bathe.
• You may use acetaminophen for pain control, but do not use aspirin or ibuprofen.
• If you are wearing an eye shield, do not remove it until your doctor gives you the go-ahead.
• Do not do things that require close eye movement such as reading and playing hand-held video games. You may watch TV.
• Do not bend forward or lower your head until the hyphema clears

up. Your doctor will tell you when you can resume lifting or engaging in strenuous activities.
- Wearing protective eye guards helps prevent hyphema and other sports-related eye injuries. This is especially important when playing racquet sports.

Seek Care Immediately If . . .
- There is more blood in your eye than before, you have trouble seeing, or your eye pain gets worse. These may be signs that your eye is starting to bleed again.
- You become nauseated or start to vomit.
- You feel dizzy or light-headed.

Hypoglycemia

See Low Blood Sugar

Hypoglycemia, Diabetic

See Insulin Reaction

Hypokalemia

See Low Potassium

Hypothermia

WHAT YOU SHOULD KNOW

In hypothermia (HI-po-THER-me-uh), your temperature drops so far below normal that the body can no longer function normally. Although you are most likely to develop this condition in freezing weather, it can also happen when the air is merely cold. Left uncorrected, it can be fatal.

Hypothermia is most common among older people and babies, whose bodies are not quick to adjust to temperature changes.

Causes
Prolonged exposure to cold will eventually cause body temperature to fall. It will fall faster if the weather is windy or your body is wet. Alcohol and certain drugs can encourage hypothermia.

Signs/Symptoms
Typical warning signs are confusion, shivering, and weakness or drowsiness. Eventually, the fingers and toes turn purple, muscles stop

functioning normally, and breathing slows. Ultimately, you may lose consciousness.

Care

Someone will need to take you to the hospital. While waiting for help to come, follow the directions below.

WHAT YOU SHOULD DO

- Before going to the hospital, try to rewarm yourself. Cover yourself with a blanket, take a warm (not hot) bath, or drink hot chocolate or warm soup.
- Do not drink alcohol; it can make hypothermia worse.
- In cold weather:
  —Wear several loose layers of warm, windproof clothing.
  —Wear a hat and scarf to help retain heat in your head and neck.
  —Stay dry. Moisture from sweating, rain, or melting snow can reduce the protective value of clothing.
  —Avoid going out in extremely cold weather.
- Wear warm clothing indoors during cold weather. Use extra blankets because hypothermia can occur when you sleep.
- Eat well-balanced meals and get plenty of rest. Stay as active as possible. Do not drink alcohol because it causes the body to lose heat faster.
- If you are over 60 years of age:
  —If you live alone, have a neighbor, relative, or friend call or check-in on you every day during cold weather.
  —Your body temperature may become dangerously low without your realizing it. Check your temperature every now and then, especially in cold weather. If you have trouble reading the thermometer, ask a friend or relative to read it for you. Normal temperature is 98.6 degrees F or 37 degrees C.

Call Your Doctor If . . .
- Your body temperature falls at all in cold weather.

Impetigo

WHAT YOU SHOULD KNOW

Impetigo (IM-peh-TIE-go) is a skin infection that usually attacks the face, arms, and legs. It is more common in children than adults. With treatment, the infection should disappear in 7 to 10 days.

Causes
This is a bacterial infection that can be spread from person to person.

Signs/Symptoms
The infection causes an itchy red rash with water- or pus-filled blisters. The blisters break and form yellow crusts.

Care
The doctor may prescribe an antibiotic to treat the infection. The rash should be kept clean and dry.

WHAT YOU SHOULD DO

- If your doctor prescribes an antibiotic, take all of the medication, even if you feel better. If you stop treatment too soon, some of the bacteria may survive and re-infect you.
- Soak and gently scrub the sores with mild soap and water. Break any blisters and remove all crusts several times a day until the sores heal. Applying cloths soaked in Burow's solution (available at drug and grocery stores) several times a day may make the sores dry faster.
- Wash your hands thoroughly with soap and water after scrubbing the sores and before touching food, your eyes, or other people. Wash bedding, towels, and clothes that have touched the sores. Do not share washcloths, towels, or bedding with family members.
- Keep hands clean and nails short. Do not touch or scratch the sores.
- You may return to school or work 24 hours after starting treatment.

Call Your Doctor If . . .
- The sores become worse or spread, or if they do not begin to heal within 3 days after treatment begins.
- A high temperature develops.
- You note any problems (such as rash, swelling, stomach ache) that may be related to the medicine.

Implanted Venous Access Ports

WHAT YOU SHOULD KNOW

These ports are used to deliver a variety of medications and nutritional liquids directly into one of the body's major veins. Delivery of fluids to the port requires a special type of needle (Huber needle) that is bent at a 90-degree angle. The most uncomfortable part of the procedure is penetration of the skin above the port. This discomfort is only temporary, since the skin will eventually become less sensitive from frequent punctures.

WHAT YOU SHOULD DO

- When you need to access the port at home, be sure that you, or the person doing it, washes his or her hands thoroughly.
- Wash the port area with soap and water, then clean it with povidine-iodine and alcohol. If you are allergic to povidine-iodine, use alcohol alone.
- Connect the extension tube to the needle and a 10-milliliter syringe filled with normal saline. Force the air out of the tubing by flushing it with a small amount of the normal saline. Clamp the tubing.
- Hold the port with the thumb and forefinger and insert the needle until the tip touches the back of the port surface. Do not tilt or rock the needle. Secure the needle with a clear or gauze bandage and tape.
- Open the clamp and pull back on the syringe until you get a blood return. Then flush the port with the normal saline to be sure that fluid flows through the system. Clamp the tube and remove the syringe.
- Next, connect the tubing or syringe containing the fluids or medicine to be administered. Open the clamp and infuse the fluids or medicine.
- When you are finished, clamp the extension tube, remove your tubing or syringe and connect a 10 milliliter syringe filled with normal saline to the extension tube. Open the clamp and flush the port with the normal saline. Clamp the extension tubing and remove the syringe.
- Flush the system with 5 milliliters of heparinized saline solution (you'll receive instructions) and remove the syringe. Put a small gauze bandage over the port.

Call Your Doctor If . . .

- You notice redness, swelling, or tenderness in the port area.
- You develop swelling in the face and neck, and feel pain in the shoulder, arms, and neck.

Infant Colic

See Colic

Infectious Mononucleosis

See Mononucleosis

Infectious Polyneuropathy

See Guillain-Barré Syndrome

Inflamed Colon

See Colitis

Influenza

See Flu in Adults

Influenza in Children

See Flu in Children

Ingrown Nail

WHAT YOU SHOULD DO

An ingrown nail develops when the sharp edge of a fingernail or toe-nail grows into the skin next to it. The big toenail is most often affected. With proper care, the nail may return to normal in 1 to 2 weeks.

Causes

The usual culprits are tight-fitting shoes that force a nail into the skin. Incorrectly trimmed toenails can also cause the problem.

Signs/Symptoms

First, you may feel tenderness and see swelling as the nail pushes on the skin. Once the nail pierces the skin, you will see redness and more swelling, and you may feel sharp pain. With time, skin will grow over the nail.

Care

If a nail has been ingrown for a long time, the doctor may have to burn away the overgrown skin. If that does not work, you may require surgery; however, the need for surgery is fairly rare.

WHAT YOU SHOULD DO

• If the problem has developed recently, you can lift the edge of the nail away from the sore skin by wedging a small piece of cotton under the corner of the nail.
• Soak the whole foot or hand in warm water for 20 minutes every day, 2 to 3 times a day. If the nail is infected you may need to soak it in an antibiotic liquid.
• Keep the nail area clean and dry.

- To prevent the problem in the future, cut nails straight across. Do not round them with a file or cut them in a semicircle.
- Wear shoes that fit well.

Call Your Doctor If . . .
- The toe or finger is not better in 7 days.
- Pain, redness, or swelling gets worse, or the wound feels warm.
- You develop a high temperature.

Inhalation Injury

See Smoke Inhalation

Insect-Sting Allergy

WHAT YOU SHOULD KNOW

If you are allergic to insects, a sting can produce uncomfortable or even life-threatening symptoms. In susceptible people, a sting causes the body to produce a flood of histamine, a chemical that may cause swelling, itching, and rash. In a severe reaction, you may even have trouble breathing.

Signs/Symptoms
A typical allergic reaction includes a red lump, pain, swelling, itching, and a rash. You may also run a fever, develop a headache, feel dizzy, or faint. Some people develop an upset stomach and throw up. Really dangerous symptoms include tightness in your chest or throat, and trouble breathing.

Care
If you experience chest pain, a tight throat, or trouble breathing and do not have emergency medicine, **get to the hospital right away**.

People with a severe allergy to insect bites are usually prescribed an emergency kit containing epinephrine (eh-pih-NEF-rin). A shot of this drug is needed as soon as the bite occurs.

WHAT YOU SHOULD DO

- If you are allergic to bug bites and stings, carry a card, or wear a medical necklace or bracelet identifying your allergy. The card or tag should list your name, your doctor's name and phone number, and type of allergy you have. Also be sure to carry an emergency kit with you at all times and make certain that both you and your family know how to use it.

- If you are stung:
  - —Stay calm. Get medical help immediately. If you can't reach your doctor, **call 0 (operator) or 911,** or go to the nearest emergency room.
  - —Take the insect's stinger out by scraping it off with your fingernail or a knife blade. Do not squeeze it. Apply a paste of meat tenderizer and water to the bite while seeking medical care.
  - —If you have a self-treatment kit, inject the epinephrine immediately, without waiting for symptoms to start. Then see your doctor to make sure the danger has passed.
- To keep from getting stung:
  - —If you are caught in or near a swarm of bees or wasps, move away slowly. Don't swat at them. Never strike, stir up, or throw anything at a wasp nest or beehive.
  - —Stay away from places that may attract stinging insects. Yellow jackets nest in the ground and hornets in trees and bushes. Every type of stinging insect is attracted to flowers. Bees are more likely to sting in gloomy weather than on bright sunny days.
  - —Stay away from wood piles. Be very careful when gardening or mowing the lawn. Also take precautions in picnic areas, orchards, beaches, and other places where there are exposed foods, fragrances, and bright colors.
  - —Use insect repellent on skin and clothing when you are outside.
  - —Do not wear hair sprays, aftershave lotions, perfumes, suntan lotions, and other scented cosmetics when outdoors. Floral odors are especially attractive to bees and wasps.
  - —Do not wear floppy, bright-colored, or flower-print clothing outdoors.
  - —Protect yourself outdoors by wearing long sleeves, slacks, shoes, and socks. Wear gloves when gardening or doing other outdoor chores.
  - —Check window screens for openings where insects can get in. Look around outside your home for insect nests. Keep your car windows closed when driving.
  - —Keep an insecticide spray that kills stinging insects handy at home, in your car, and whenever you are outdoors.
  - —Never drink from a bottle or can that might have a hidden insect inside. Check objects for insects before touching, sitting, or brushing against them.

Call Your Doctor If . . .

- You have been bitten or stung and your skin is swelling, itching, and has a rash; but you are **not** having trouble breathing.

• You have taken a shot of epinephrine after being bitten or stung, even if symptoms fail to appear.

Seek Care Immediately If . . .
• You are having trouble breathing, feel chest pain, or have a tight throat, even if you have taken a shot of epinephrine. **THIS IS AN EMERGENCY. Call 911 or 0 (operator)** to get to the nearest hospital or clinic. **Do not drive yourself!**

Insect Stings

WHAT YOU SHOULD KNOW

Most insect stings leave a painful or itchy red lump that may have a tiny hole in the center. Sometimes the stinger remains in the skin. Unless you are allergic to the stings, most cause no problems.

Causes
Mosquitoes, fleas, ticks, chiggers, bedbugs, ants, bees, wasps, spiders, or other insects all can leave annoying bites.

Signs/Symptoms
Typically, you'll find a red lump, often accompanied by pain, swelling, itching, or a rash. You may also have a fever, headache, or dizziness; and you may feel nauseated or throw up. If you develop chest pain, a tight feeling in your throat or chest, and trouble breathing **seek care immediately**. These are signs of a dangerous, even life-threatening, allergic reaction.

Care
If necessary, the doctor can recommend medicine for minor pain, swelling, or itching. Symptoms of an allergic reaction demand emergency treatment at a hospital. (See "Insect-Sting Allergy.")

WHAT YOU SHOULD DO

• Take the stinger out by scraping it off with your fingernail, the edge of a credit card, or a knife blade. Do not squeeze it.
• Wash the sting with soap and water, then put ice on it.
• Raise and rest the area of the sting.
• To help reduce swelling and itching, soak a clean washcloth or towel in cold water, wring it out, and put it on the sting. Leave it on for 10 to 20 minutes out of every hour.
• After 24 to 48 hours, a warm compress can be used to soothe the area and reduce swelling.

- To relieve pain, make a paste with water and either meat tenderizer or baking soda and rub it on the bite or sting for 5 minutes.
- To further reduce the itching and swelling, use over-the-counter medicines such as diphenhydramine elixir (be sure not to drink or drive while taking this medication) or hydrocortisone cream. If you are using calamine lotion with diphenhydramine do not take diphenhydramine by mouth at the same time.
- If you are allergic to insect stings and have a self-treatment kit, give yourself the shot of epinephrine (eh-pih-NEF-rin) immediately, without waiting for the rash, itching, or swelling to start. Then call your doctor right away to make sure you are out of danger.
- To keep from getting bitten or stung again follow the directions listed under "Insect-Sting Allergy."

Call Your Doctor If . . .
- Your symptoms do not improve in a few days.
- The area beyond the bite or sting becomes red, warm, tender, and swollen. These are signs of infection.
- You have a high temperature.

Seek Care Immediately If . . .
- You have symptoms of an allergic reaction (wheezing or trouble breathing, chest pain, fainting, raised red patches on the skin that itch, upset stomach, vomiting, cramping, or diarrhea). **THIS IS AN EMERGENCY!**

Insulin Reaction

WHAT YOU SHOULD KNOW

Insulin is used to reduce the amount of sugar in your blood. However, if your sugar level drops *too* low, you'll develop the symptoms of hypoglycemia, a potentially serious condition that is most common among insulin-dependent diabetics. The problem is often called an insulin reaction. Fortunately, prompt treatment will cure it.

Causes
You can drive down your blood sugar too far by missing a meal, eating too little, eating late, or exercising more vigorously than usual without eating extra food. Hypoglycemia can also be triggered by an infection, excessive doses of insulin, alcohol, and certain medicines.

Signs/Symptoms
Mild Signs Include: Headache, hunger, sweating, nervousness, problems staying focused, mood changes, and weakness.

Moderate Signs Include: Heavy sweating, increasing weakness, heart palpitations, memory loss, double vision, problems walking, and numbness in the area of the mouth and (possibly) the fingers.

Severe Signs Include: Seizures, fainting, muscle twitching, and passing urine unexpectedly.

Care
For mild hypoglycemia, you should drink a small glass of fruit juice, eat hard candy, or take a sugar tablet. A severe attack is an emergency. Make sure your family and friends know the signs and will get you to an emergency room if an attack occurs. They should **call 911 or 0 (operator)** for help.

WHAT YOU SHOULD DO

- If you have been treated at a hospital or doctor's office, a friend or relative will need to drive you home.
- In the future, check your blood sugar before driving.
- Make sure to keep your blood sugar at the level recommended by your doctor. If your blood sugar drops below this level, you must eat immediately. Call your doctor if you need more information on monitoring your blood sugar at home.
- Take orange or apple juice, sugar, or candies if you have any symptoms of low blood sugar. If you have time, check your blood sugar first.
- Keep sugar (such as candies) and glucagon in your car and home.
- Warn friends and family not to make you swallow anything if you pass out.
- Check with your doctor before you resume exercise.
- Eat regular meals and snacks using the diet suggested by your doctor.
- Do not drink alcohol. Alcohol may lower your blood sugar.

Call Your Doctor If . . .
- Your symptoms are not relieved by eating.
- You have repeated attacks of low blood sugar.

Seek Care Immediately If . . .
- You cannot get something to eat and you feel you are going to pass out. **THIS IS AN EMERGENCY!**

Intravenous Pyelogram

WHAT YOU SHOULD KNOW

An intravenous (IN-truh-VEEN-us) pyelogram (PIE-uh-lo-gram)—
also called an IVP—is a test that uses contrast dye to outline the kidneys, ureters (tubes that carry urine from the kidney to the bladder),
and bladder on an x-ray. The dye is administered through a vein.

Risks

The dye used in the test sometimes causes an allergic type of reaction.
However, if you follow your doctor's directions, you are not likely to
have problems.

IF YOU'RE HEADING FOR THE HOSPITAL . . .

Before You Go

• The day before your test, drink extra liquids.
• Your doctor will tell you when you must stop eating and drinking.
  DO NOT eat or drink after that time.
• You may be given a laxative to clean out your bowel. It should be
  taken the night before your test. You may also need an enema (EN-
  uh-muh) to clean out the bowel.

What to Expect While You're There

You may encounter the following procedures and equipment during
your stay:
• **Taking Your Vital Signs:** These include your temperature, blood
  pressure, pulse (counting your heartbeats), and respirations (counting your breaths). A stethoscope (steth-uh-scope) is used to listen to
  your heart and lungs. Your blood pressure is taken by wrapping a
  cuff around your arm.
• **During the Intravenous Pyelogram . . .**
  —You will need to lie on your back. An x-ray of your kidneys,
    ureters, and bladder may first be taken without dye.
  —A needle will be put into a vein in your arm or hand, and dye (also
    called contrast material) will be injected. You may feel warm
    and notice a salty taste in your mouth when the dye goes into
    your vein.
  —The first x-ray will be taken about 1 minute after the dye is
    injected. More x-rays will be taken after 5, 10, 15, 20, and 30 min-
    utes. Sometimes "moving" pictures called tomographs (TOME-
    o-graphs) are taken.
  —A band may be put across your abdomen and pulled tight. The

pressure closes off the ureters. This helps your doctor see how your kidneys are working.

—At the end of the test, you may be asked to urinate. Another x-ray will be taken to see if urine has stayed in your bladder.

—The test usually takes about 45 minutes to 1 hour.

After You Leave

• You should drink plenty of fluids (6 to 8 glasses a day) and resume your normal diet.

• You may resume your regular activities when you feel up to it.

Seek Care Immediately If . . .

• You have specks of blood in your urine.

• You are urinating less than usual, have nausea, or begin vomiting.

Ipecac

See Syrup of Ipecac

Iritis

WHAT YOU SHOULD KNOW

Iritis (eye-RYE-tis) is an irritation of the iris in your eye. It may appear suddenly without warning or may develop over a period of time. The problem usually affects only one eye and, with treatment, should clear up in a week or two.

Causes

Iritis usually starts as an infection in another part of the body that moves to the eye. It sometimes occurs as a result of a disease or an eye injury. Often the cause is unknown.

Signs/Symptoms

Typical symptoms include eye pain, redness, and blurred vision. Your eyes may tear more than usual, and you may develop an increased sensitivity to bright light.

Care

Your doctor may prescribe medicine to relieve the pain and irritation and treat any infection.

WHAT YOU SHOULD DO

- To ease the pain, apply a clean, warm or cool washcloth to your eye several times a day for 10 to 20 minutes.
- To help reduce pain and sensitivity to light, wear dark glasses, even when indoors, until treatment is finished.
- Your doctor may suggest you rest as much as possible for the first week or two after treatment begins. Sometimes bedrest is necessary.
- You may use over-the-counter medicines such as acetaminophen or ibuprofen to relieve pain. Take them exactly as directed.

Call Your Doctor If . . .
- You have any problems that may be related to the medicine you are taking.

Seek Care Immediately If . . .
- You have severe, throbbing eye pain and headaches.
- Your vision suddenly becomes blurred.
- You see halos around lights.
- Your eyeball is painful and hard to the touch.
- You become nauseated or start to vomit.

Irritable Bowel Syndrome

WHAT YOU SHOULD KNOW

Irritable bowel syndrome, also known as spastic colon or mucous colitis, is a problem that keeps stool from moving through the bowel (intestine) normally. The stool may move too slowly or too fast.

Causes
Not known for sure. The problem may occur because of stress, anxiety, or depression, or may be brought on by eating. However, it may not be possible to find out which food is the cause.

Signs/Symptoms
Often, the chief symptom is cramp-like pain that may go away when you move your bowels, or diarrhea that starts without warning. You also may not be able to move your bowels, or have pain when you do because the stool is hard and dry. Other symptoms include: headache, backache, or feeling sick to your stomach. You may not want to eat and may lose weight. You may feel tired, depressed, or anxious, or find it hard to think.

Care

May include tests to study your stool, an x-ray of your intestines, and an examination of your rectum. Medicines may be given to reduce any cramping you may feel or to relieve anxiety, gas, diarrhea, or constipation.

WHAT YOU SHOULD DO

- Your doctor may recommend over-the-counter medications to control your symptoms:
  —A stool softener to make the stool easier to pass, or—
  —Antidiarrhea medicine if the problem takes this form.
- Try to identify any foods that may cause flare-ups and avoid eating them. You may find it helpful to keep a diary of everything you eat and drink.
- Increasing fiber in your diet may help relieve symptoms. Good choices are whole grain breads, oatmeal or bran cereals, and fresh vegetables and fruits.
- Get plenty of rest.
- Try to reduce the amount of stress in your daily life. Take a short time-out period from stressful situations that occur during the day. Close your eyes and breathe deeply. Tense the muscles of your face, hold for a few seconds, then relax. Repeat this procedure with the muscles in your neck, shoulders, hands, stomach, back, and legs.
- Exercise at least 3 times a week.
- Don't smoke or use drugs or alcohol to relieve stress.

Call Your Doctor If . . .

- You have a high temperature.
- Your stool is black or contains blood or mucus.
- You lose 5 or more pounds without dieting.
- Your symptoms don't improve despite treatment.

Ischemic Heart Disease

See Coronary Artery Disease

IVP

See Intravenous Pyelogram

Jammed Finger

See Mallet Finger

Jaundice, Newborn

See Newborn Jaundice

Jaw Dislocation

See Dislocated Jaw

Jaw Fracture

See Broken Jaw

Ketoacidosis

See Diabetic Ketoacidosis

Kidney Failure, Acute

WHAT YOU SHOULD KNOW

Acute kidney failure (known medically as acute renal failure) is a very dangerous illness. The kidneys filter waste products from the blood and maintain the body's balance of fluid and minerals, discarding the waste in the urine. If this filtering process stops, poisons will build up in the blood. The disease may begin quickly and go away after treatment, or it may come and go repeatedly, creating a long-term problem.

Causes
The kidneys can be disrupted by blood infection, kidney injury, kidney stones, heart or liver disease, some medicines, dehydration, or a blockage in the arteries or veins that serve the kidneys.

Signs/Symptoms
Likely symptoms include reduced urination, nausea, vomiting, diarrhea, sleepiness, irritability, and loss of appetite. In addition, your skin may become dry and itchy, and bruise easily.

Care
You will need a stay in the hospital for tests and treatment.

Risks
Acute renal failure can be fatal. But prompt treatment lowers the risk of serious illness or death.

IF YOU'RE HEADING FOR THE HOSPITAL . . .

What to Expect While You're There

You may encounter the following procedures and equipment during your stay:

- **Taking Vital Signs:** These include your temperature, blood pressure, pulse (counting your heartbeats), and respirations (counting your breaths). A stethoscope is used to listen to your heart and lungs. Your blood pressure is taken by wrapping a cuff around your arm.

- **Foley Catheter:** This tube is threaded into your bladder so care givers can take exact measurements of the amount of urine your kidneys are producing.

- **KUB** (kidney-ureter-bladder) **X-ray:** This is a picture of your kidneys and ureters, the tubes that carry urine from the kidneys to your bladder. The doctor will use it to see if your kidneys or tubes are blocked.

- **Renal Ultrasound:** A painless test done while you are lying down. A device that projects sound waves will be used to build a picture of your kidneys on a TV-like screen.

- **Dialysis** (die-AL-uh-sis): You may be hooked up to a dialysis ("artificial kidney") machine. Dialysis washes your blood and removes extra water, chemicals, and waste products.

- **Blood:** Usually taken from a vein in your hand or from the bend in your elbow and sent to a laboratory for testing.

- **IV:** A tube placed in your vein for giving medicine or liquids. It will be capped or have tubing connected to it.

- **ECG:** Also called a heart monitor, an electrocardiograph (e-LEC-tro-CAR-dee-o-graf), or EKG. The patches on your chest are hooked up to a TV-type screen or a small portable box (telemetry unit). This screen shows a tracing of each heartbeat. Your heart will be watched for signs of injury or damage due to the problem with your kidneys.

- **Oxygen:** Your body may need extra oxygen at this time. It is given either by a mask or nasal prongs. Tell your doctor if the oxygen is drying out your nose or if the nasal prongs bother you.

- **Pulse Oximeter:** While you are getting oxygen, you may be hooked up to a pulse oximeter (ox-IM-uh-ter). It is placed on your ear, finger, or toe and is connected to a machine. It measures the oxygen in your blood.

- **Strict Intake/Output:** Your nurses will carefully monitor the amount of liquid you are getting and how much you are urinating.

- **Daily Weight:** You will be weighed daily.

- **Eating/Drinking:** If you have been throwing up, your stomach will

need rest. Because you will not be able to eat or drink until the vomiting has stopped, you will be fed all the vitamins and liquids you need through an IV.
- **Diet:** When you are able to eat, your doctor may put you on a special diet.
- **Activity:** You may need to rest in bed until you are feeling better.
- **Medicines:** May be given in your IV, as a shot, or by mouth. You may be given pain medication. If you have an infection, you'll also receive antibiotics.

After You Leave
- If your doctor prescribes an antibiotic, continue to take it until you have finished all the medicine, even if you feel well. If you stop too soon, some germs may survive, and the infection may come back. Take all medications exactly as directed.
- Your doctor may ask you to keep a daily record of your weight.
- Follow your doctor's advice about resting, eating and drinking liquids. You may be asked to write down the amount of liquid you drink, and how much you urinate.
- You may get information about acute renal failure from the **National Kidney Diseases Information Clearinghouse**, Box NKUDIC, Bethesda, MD 20893, (301) 468-6345, or by calling the **National Kidney Foundation** at 1-800-622-9010.

Call Your Doctor If . . .
- You are not eating or drinking, or are losing weight.
- You feel irritable or confused.
- You have a high temperature.
- You are urinating less.
- You have trouble breathing.
- Your muscles ache.

Seek Care Immediately If . . .
- You have chills, fever, nausea, or vomiting.
- You have an extremely high temperature.
- You are sleeping more than usual, and it's hard to wake up.
- You have blood in your stool or urine.
- You have blood coming from your nose, mouth, or ears for no clear reason.

Kidney Failure, Chronic

Kidney Failure, Chronic

WHAT YOU SHOULD KNOW

Kidney failure, also known as chronic renal failure (CRF), is a serious, long-term disease of the kidneys. In CRF, the kidneys lose some of their ability to filter body wastes from the blood and dispose of them in the urine.

Chronic renal failure may come on slowly and get worse with time; or problems may start suddenly in your kidneys, then get better with treatment. You may need care over a long period of time.

Causes
The kidneys' performance can be disrupted by high blood pressure, kidney disease, other diseases that affect the kidneys (such as diabetes and lupus), infection or blockage of the urinary system, and some medicines. In some cases, there may be a blockage in arteries leading to the kidneys.

Signs/Symptoms
Typically, you'll notice that you are urinating less than usual. You're likely to experience nausea, vomiting, and tiredness. You may develop shortness of breath, become irritable, notice a bad taste in your mouth, and lose your appetite. Other signs are confusion, headache, muscle aches, and numbness in the feet and legs. Your skin may become dry and itchy, and tend to bruise easily.

Care
Your doctor will run tests on your blood and urine. You will need rest, medicine, and a special diet. You may need a stay in the hospital for tests and treatment.

Risks
Left untreated, chronic renal failure can get worse and lead to death. If you suspect this problem, check with your doctor immediately.

WHAT YOU SHOULD DO

• Take any medicine prescribed by your doctor exactly as directed. If you feel it is not helping, call your doctor, but do not stop taking it on your own. If you are taking an antibiotic, finish the entire prescription even if you feel well. Ending treatment too soon can allow some of the germs to survive and re-infect you.
• Write down your weight daily.
• Follow your doctor's advice about resting, eating, and drinking liq-

uids. You may be asked to write down how much liquid you drink and how much you urinate. Your doctor may also put you on a special diet.

• For more information on kidney disease, contact the **National Kidney Diseases Information Clearinghouse**, Box NKUDIC, Bethesda, MD 20893, (301) 468-6345, or call the **National Kidney Foundation**, 1-800-622-9010.

Call Your Doctor If . . .
• You can't eat or drink and find that you are losing weight.
• You feel confused and irritated.
• Your urine output for a day is considerably less than normal.
• You are having breathing problems or muscle aches.
• You develop vomiting or diarrhea.

Seek Care Immediately If . . .
• You have a high temperature.
• You are sleeping more than usual, and find it hard to wake up.
• You notice specks of blood in your urine or stool.
• Blood is coming from your nose, mouth, or ears for no clear reason.
• You have a bad headache or a seizure.

IF YOU'RE HEADING FOR THE HOSPITAL . . .

What to Expect While You're There
You may encounter the following procedures and equipment during your stay:
• **Taking Your Vital Signs:** These include your temperature, blood pressure, pulse (counting your heartbeats), and respirations (counting your breaths). A stethoscope (steth-uh-scope) is used to listen to your heart and lungs. Your blood pressure is taken by wrapping a cuff around your arm.
• **Oxygen:** Your body may need extra oxygen at this time. It is given either by a mask or nasal prongs. Tell your doctor if the oxygen is drying out your nose or if the nasal prongs bother you.
• **Pulse Oximeter:** While you are getting oxygen, you may be hooked up to a pulse oximeter (ox-IM-uh-ter). It is placed on your ear, finger, or toe and is connected to a machine that measures the oxygen in your blood.
• **KUB (kidney-ureter-bladder) X-ray:** A picture of your kidneys and ureters (the tubes that carry urine from the kidneys to the bladder). The doctor will check the x-ray for blockages.
• **Renal Ultrasound:** A painless test in which sound waves are used

to make a picture of your kidneys on a TV-like screen. The test is performed while you are lying down.

- **Foley Catheter:** A tube inserted to drain the bladder.
- **Blood:** Usually taken from a vein in your hand or from the bend in your elbow and sent to a laboratory for testing.
- **IV:** A tube placed in your vein for giving medicine or liquids. It will be capped or have tubing connected to it.
- **Dialysis (die-AL-uh-sis):** You may be hooked up to a dialysis machine, also known as an "artificial kidney machine." It filters your blood and removes extra water, chemicals, and waste products.
- **ECG:** Also called a heart monitor, an electrocardiograph (e-LEC-tro-CAR-dee-o-graf), or EKG. Patches on your chest will be hooked up to a TV-type screen or a small portable box (telemetry unit). This screen shows a tracing of each heartbeat. Your heart will be watched for signs of injury or damage that could be related to your illness.
- **Strict Intake and Output:** Caregivers will closely watch how much liquid you are getting and how much you are urinating.
- **Weight:** You will be weighed daily.
- **Eating/Drinking:** If you have been vomiting, your stomach will be given a rest. You will get all the liquids and vitamins you need through your IV until you can eat normally.
- **Diet:** When you are able to eat, you may be put on a special diet. Your doctor will talk to you about foods you can take.
- **Activity:** You may need to rest in bed until you are feeling better.
- **Medicine:**
  —**Pain medicine** may be given in your IV, as a shot, or by mouth. If the pain does not go away or comes back, tell a doctor right away.
  —**Antibiotics** may be given by IV, in a shot, or by mouth to fight infection.
  —**Other medicines** may be used to control high blood pressure, nausea and vomiting, stomach acid, or constipation. Vitamins and minerals may also be necessary.

Kidney Stones

WHAT YOU SHOULD KNOW

Kidney stones are rock-like concretions of minerals that form in the kidney. There may be more than one stone, and they may be large or small. Men get kidney stones more often than women do.

Causes

An illness called gout can cause kidney stones, as can a blockage of urine or a large amount of calcium in the urine. Too much calcium from food, vitamins, or other sources can contribute to formation of the stones.

Signs/Symptoms

Typical symptoms include sharp mid-back pain, blood in the urine, painful urination, nausea, and vomiting.

Care

To help the stone pass, drink 3 quarts of water (the equivalent of 8 soda-size cans), each day. A heating pad set on "low" may help ease the pain. Your doctor may also prescribe pain medicine. If the stone doesn't pass naturally, you may need to be hospitalized

Risks

Kidney stones can cause long-term kidney problems that in rare cases can be fatal. But with proper treatment, serious problems are unlikely.

WHAT YOU SHOULD DO

- You may take over-the-counter aspirin, acetaminophen or ibuprofen. If your doctor prescribes another medicine to lessen pain, take it exactly as directed.
- Drink at least 8 to 10 glasses of water every day. This helps flush the stone through the urinary tract and will also help prevent other stones from forming.
- It is important that you strain your urine through a special strainer or through a piece of thin cloth every time you go to the bathroom so that you can catch the stone when it passes through your bladder. You may find it easier to urinate into a glass jar; when the stone passes, you'll be able to see it at the bottom of the jar. Save the stone and take it to your doctor for analysis.
- Keeping active may help the stone pass. Do not stay in bed; walk as much as possible.
- Stay home from work until the stone passes if you have a job in which sudden pain might be dangerous (for example, working around machinery, climbing ladders, or working on girders or roofs).
- You may need to change your diet, depending on the chemicals in your stone. Your doctor will prescribe the right diet after tests on the stone are completed.

Call Your Doctor If . . .
• You have any problems that may be related to the medicine you are taking.

Seek Care Immediately If . . .
• You have severe pain.
• You have nausea or start to vomit.
• You have a high temperature.
• You have stinging or burning when you pass urine, or feel a frequent urge to urinate. These are signs of infection.

IF YOU'RE HEADING FOR THE HOSPITAL . . .

What to Expect While You're There
You may encounter the following procedures and equipment during your stay:
• **Taking Your Vital Signs:** These include your temperature, blood pressure, pulse (counting your heartbeats), and respirations (counting your breaths). A stethoscope is used to listen to your heart and lungs. Your blood pressure is taken by wrapping a cuff around your arm.
• **IV:** A tube placed in your vein for giving medicine or liquids. It will be capped or have tubing connected to it.
• **Pain Medicine:** May be given by IV, shot, or by mouth. If the pain does not go away or comes back, tell a doctor right away.
• **Blood:** Usually taken from a vein in your hand or from the bend in your elbow and sent to a laboratory for testing.
• **Urine:** You will be asked to save your urine. It will be tested for blood and strained to catch any stones you may pass.
• **Abdominal X-ray:** This standard x-ray provides the doctor with a picture of the organs in your abdominal area.
• **Pelvic/Kidney Ultrasound:** This painless test is done while you are lying down. A dab of jelly-like lotion is placed on your belly. The person doing the test will gently move a small handle through the lotion and across your skin. A view of the internal organs appears on a TV-like screen attached to the handle.
• **IVP:** Also called intravenous pyelogram (in-truh-VEEN-us PIE-uh-lo-gram). In this test, dye injected through a vein is used to make an x-ray picture of your kidneys. You may feel warm after the dye is put in your IV.
• **CT Scan:** Also called a "CAT" scan. This x-ray uses a computer to make pictures of your kidneys.
• **Shock-Wave Lithotripsy** (LITH-oh-TRIP-see): This device sends

shock waves inside your body to break up the stone. The procedure is painless.
• **Surgery:** If the stone doesn't pass or lithotripsy doesn't work, you may need an operation to remove the stone.

Knee Arthroscopy

WHAT YOU SHOULD KNOW

Arthroscopy (arth-ROS-co-PEE) is an examination of the inside of a joint, such as a knee, using a surgical tool called an arthroscope (ARTH-row-scope) that is inserted into the joint through a small incision. An arthroscope is a small, soft tube with a light and lenses on the tip. Your doctor will perform this procedure if there's a possibility that your knee joint may be injured or diseased, or if you need to have bone or cartilage removed or tendons or ligaments repaired. After the arthroscopy, you may have some pain and swelling for a few days.

Risks
There is a chance that the procedure will cause bleeding, infection, or injury to another part of your knee. A problem in a leg vein could cause a blood clot to form.

IF YOU'RE HEADING FOR THE HOSPITAL . . .

Before You Go
• You will need to stop eating and drinking in preparation for this procedure. The doctor will tell you exactly when to begin fasting.

What to Expect While You're There
You may encounter the following procedures and equipment during your stay:
• **Taking Your Vital Signs:** These include your temperature, blood pressure, pulse (counting your heartbeats), and respirations (counting your breaths). A stethoscope is used to listen to your heart and lungs. Your blood pressure is taken by wrapping a cuff around your arm.
• **IV:** A tube placed in your vein for giving medicine or liquids. It will be capped or have tubing connected to it.
• **During Your Arthroscopy . . .**
  —You will be taken to the operating room. The hair around your knee will be shaved and the area will be scrubbed with soap and water.
  —You will need to lie still and move as little as possible during the procedure. Your doctor will give you numbing medicine, so you

will feel little pain. You may be put to sleep with anesthetic medication.

—An elastic bandage will be wrapped tightly around your right leg and foot. This helps drain blood from your leg. You may have a rubber cuff put around your right thigh to slow down the blood flow into your knee. Sometimes liquid is pumped into the knee joint to further decrease blood flow to the knee.

—Your doctor will make a small hole in the skin over your knee and put the arthroscope through it. The arthroscope may have to be inserted into a second area in your knee. During this part of the procedure, you may feel pressure or a thumping sensation.

—Your doctor may fix or remove tissue in the knee joint.

—When the arthroscope is taken out, your doctor will close the hole with sutures (a type of thread) and put a bandage on the wound.

—Your arthroscopy will take about 30 to 45 minutes. You may be given medicine to ease the pain.

After You Leave

• When you leave the hospital, you may still be drowsy from the medicine. Do not drive during this period.

• Stay off your feet as much as possible for 24 to 48 hours. Keep your leg raised on 2 pillows whenever possible for the next 2 days.

• For the first 24 hours, apply an ice pack to the area to reduce pain and swelling. Put ice in a plastic bag and place a towel between the bag of ice and your skin or the bandage. Keep the ice pack on your knee for up to 2 hours at a time.

• You will need to walk with crutches for one week; put as much weight on your knee as comfort permits.

• Keep your dressing dry and clean. After 4 days, remove the wrap and dressing.

• After your bandage is off, you may bathe or shower as usual. Wash the incision gently with soap and water.

• To prevent development of blood clots, move your legs often while resting in bed.

• You may begin drinking or eating as soon as you are up to it.

• Resume work and normal activity as soon as possible.

• Avoid vigorous exercise such as jogging or bicycling for 6 weeks after the procedure.

Call Your Doctor If . . .

• Swelling, drainage, or bleeding gets worse in the area of the incision.

• You develop signs of infection such as a headache, muscle aches, dizziness, or a generally ill feeling.
• You suffer really bad pain that is not helped by medicine.

Knee Injury

WHAT YOU SHOULD KNOW

Knee injuries can take the form of a sprain or a strain. Sprains result from suddenly stretching or tearing the ligaments that hold the bones together. A strain is an injury to the muscles or the tendons that connect the muscles to the bones. In most cases, either type of injury will take about 6 to 8 weeks to heal.

Causes
Sprains are usually caused by an accident, such as tripping, falling, or twisting the knee. Strains usually result from over-use.

Signs/Symptoms
Typically, there will be pain, tenderness, swelling, or bruising of the injured area. If the injury is serious, you may have trouble moving the knee.

Care
You'll probably need to wear a splint or ace bandage to keep the knee from moving. The doctor may take an x-ray of the area; and if you also injured the skin, you may need a tetanus shot.

WHAT YOU SHOULD DO

• Stay off your feet for 24 hours. After that, you can gradually increase the amount you use your injured knee when walking, as long as it doesn't hurt too much.
• Use crutches or a cane until it is no longer painful to put weight on the knee when you stand.
• Put ice on the injury for 15 to 20 minutes each hour for the first 1 to 2 days. Place the ice in a plastic bag and place a towel between the bag of ice and your skin.
• After the first 1 to 2 days, you may put heat on the injury to help ease the pain. Use a heating pad (set on low), a whirlpool bath, or warm, moist towels for 15 to 20 minutes every hour for 48 hours.
• To rest your knee and allow it to heal, wear your splint or elastic bandage (ace wrap) as directed by your doctor.
• You can loosen or tighten the splint or bandage to make it more comfortable. It should be tight enough to provide support, but not so

tight that it causes numbness or tingling in your toes. If you are wearing an ace bandage, take it off and rewrap it once a day.
- You may take over-the-counter medications to relieve the pain. If the doctor prescribes any medicine, take it exactly as directed. If it makes you drowsy, don't drive.
- If you have been given a tetanus shot, your arm may get swollen, red, and warm to the touch at the shot site. This is a normal reaction to the medicine.

Call Your Doctor If . . .
- The bruising, pain, or swelling grows worse.
- The skin on your lower leg turns white or blue and feels cool to the touch.

Knee Joint Replacement

WHAT YOU SHOULD KNOW

In knee joint replacement (also called total knee replacement), the surgeon removes a badly damaged knee joint and installs an artificial one. Medically, the new joint is known as a prosthesis (prahs-THEE-sis), an artificial or man-made device made of metal or a mixture of metal and plastic. The surgery is performed to relieve pain and restore movement in people who have severe osteoarthritis or rheumatoid arthritis of the knee, or disabling injuries to this important joint. Most knee replacements are totally successful. If you have this operation, allow at least 3 to 5 months to recover your strength and energy.

Risks
Without treatment, the pain and stiffness may continue and get worse.

IF YOU'RE HEADING FOR THE HOSPITAL . . .

Before You Go
- Your doctor will tell you when on the night before surgery you must stop eating and drinking. Follow these directions exactly.
- You may take pills with a sip of water the morning of surgery.
- Follow your doctor's instructions about when to stop taking aspirin or ibuprofen before the operation.
- To assure a good night's rest, you may be given a sleeping pill to take the night before surgery.

When You Arrive
- You will be taught how to cough and breathe deeply to reduce your chances of getting a lung infection after surgery.

- Before surgery, you may be taught special exercises to help make your knee stronger. You will also learn how to roll from side to side after the surgery and how to use a trapeze bar to move yourself around in bed.
- An anesthesiologist (AN-is-THEE-se-OL-o-gist) will put you to sleep just before the operation. This doctor may come and talk to you the day before surgery.
- You may need to have your knee cleaned with a special liquid before going to the operating room. The medication in this liquid may make your skin yellow, but will come off easily.

What to Expect While You're There
You may encounter the following procedures and equipment during your stay.

- **Taking Your Vital Signs:** These include your temperature, blood pressure, pulse (counting your heartbeats), and respirations (counting your breaths). A stethoscope is used to listen to your heart and lungs. Your blood pressure is taken by wrapping a cuff around your arm.
- **Oxygen:** May be given to you during surgery. You may also need extra oxygen as you are waking up after the operation.
- **Pulse Oximeter:** You may be hooked up to a pulse oximeter (ox-IM-uh-ter). This device is placed on your ear, finger, or toe and is connected to a machine that measures the oxygen in your blood.
- **Blood:** Usually taken from a vein in your hand or from the bend in your elbow and sent to a laboratory for testing.
- **IV:** A tube placed in your vein for giving medicine or liquids. It will be capped or have tubing connected to it.
- **Chest X-ray:** This is a picture of your lungs and heart. The doctors use it to see how your heart and lungs are doing before surgery.
- **Before Surgery:** You may be given medicine to make you sleepy before you are taken to the operating room.
- **ET Tube:** During surgery, you may have a tube placed in either your mouth or nose. This tube goes into your trachea (windpipe). The ET tube serves two purposes: It protects your trachea during surgery and it allows your doctor to give you oxygen when you need it. After the tube is taken out, you may have a sore throat for a while.
- **After Surgery:** You will be taken to a special unit until you wake up. When you wake up or are close to waking up you will be taken back to your room. You will have a bandage and maybe a splint over your knee where the operation was performed.
- **Activity:** You will need to rest in bed until your doctor says you may get up. Otherwise you may damage your knee.

- **ECG:** Also called a heart monitor, an electrocardiograph (e-LEC-tro-CAR-dee-o-graf), or EKG. The patches on your chest are hooked up to a TV-type screen or a small portable box (telemetry unit). This screen shows a tracing of each heartbeat. Your heart will be watched to make sure your body is handling your surgery well. It will also be monitored for signs of injury or damage during surgery.
- **Turning:** You must turn in a special way after surgery and you will need to use pillows between your legs to keep the one that was operated on from moving in the direction of the other leg.
- **Physical Therapy:** Sometime after surgery, a physical therapist will teach you special exercises to strengthen the knee and improve its movement.
- **Pressure Stockings:** After the operation, you may need to wear these special stockings on both legs or on just the leg that was operated on. You may be given stockings that tighten first on one leg and then the other, or you may wear a special pair of tight socks. These are needed during long periods of immobility to keep the blood from pooling in the legs and causing clots.
- **Medicines:**
  —**Antibiotics** may be prescribed to prevent infection following the surgery. They may be given by IV, in a shot, or by mouth.
  —**Blood Thinners** such as heparin, warfarin, or aspirin may be given to prevent blood clots, especially if you will be resting in bed for a long time.
  —**Pain Medicine** may be given in your IV, as a shot, or by mouth. If the pain does not go away or comes back, tell a doctor right away.
  —**Anti-Nausea Medicine** may be prescribed if your pain medication upsets your stomach or makes you vomit.

After You Leave
- Always take your medicine as directed by your doctor. If you feel it is not helping, call your doctor, but do not stop taking it on your own.
- If your doctor has prescribed antibiotics, finish all the medication even if you feel well. Ask your doctor if you need to take antibiotics before seeing your dentist.
- If you are taking medicine that makes you drowsy, do not drive or use heavy equipment.
- You will need to use crutches for walking for the first 6 to 12 weeks. Then you may slowly start walking without crutches or a cane.
- You may also need to wear a knee brace or splint for a while to protect your knee and keep it from moving too much while it heals. You

may take it off to shower or bathe. If your toes feel numb and tingly, loosen it.
- For the next 3 months, you must be careful about how you move or place your leg.
  —Do not cross your legs when you are sitting, lying, or standing.
  —Keep your leg facing forward at all times, even in bed. Never turn your knee outward or inward.
  —Put a pillow between your legs when you lie down on the side opposite the operation.
- Do not sit on low chairs, low stools, or low toilet seats. Do not use reclining chairs. You may need a firm cushion to raise chair seats. You may want to rent or buy a raised toilet seat. This will help to prevent you from putting too much strain on the knee.
- Sit only in chairs that have arms. When you get up from a chair, move to the edge, then hold the chair arms and push yourself up. While getting up, keep the leg that was operated on in front of the other one and push up with the good leg.
- After you've recovered, it is usually all right to swim, play golf, walk, and bicycle; but avoid exercises that repeatedly jar the knee joint, such as tennis and jogging.
- Do not drive until your doctor gives you the go-ahead.
- Until you are completely back on your feet, you may need to wear support socks to help reduce swelling in your legs.

Call Your Doctor If . . .
- You have fever, swelling, or redness at your surgery site.
- The pain in your knee increases or you have trouble moving around.

Seek Care Immediately If . . .
- You fall and injure the knee.
- You suddenly have trouble breathing.
- Your leg or toes feel numb, tingly, or cool to the touch, or turn pale or blue.

Knee Sprain or Strain

See Knee Injury

Labor, Early Signs of

See Early Labor Signs

Labyrinthitis

WHAT YOU SHOULD KNOW

Labyrinthitis (LAB-uh-rin-THIE-tis) is an inflammation of the inner ear canal that helps you control your balance. Labyrinthitis is not a serious illness and produces no long-term problems. With treatment, the problem should clear up in 1 to 6 weeks.

Causes
Labyrinthitis is usually caused by a viral infection. Other causes include bacterial infection, head injury, allergies, and certain medicines. Sometimes no cause can be found.

Signs/Symptoms
The signature symptom is dizziness (vertigo) that gets worse when you move your head. You may have a spinning sensation, feel nauseated, hear ringing in your ears, or suffer hearing loss. You may not be able to control the movement of your eyes, and your balance may be affected.

Care
Resting quietly may help. For some infections, the doctor may prescribe antibiotics. For stubborn cases, surgery may be needed.

WHAT YOU SHOULD DO

- Rest in bed. Keep your head as still as possible until the dizziness clears up. Walk with help until you are sure you can walk without falling. Slowly resume your normal activities.
- Reduce your salt and fluid intake. Do not add extra salt to foods. Avoid carbonated beverages that contain sodium.
- Stay at home and do not drive or work around machinery until the dizziness disappears.

Call Your Doctor If . . .
- You develop a high temperature.
- You notice decreased hearing in either ear.
- You develop vomiting that will not stop.
- You have new or unexplained symptoms that may be caused by your medicine.

Seek Care Immediately If . . .
- You begin to have seizures or fainting spells.

Lacerations

Laceration is the medical term for a cut. It may be large or small and may bleed a lot or a little. If a laceration bleeds a great deal with no sign of stopping, it needs to be closed with stitches. You may also need stitches to keep the wound from becoming infected and to reduce the scarring that may develop after it has healed. If the wound is too old, stitching it may not be possible. Some lacerations actually heal better without stitches.

The healing time for a laceration depends on its location. For instance, a cut on the leg usually heals more slowly than one on the head. Stitches are usually removed within 5 days to 2 weeks. The cut will continue to heal for up to 6 months.

Causes
Typically, a blow from a sharp object sustained in a fall or an accident.

Signs/Symptoms
Symptoms include bleeding, pain, numbness, and swelling of the injured skin.

Care
The doctor will clean the laceration and examine it carefully. If it is very painful, you may be given numbing medicine before any procedures are performed. If stitches are necessary, your doctor will tell you how to take care of them. You will need to see your doctor again to have them removed. You may also need a tetanus shot if you have not had one in a long time.

WHAT YOU SHOULD DO

• Keep your bandage clean and dry. If the bandage gets wet and needs to be changed, unwrap it slowly and carefully. If it sticks or starts to hurt, use water to loosen it gently. Pat the area dry with a clean towel before putting on another bandage. Keep the wound bandaged until your doctor instructs you to stop.
• If possible, keep the wound lifted above the level of your heart for 24 to 48 hours. This reduces pain and swelling and helps healing.
• Clean the wound gently 3 to 4 times a day:
  —Flush an open wound thoroughly with clean water. Wash the area around the wound with soap and water or a cotton swab dipped in a mixture of half water and half hydrogen peroxide.

—If you have a cut on your mouth or lip, rinse your mouth after meals and at bedtime. Ask your doctor what to use as a rinse.
• If you have a scalp wound, you may wash your hair gently after you get home. Keep your hair dry until the day you are to have your stitches removed, then wash it gently before seeing the doctor.
• Do not soak the wound or go swimming. If the wound is on your hand or lower arm, avoid washing dishes.
• If you are given a tetanus shot, your arm may get swollen, red, and warm to the touch at the site of the shot. This is a normal reaction to the medicine.

Call Your Doctor If . . .
• The wound keeps bleeding.
• You have a high temperature.
• Pain in the wound gets worse and won't stop.
• You have signs of infection (redness, swelling, pus, a bad smell, or red streaks leading from the wound).
• You have numbness or swelling below the wound, or you cannot move the joint below the wound.

Laminectomy

See Lumbar Laminectomy

Laryngitis

WHAT YOU SHOULD KNOW

Laryngitis (LAIR-in-JIE-tis) is an irritation and swelling of the voice box and the area around it. It may cause your voice to change, or you may lose your voice entirely for a short while. The problem is most common in late fall, winter, or early spring. With or without treatment, you should be well in 7 to 14 days.

Causes
Laryngitis is usually caused by a virus or by bacteria. People who smoke, have allergies, or strain their voices by yelling, talking, or singing may also come down with the problem.

Signs/Symptoms
The classic symptoms are a hoarse, low voice, and a scratchy throat. You also might lose your voice, develop a sore throat, come down with a fever, feel you have a lump in your throat, or feel very tired.

Care

Your doctor may prescribe an antibiotic to treat any infection.

WHAT YOU SHOULD DO

- Do not use your voice for several days. Either speak very softly or write notes until you can talk normally.
- Use a cool-mist humidifier (vaporizer) to increase air moisture and help relieve the tight feeling in your throat. Hot, steamy showers can also help.
- Do not drink alcohol or smoke until your voice is back to normal.
- Get plenty of rest.
- Drink extra fluids, such as water, fruit juice, and tea.

Call Your Doctor If . . .

- You develop a high temperature.
- Hoarseness lasts longer than 7 days.
- You have bleeding from the throat.
- Your throat feels worse.
- You have large, tender lumps in your neck.

Seek Care Immediately If . . .

- You have difficulty breathing.
- You have trouble swallowing and begin to drool.

Laryngotracheobronchitis

See Croup

Leg Fracture

See Broken Leg

Lice, Head

See Head Lice

Lice, Pubic

See Crabs

Ligament Sprain

See Sprained Ligament

Lightning Strike

WHAT YOU SHOULD KNOW

A lightning strike sends a strong electrical charge either through the body or over its surface. If it hits you or something close to you, lightning can cause serious injury. You may get burned if you have any metal on your body (a belt buckle, a zipper, or coins, for example). After a mild lightning injury, you will usually feel better within hours or days. A severe injury, however, can cause lasting damage to the brain, nerves, eyes, or ears, and may even be fatal.

To avoid being struck by lightning, stay away from anything made from metal, such as wire fences, umbrellas, pipelines, metal clotheslines, and golf clubs, during an electrical storm. Also avoid standing near trees, in a clearing, or on a hilltop.

Signs/Symptoms

In some cases, you may be hit by lightning and not even know it. A mild strike may cause pain, headache, confusion, tingling, numbness, or weakness, sometimes accompanied by difficulties with vision, hearing, and memory. In a severe strike, the blast of electricity may tear the clothing or shoes from your body. Burns may not be visible at first, but may appear hours later. You may have broken bones, and if the heart is severely injured, it may stop.

Care

For anything more than a mild injury, **call 911 or 0 (operator) for help.** A severe lightning injury is an **EMERGENCY.** The victim may need CPR if the heartbeat or breathing has stopped. Hospitalization is needed for tests and treatment.

Even if the injury is mild, you should check with your doctor. You may need medicine for pain and swelling, and the doctor may feel you need a tetanus shot.

IF YOU'RE HEADING FOR THE HOSPITAL . . .

What to Expect While You're There

You may encounter the following procedures and equipment during your stay:

- **Taking Vital Signs:** These include your temperature, blood pressure, pulse (counting your heartbeats), and respirations (counting your breaths). A stethoscope is used to listen to your heart and lungs. Your blood pressure is taken by wrapping a cuff around your arm.
- **Oxygen:** Your body may need extra oxygen at this time. It is given

either by a mask or nasal prongs. Tell your doctor if the oxygen is drying out your nose or if the nasal prongs bother you.

• **Pulse Oximeter:** While you are getting oxygen, you may be hooked up to a pulse oximeter (ox-IM-uh-ter). It is placed on your ear, finger, or toe and is connected to a machine. It measures the oxygen in your blood.

• **IV:** A tube placed in your vein for giving medicine or liquids. It will be capped or have tubing connected to it.

• **Blood:** Usually taken for tests from a vein in your hand or from the bend in your elbow.

• **Blood Gases:** For this test blood is taken from an artery in your wrist, elbow, or groin. It is tested to see how much oxygen it contains.

• **Chest X-ray:** This picture of your lungs and heart will help the doctor find any damage that may have occurred.

• **CT Scan:** (Also called a "CAT" scan.) This computerized x-ray is also used to detect internal injuries.

• **ECG:** (Also called a heart monitor, an electrocardiograph [e-LEC tro-CAR-dee-o-graf], or EKG.) Patches on your chest are hooked up to a TV-type screen or a small portable box (telemetry unit). This screen shows a tracing of each heartbeat. The heart is controlled by electrical currents, so the doctor will watch it closely.

• **EEG:** (Also called an electroencephalogram [e-LEC-tro-en-SEF-uh-lo-gram].) This is a brainwave study. Electricity can have drastic effects on the brain, so this test will also be carefully examined.

• **ET Tube:** A tube inserted through either the mouth or nose and down into the windpipe. It is often hooked up to a breathing machine. You will not be able to talk while the tube is in place.

• **Ventilator:** A special machine used to help with breathing.

• **Foley Catheter:** A tube put into the bladder to drain the urine. The catheter will be removed when you can urinate on your own.

• **Strict Intake/Output:** Care givers will carefully watch how much liquid you are getting and how much you are urinating.

• **Neuro Signs:** Care givers will look at your eyes, see how easily you awaken, and check your memory to help them determine how well your brain is functioning.

After You Leave

• Your doctor may ask you to see an eye or an ear doctor. You may need to make an appointment with a neurologist who will check you for long-term damage to your brain or nerves.

• To lessen pain and swelling of burns, keep the injured area raised above the level of your heart as much as possible. Do not use the injured area too much until it heals.

- If you have a bandage, keep it clean and dry.
- To change the bandage:
  —Unwrap it slowly and carefully. If it sticks, soak it in warm water.
  —Rinse the wound off and pat it dry with a clean towel.
- Your doctor will tell you how long to leave the bandage on.
- Clean the wound 2 to 3 times a day with mild soap and water or a solution of half hydrogen peroxide and half water.
- To clean mouth and lip wounds, rinse your mouth after meals and at bedtime with a product suggested by your doctor. Do NOT swallow the mixture.
- For scalp wounds:
  —You may wash your hair gently after you get home.
  —After that, keep your hair dry until the day you have your stitches removed.
- Ask your doctor when to return for a wound check and when to have your stitches removed.
- If you have an eye patch, leave it on until your doctor says it is safe to remove it.
- If you are given a tetanus shot, your arm may get swollen, red, and warm to the touch at the site of the injection. This is a normal response to the medicine in the shot.

Call Your Doctor If . . .
- You have increasing pain, blurred vision, trouble hearing, worsening headaches, numbness or tingling in your arms or legs, or increasing weakness—even long after the injury. Some of these problems may not show up right away.
- You develop a rapid heartbeat, your heart skips beats, or you have chest pain.

Seek Care Immediately If . . .
- You cannot move your arms or legs, lose your vision, lose consciousness, or have sudden or severe headaches.

Low Back Pain

See Back Pain

Low Blood Sugar

WHAT YOU SHOULD KNOW

If there isn't enough sugar in your blood to give your muscles and brain cells the energy they need to work, the condition is known as low blood sugar, or hypoglycemia.

Causes
Skipping meals and over-exercising can trigger hypoglycemia. The problem can also be caused by an oversupply of insulin, the natural hormone that helps transport sugar from your blood to your muscle and tissue cells. Hypoglycemia is also associated with stomach surgery, certain medicines, alcohol, liver disease, pregnancy, and high fever.

Signs/Symptoms
The problem is usually signaled by sweating, shaking, hunger, weakness, faintness, and nervousness, often accompanied by a headache. Other possible symptoms include confusion and sometimes even convulsions.

WHAT YOU SHOULD DO

- Your symptoms can be controlled by changes in your diet:
  —Eat 6 or 7 small meals a day at regular intervals. Don't skip meals.
  —Eat foods low in carbohydrates (starch and sugar) and high in protein.
  —Fruits, vegetables, cereals, potatoes, and breads should contribute the carbohydrates in your diet.
  —Between meals, eat snacks such as eggs, chicken, nuts, cheese, or skim milk.
  —Avoid eating sugar, sweetened desserts, jelly, jams, honey, syrup, candy, sweetened fruits, and soft drinks.
- Alcoholic beverages can trigger hypoglycemia, particularly when taken on an empty stomach. Be very careful about your intake if you are prone to low blood sugar.
- If you have frequent attacks, don't drive or operate heavy machinery.

Call Your Doctor If . . .
- You develop the symptoms of low blood sugar.

Lower GI Endoscopy

See Colonoscopy and Sigmoidoscopy

Low Potassium

WHAT YOU SHOULD KNOW

Potassium plays a crucial role in the body, regulating heartbeat and other critical functions. Low levels of potassium—known medically as hypokalemia (HI-poh-kah-LEE-me-uh) can be dangerous and potentially fatal.

Causes

Among the many causes of hypokalemia are vomiting, diarrhea, and kidney disease. Potassium supplies can also be depleted by certain medicines (especially water pills), heavy sweating during exercise, and lack of sufficient potassium in your diet.

Signs/Symptoms

You're likely to develop muscle cramps and weakness, accompanied by thirst and a great deal of urination. Your heart may begin to skip beats— **a very dangerous sign.**

Care

If your potassium is not too low, you may be able to clear up the condition by eating high-potassium foods such as potatoes with skin, bananas, and spinach. In some cases, you may have to take potassium supplements in pill or powder form. If your potassium is extremely low, you may need to be hospitalized so that you can be given blood tests and intravenous potassium.

Do's and Don'ts

If you are taking digitalis for a heart problem or are on water pills, make sure to get your blood tested regularly.

WHAT YOU SHOULD DO

- Be careful to take all your medicines exactly as directed. If you suspect that any of them are causing a problem, let your doctor know about it immediately; but don't stop taking them on your own.
- Along with your normal diet, eat foods that have potassium in them.

- You may continue your normal activities when you feel better.
- Learn to count your pulse at your wrist or your neck, especially if you are taking water pills or digitalis.
- Teach your relatives how to count your heartbeats also.

Call Your Doctor If . . .
- You feel weak or faint.
- You cannot stop vomiting or have lasting diarrhea.

Seek Care Immediately If . . .
- You cannot move your arms or legs.
- Your heart is skipping beats or you have chest pain. This may be life-threatening. Call **911 or 0 (operator)**. **DO NOT** drive yourself to the hospital.

Lumbar Laminectomy

WHAT YOU SHOULD KNOW

A lumbar laminectomy (LAM-in EC-tow-me), also called a discectomy is the removal of a disc (or a piece of it) from the lower (lumbar) part of your spine. A disc, which functions as a shock absorber between the bones in the spine (vertebrae), is a tough sac filled with a jelly-like substance. The disc is usually removed when the cover of the sac weakens and the contents leak or bulge out. When this happens, the disc may press on a nerve or the spinal cord, causing back pain.

Choices
There are several ways of doing this operation; and there are a variety of alternative treatments for back problems, ranging from physical therapy to acupuncture. Be sure to ask the doctor for all the options that may work for you.

Risks
Without treatment, your back problem could get worse. If the disk damages a nerve, you could have trouble moving.

IF YOU'RE HEADING FOR THE HOSPITAL . . .

Before You Go

• Rest as much as possible to reduce your pain. You may get up to go to the bathroom.

• Do not lift heavy objects.

• You may find that sleeping on your side with your knees and hips bent is more comfortable than sleeping on your back or stomach.

• A few days before the operation, your doctor will probably tell you to stop taking over-the-counter pain killers such as aspirin or ibuprofen.

• Before the surgery, you may need to talk to the anesthesiologist (AN-is-THEE-se-OL-o-gist) who will put you to sleep during the operation.

• You may be given a sleeping pill the night before surgery.

• You will need to stop eating and drinking sometime before the operation; your doctor will tell you exactly when this is necessary.

• If you take pills, swallow them with only a sip of water on the day of surgery.

• You may need to have the skin on your back cleaned with soap before going to surgery. The soap may make the skin yellow, but the stain will come off easily.

What to Expect While You're There

You may encounter the following procedures and equipment during your stay.

• **Taking Your Vital Signs:** These include your temperature, blood pressure, pulse (counting your heartbeats), and respirations (counting your breaths). A stethoscope is used to listen to your heart and lungs. Your blood pressure is taken by wrapping a cuff around your arm.

• **Oxygen:** Your body may need extra oxygen at this time. It is given either by a mask or nasal prongs. Tell your doctor if the oxygen is drying out your nose or if the nasal prongs bother you.

• **Pulse Oximeter:** You may be hooked up to a pulse oximeter (ox-IM-uh-ter). It is placed on your ear, finger, or toe and is connected to a machine that measures the oxygen in your blood.

• **IV:** A tube placed in your vein for giving medicine or liquids. It will be capped or have tubing hooked up to it.

• **Blood:** Usually taken from a vein in your hand or from the bend in your elbow and sent to a laboratory for testing.

• **Chest X-ray:** This picture of your lungs and heart is used to check for problems before and after surgery.

- **ECG:** Also called a heart monitor, an EKG, or an electrocardio-graph (e-LEC-tro-CAR-dee-o-graf). The pads on your chest are hooked up to a TV-type screen or a small portable box (telemetry unit). This screen shows a tracing of each heartbeat. Your heart will be watched for signs of injury or damage that could be related to the operation.
- **ET Tube:** This tube is inserted through the mouth or nose and ad-vanced into the windpipe. It is often hooked up to a breathing ma-chine. While the tube is in place, you will not be able to talk.
- **Breathing Deeply and Coughing:** After surgery, it is important to do this often to prevent a lung infection.
- **Blood Transfusion:** May be given to you if you need more blood.
- **Neuro Signs:** After surgery, nurses routinely check your eyes, see how easily you awaken, and test your memory to make sure your nervous system is functioning normally.
- **Activity:** After surgery, you will be encouraged to turn from side to side while lying in bed. When you turn, keep a pillow between your legs and move your whole body at the same time. Your doctor can show you how to do this. Do not sit except when using the toilet. You may be asked to walk as early as the day after surgery, but do not get out of bed until you are given the go-ahead.
- **Pressure Stockings:** You may need to wear these special stockings for a while after the operation. They prevent blood from collecting in your legs and causing clots.
- **Cold and Heat:** Place a cool towel or heating pad (set on low) on the area that hurts to ease the pain. Do not lie on the heating pad; it can burn you if you do.
- **Strict Intake and Output:** Nurses will carefully watch how much liquid you are getting and how much you are urinating.
- **Medicines:**
  - **Before surgery,** you may be given medicine to make you sleepy before you are taken to the operating room.
  - **Pain medicine** may be given in your IV, as a shot, or by mouth. If the pain does not go away or comes back, tell a doctor right away.
  - **Antibiotics** may be given by IV, in a shot, or by mouth to fight infection.
  - **Anti-nausea medicine** will be given if you are troubled with vomiting after the operation. This will help prevent you from losing so much water that your body becomes dehydrated.

After You Leave

- Be sure that you have a firm mattress. When lying on your back, place 2 or 3 pillows under your knees and the lower part of your legs to elevate them. When lying on your side, bend your knees and use a small pillow under your head and neck to keep from straining your shoulders, neck, and arms. DO NOT lie on your stomach.
- Move your legs often when resting in bed to keep from getting clots in your legs.
- You may use an electric heating pad (set on low) or a warm towel to ease the pain at the site of the surgery. Do not lie on the heating pad or use it when you are sleeping; you could burn yourself.
- When you sit down, put your feet on a footstool so your knees are at the level of your hips or higher.
- When you stoop down to pick things up from the floor, bend your knees and keep your back straight. Do not bend from the hips.
- Do not get up and move around too much at first. Limit the number of times you go up and down stairs each day.
- During the first weeks after surgery, ride in a car as little as possible; the motion of the car may cause your back to hurt. Your doctor will tell you how soon you may start driving again.
- Do not carry or lift anything heavier than 5 pounds until your doctor says it is all right to do so.
- Your doctor will tell you when you can resume strenuous physical activity.
- You may resume having sex as soon as it does not cause pain.
- You may shower or bathe after the site of your surgery (incision) has healed. Have a family member check your incision every day for drainage or redness.

Call Your Doctor If . . .

- Redness or yellow drainage appears at the incision.
- Pain at the incision site increases.
- You develop signs of infection such as headache, muscle aches, dizziness, a generally ill feeling, and fever.
- You feel weakness, numbness, or pain in your back, buttocks, or legs.

Seek Care Immediately If . . .

- You suddenly have trouble breathing or get a really bad chest pain.
- You cannot control your bladder or bowels.

Lumbar Puncture

See Spinal Tap

Lung, Collapsed

See Collapsed Lung

Lyme Disease

WHAT YOU SHOULD KNOW

Lyme disease is an infection spread by ticks. It starts as a small bump from the bite and may turn into a rash after a few days or weeks. If not treated early, it may spread to other parts of the body.

Causes

A recently discovered germ named *Borrelia burgdorferi* is the cause. It is spread only by tick bites, and cannot be passed from one person to another. The ticks that spread Lyme disease usually live on deer, rabbits, and mice, but also can be found on dogs. Infections are most frequent in the late spring and summer. You can get sick anywhere from 3 days to a month after being bitten. Some people don't remember the bite.

Signs/Symptoms

Soon after an infected bite, a small red bump appears and then grows bigger, usually with a clear area in the middle that looks like a bull's-eye. You may develop other symptoms that seem like the flu, including muscle pain, headache, stiff neck, fever, chills, and tiredness. Weeks, months, or even years later, you may develop joint pain and eye, heart, or nerve problems.

Care

The doctor may need to order blood tests to make sure you have the disease. Antibiotics are prescribed to cure the infection. Medicine for pain, irritation, and swelling may be given, if needed. Early treatment is important. The sooner you are treated, the better your chances of full recovery.

WHAT YOU SHOULD DO

- Take antibiotics exactly as directed until they are all gone. Don't stop taking them when you begin to feel better. Some of the germs may still be alive.
- Rest in bed until you feel well. You may then go back to work or school.
- To avoid tick bites:
  —During tick season, stay out of woods and fields likely to have ticks, if possible.
  —In the woods, wear long pants, socks pulled up over the bottom of your pants legs, and shirts with long sleeves. Keep your shirt tucked in. Use a lotion or spray to keep bugs and ticks away.
  —Check for ticks every 2 to 3 hours while you are out and again after you go inside. Be sure to check your head, neck, armpits, and crotch. Also check your pets for ticks and have them wear tick collars.
  —If you find a tick, take it off with a pair of tweezers. Don't use your fingers. Hold the tick behind the head and slowly pull it out. Ticks that are taken off within 18 hours are not likely to cause Lyme disease.

Call Your Doctor If . . .
- You get any new symptoms.
- You have a rash, itching, or swelling after taking your medicine.

Seek Care Immediately If . . .
- You get a stiff neck, really bad headache, shortness of breath, or a fast heartbeat.

Lymphadenopathy

See Swollen Lymph Nodes

Mallet Finger

WHAT YOU SHOULD KNOW

A mallet finger (also called a jammed finger) occurs when the tendon in the finger is stretched or torn, or the bone attached to the tendon is broken off. (Tendons are the tissues that connect muscle to bone.) It may take from 4 to 8 weeks for the injury to heal.

Causes

Jamming the end of the finger against an object or hitting it on something is the usual cause. The injury often results when a ball hits the end of a straight finger.

Signs/Symptoms

Swelling, pain, and redness of the injured area are typical signs. You will also have difficulty moving the finger. The fingertip often will droop.

Care

You may need to have your finger x-rayed; and you will probably need to wear a splint to prevent the finger from moving while it heals. Surgery is sometimes necessary.

WHAT YOU SHOULD DO

- Apply ice to the injury for 15 to 20 minutes each hour for the first 1 to 2 days. Put the ice in a plastic bag and place a towel between the bag of ice and your skin.
- After the first 1 to 2 days, you may put heat on the injury to help ease the pain. Use a heating pad (set on low), a whirlpool bath, or warm, moist towels for 15 to 20 minutes every hour for 48 hours.
- For the first 48 hours, keep your arm lifted above the level of your heart whenever possible to reduce pain and swelling.
- If you are given a finger splint, continue to wear it until your doctor says you no longer need it.
  —You may remove the splint each day to wash your finger.
  —When your splint is off, do not try to bend the tip of your finger.
  —Put the splint back on as soon as possible. If your finger is numb or tingling, the splint is probably too tight. You can loosen it for comfort.
- Several times a day, move the part of the finger not covered by the splint.
- Over-the-counter medications may be used for pain.
- If you have been given a tetanus shot, your arm may get swollen, red, and warm to the touch at the site of the shot. This is a normal reaction to the medicine.

Call Your Doctor If . . .

- The pain or swelling is getting worse.
- The finger becomes more swollen and turns very red.
- The finger feels numb, tingly, or cold, or turns white or blue.
- You lose your splint.

Mammogram

WHAT YOU SHOULD KNOW

A mammogram (MAM-o-gram) is an x-ray of your breasts. It can find early cancers that are too small to be noticed during a breast self-exam.

Your first mammogram should be taken between ages 35 and 39. Mammograms should be done every 1 to 2 years between ages 40 to 50. After age 50 you should have one every year. Your doctor may want you to have a mammogram earlier or more often, especially if you have relatives who have had breast cancer.

Risks

A mammogram uses about the same amount of radiation as an x-ray of your teeth—a very minor risk. On the other hand, you could die from breast cancer that is not found and treated. Regular mammograms reduce your risk of serious illness or death.

WHAT YOU SHOULD DO

• Follow your doctor's instructions for follow-up care.
• Continue to do your monthly breast self-exams.

Call Your Doctor If . . .

• You have questions or concerns about your care.

IF YOU'RE HEADING FOR THE HOSPITAL . . .

Before You Go

• You may feel nervous, scared, or upset before having a mammogram. Let your doctor and the technician doing the mammogram know that you have these concerns.
• Do not put deodorant, powder, or lotion on your breasts or under your arms before the test. These may prevent the x-rays from turning out correctly.
• Wear a two-piece outfit, since you will have to remove clothing from the waist-up. You will wear a hospital gown during the test. Do not wear jewelry around your neck.

When You Arrive

• Tell the technician doing the mammogram if you have breast implants. Extra care is needed to do the test.
• You will sit or stand next to a small x-ray table. The caregiver doing the test will help you place one of your breasts on the x-ray plate. Your breast will be moved until the correct position has been found.

- Your breast will be gently flattened between 2 plastic plates for a few seconds. Flattening of your breast is important to find lumps. It may feel uncomfortable, but should not hurt.
- You will be asked to hold your breath while the x-ray is taken. Another x-ray will be taken of the same breast after the position of the x-ray machine has been changed.
- Your other breast will be x-rayed the same way.
- The mammogram will take about 10 to 15 minutes. If you have breast implants, it will take 20 to 30 minutes.
- You can return to normal activities when the test is done.
- You will get the test results in a few days.

Mandibular Fracture

See Broken Jaw

Marine-Life Stings and Bites

WHAT YOU SHOULD KNOW

Among the many marine animals with painful stings or bites are the eel, jellyfish, man-of-war, stingray, stonefish, lionfish, scorpionfish, octopus, sea urchin, and coral. Some stings are poisonous and even deadly, so it's important to have a bad sting checked by a doctor.

Signs/Symptoms
Possible symptoms include pain, swelling, redness, itching, or blisters at the site of the bite or sting. You may also become nauseated or vomit. Other possible symptoms include a headache, chills, fever, sweating, and tingling or numbness. Difficulty breathing, fainting, and seizures are signs of a life-threatening sting.

Care
If the wound is small and doesn't cause a lot of problems, you can take care of it at home. Clean the area, pat it dry, and try not to scratch it. For more troublesome wounds, go to the doctor. You may need a tetanus shot and medicine for infection, pain, or swelling.

   If you have trouble breathing, become faint, have convulsions, or develop a tight feeling in your chest or throat, you will probably need hospitalization. You may also need to be put in the hospital if the wound is large or infected, or if you lost a lot of blood.

WHAT YOU SHOULD DO

- Try to keep the wound raised above the level of your heart to reduce pain and swelling. Do not use the wounded area too much until it starts healing.

- Your doctor will tell you how long to leave the bandage on. Keep it clean and dry.
- To change the bandage, unwrap it slowly and carefully. If it sticks to the wound, soak it in lukewarm water. Rinse the wound off and pat dry with a clean towel.
- Clean the wound 2 to 3 times a day either with a solution of half hydrogen peroxide and half water or with mild soap and water.
- Return for a wound recheck in a few days.
- If you get stitches, your doctor will tell you when to have them removed.
- If you are given a tetanus shot, your arm may get swollen, red, and warm to the touch at the site of the injection. This is a normal reaction to the medicine in the shot.
- To keep from getting stung again:
  —Be alert for potentially dangerous marine creatures whenever going into the water.
  —When swimming in the ocean, do not touch the marine life unless you can identify it and are sure it can do you no harm.
  —Do not dive or swim in the ocean alone.

Call Your Doctor If . . .
- Your wound does not stop bleeding.

Seek Care Immediately If . . .
- You show signs of infection (increased pain or soreness, swelling, redness, pus, a bad smell, or red streaks coming from the wound).
- You have a high temperature.
- You have numbness or swelling below the wound, or you cannot move the joint below the wound.
- You become dizzy or weak, have trouble breathing, or develop diarrhea, headaches, or seizures. You may be having an allergic reaction to the bite.

Mastitis

WHAT YOU SHOULD KNOW

Mastitis (mass-TIE-tis) is a breast infection that occurs in nursing mothers. It is not a serious problem, but without care it can cause pain. Mastitis occurs most often during the 3rd or 4th week of breastfeeding.

Causes
Cracked nipples, a plugged milk tube, or a part of the breast that has not been emptied of milk can cause mastitis. The infection is in the breast tissue and not in your milk. It usually involves one breast.

Signs/Symptoms
The first signs of mastitis are redness, pain, swelling, and hardness in an area of your breast. You may also have fever, chills, headache, flu-like pain, nausea, and vomiting. Your breast could feel hot to the touch.

Care
Your doctor will give you a kind of medicine called an antibiotic to treat your breast infection. Take it until it is all gone, even if your breast feels better. You do not need to stop breastfeeding. The medicine and infection will not hurt your baby.

WHAT YOU SHOULD DO

- Take your medicine as directed by your doctor.
- Before breastfeeding:
  - —Fifteen minutes before nursing, put warm moist heat to your sore breast. Use a washcloth or small towel dipped in semi-hot water. Wring it out and put it in a plastic bag.
  - —Hold the bag to your breast for 15 to 20 minutes. Do this again after breastfeeding. Warm heat opens the milk tubes to help your milk come down. The heat may also help your breast pain.
  - —Wash your hands and nipples with soap and water. Begin nursing on the sore breast to keep it emptied. Nurse your baby on both breasts every 1 to 3 hours both day and night.
- Your doctor may suggest you use over-the-counter medicine such as acetaminophen for fever or pain.
- Keep your nipples clean and dry between feedings. Don't let your baby chew on your nipples instead of sucking.
- Drink 8 glasses (soda-can size) of water or fruit juices daily.
- Rest until your fever is gone and your breast is not sore.
- Wear a nursing bra that is not tight, but feels good and supports your breasts.
- Do not sleep on your belly until your infection is gone.

Call Your Doctor If . . .
- Your fever and breast pain last more than 48 hours.
- You have a high temperature.

- You have a painful swelling or lump in your breast. This could mean you have a breast abscess (pocket of pus).
- You have swollen and tender glands in your armpit on the same side as the infected breast.
- You get sore nipples and severe, burning pain in your breast.

Measles

WHAT YOU SHOULD KNOW

Measles (ME-suls) is a viral infection that spreads very quickly to people who have never had the disease or a shot (vaccine). It infects the throat, airways, and lungs, as well as the skin. After being around someone with measles, it will take 1 to 2 weeks before you know whether you have it. The disease is also called rubeola (rue-be-O-luh).

Causes
Measles is caused by the rubeola virus. Your chances of getting the disease are greater if you have never had the measles shot (part of the MMR shot).

Signs/Symptoms
The first symptoms are a high fever, loud coughing, runny nose, and red eyes. These are followed in 2 to 4 days by the appearance of tiny, white spots in the mouth and throat. A day or two after that, a rash breaks out on the forehead, then spreads around the ears and down onto the body. The rash lasts 4 to 7 days.

Care
Antibiotics don't work against measles, but you can give acetaminophen to ease the fever. Call your child's school or daycare center right away and let them know that your child has the measles.

For advance protection against measles, make sure all your children get MMR shots. If you or a child have been around someone with measles, ask your doctor about getting a gamma globulin shot.

WHAT YOU SHOULD DO

- Do NOT give aspirin to a child with measles who is under 18 years of age. This could lead to brain and liver damage (Reye's syndrome). Be sure to check for aspirin on the label of any over-the-counter medicines you buy.
- You may give your child acetaminophen for fever.
- To relieve coughing, use a cool-mist humidifier to increase air

moisture. Do not use hot steam. You also may give your child honey, corn syrup, cough drops, or a cough medicine.

- Keep your child away from people who have never had measles or the measles vaccine.
- Your child should rest as much as possible and get plenty of sleep.
- Give plenty of fluids (water, juice, clear soups).
- Your child's eyes may be sensitive to light for a few days. Wipe the eyes often with a clean, wet cotton ball. It will also help for the child to wear sunglasses or stay in a darkened room.
- Keep the child home from school or daycare until the fever and rash are gone. This usually takes about 7 days.

Call Your Doctor If . . .
- Your child gets a high temperature after being normal for a day or two.
- Your child brings up thick, brown, green, or gray sputum while coughing, or the cough lasts for more than 4 or 5 days.
- Your child has a really bad headache.
- Your child has an earache.

Seek Care Immediately If . . .
- Your child has trouble breathing or is breathing very fast.
- Your child has a headache, drowsiness, stiff neck, and vomiting all at once.
- Your child has a seizure.
- Your child develops a very high temperature.

Measles, German

See German Measles

Ménière's Disease

WHAT YOU SHOULD KNOW

Ménière's (MEN-ee-erz) disease causes an increase in fluid and pressure in the inner ear that may affect your balance, interfere with your hearing, and make you dizzy. One ear is usually involved. The symptoms may appear every few weeks or attacks may be years apart. An attack can last anywhere from a few hours to several days. Ménière's disease can be an upsetting problem. Although there is no cure for it, medications can relieve the symptoms.

Causes

The cause of this disease is unknown.

Signs/Symptoms

Typically, you'll experience sudden dizziness (vertigo) accompanied by nausea and vomiting. You may hear ringing or buzzing in the ears, or feel that your ear is full. Other possible symptoms include loss of balance, sweating, and jerky eye movements. You may suffer increasing hearing loss with each attack.

Care

Medicine may relieve your dizziness and ear pressure. Surgery may be necessary if the medicine doesn't work.

WHAT YOU SHOULD DO

• During an attack, rest in bed until the dizziness and nausea are gone.
  —Keep your head as still as possible and do not change positions quickly.
  —Do not walk without help and do not drive, climb ladders, or work with tools or machinery.
  —Avoid glaring light.
  —Do not read.
• Do not drink a lot of fluids and avoid salty foods. Fluid build-up can make the ear problem worse.
• Be sure to get follow-up care from your doctor.

Call Your Doctor If . . .

• During treatment you have:
  —Decreased hearing in either ear
  —Vomiting that doesn't stop
  —Convulsions
  —Fainting
  —A high fever
• You develop new, unexplained symptoms.

Meningitis, Bacterial

See Bacterial Meningitis

Meningitis, Bacterial in Children

See Bacterial Meningitis in Children

Meningitis, Fungal

See Fungal Meningitis

Meningitis, Viral

See Viral Meningitis

Menopause

See Change of Life

Menstrual Cramps

WHAT YOU SHOULD KNOW

Menstrual cramps are known medically as dysmenorrhea (dis-men-oh-REE-uh). During your period, the uterus (womb) gets rid of the lining (blood and tissue) that builds up during the time between your periods. The uterus, which has muscular walls, expels the blood by tightening and pushing it out. This can cause pain in the abdomen that sometimes spreads to the back and legs. It usually goes away after 1 or 2 days.

Causes

Generally, the cramps are caused by muscles tightening in the uterus. Sometimes pain occurs when the passage between the uterus and the vagina (the cervix) opens to let blood clots through. In some cases, a woman may have an infection or growth that causes pain during her periods.

Signs/Symptoms

The problem takes the form of cramps and sharp pains in the abdomen, lower back, and legs. Sometimes nausea, vomiting, and diarrhea may occur. You may feel tired and things may easily bother you.

Care

If the pain is really bad, your doctor may need to inspect your vagina (pelvic exam) to make sure there is not another cause for the pain. The doctor may give you several different kinds of pain medicine to see which one works for you.

WHAT YOU SHOULD DO

• You may take nonprescription medicine such as aspirin, ibuprofen, naproxen and acetaminophen for menstrual cramps. Use it only as directed.

- If your doctor gives you a prescription for menstrual cramps, take it exactly as directed.
- Applying heat to your abdomen or back helps ease the pain. Do this for about 20 minutes once or twice a day. Use a heating pad set on low or a warm water bottle, or take a warm bath for 10 to 15 minutes.
- Stay as active as possible. Exercise often helps relieve pain. You don't need to stay in bed.
- Don't drink too much caffeine (cola or coffee); and try to keep away from things that cause you to feel stressed-out.

Call Your Doctor If . . .
- Your pain is not controlled with medication or lasts more than 3 days.
- You have pain with urination or bowel movements, or pain that is located on one side only.
- The medicine you are taking is causing any problems.

Seek Care Immediately If . . .
- Your pain is so bad that you can't walk.
- You have a high temperature, vomiting, diarrhea, rash, dizziness, or muscle aches during your menstrual period.

MI

See Heart Attack

Migraine Headache

WHAT YOU SHOULD KNOW

Migraine headaches typically affect one side of the head. They can last anywhere from a few hours to a few days. Some people have them weekly, others have fewer than one a year. Migraines usually begin sometime between the teen years and the age of 40, and can be classified as either "classic" or "common."

Causes
At the onset of a migraine, the blood vessels in your head first shrink, then swell, causing pain.

Tension, bright lights, loud noises, strong smells, weather changes, fatigue, missed meals, and emotional upset all may trigger a migraine. The headaches may also be brought on by many common foods and beverages, including lunch meat, hot dogs, alcohol, beans, coffee or tea, cheese, chocolate, nuts, pickles, raisins, and canned soup. Artificial sweeteners can trigger a migraine. Many women get the headaches before or during their monthly period.

Signs/Symptoms

You may know you are going to have a migraine before the headache starts. Warning signs include nausea, vomiting, and sensitivity to noise, light, or smells.

Classic migraines begin with warning signs such as flashing lights or colors. You may feel as though you are looking through a tunnel. One side of your body may feel prickly, hot, or weak. These warning signs last about 15 to 30 minutes and are followed by pain in your head.

Common migraines do not have the same warning signs. However, you may feel tired, depressed, restless, or talkative for 2 or 3 days before the headache starts.

Care

There are a number of prescription medications for migraine. They tend to work better if you take the medicine as soon as your headache starts. Discuss these and other methods of preventing migraines with your doctor.

WHAT YOU SHOULD DO

- If your doctor prescribed medicine to treat or prevent your headaches, take it exactly as directed.
- At the first sign of a headache:
  —Apply cold compresses or ice packs to your head, or splash cold water on your face.
  —Lie down in a quiet, dark room for several hours. You may sleep, meditate, or listen to music. Do not read. Rest during the attack.
- To help prevent migraines:
  —Keep a record of what you ate before each headache. Avoid foods, such as chocolate, cheese, and red wine, that seem to cause an attack. Don't skip or delay meals.
  —Try to keep your life as free of stress as possible. Learn to pace yourself. Yoga, biofeedback, or relaxation therapy may be helpful.
  —If the headaches first appeared after you began taking birth control pills, you may want to talk to your doctor about changing to a different method of birth control.

Call Your Doctor If . . .

• You have any problems that may be related to the medicine you are taking.

Seek Care Immediately If . . .

• You have a headache that gets worse or lasts more than 24 hours despite treatment.
• You develop a high temperature.
• You faint or develop weakness, numbness, double vision, difficulty with speech, or neck pain or stiffness.

Miscarriage

WHAT YOU SHOULD KNOW

Miscarriage is the loss of a pregnancy before the growing baby is born. This usually occurs within the first 20 weeks of pregnancy. There is nothing you can do to prevent a miscarriage. However, you can still get pregnant again and have a healthy baby.

Causes

It may not be known why you miscarried. A miscarriage is your body's way of dealing with a baby that was not growing normally. Health problems of the mother can lead to miscarriage. Smoking, drinking alcohol, or drug abuse can also cause miscarriage. Having sex, exercising, working, suffering a minor fall, or using birth control pills before pregnancy does not cause miscarriage. Often, no reason for the miscarriage can be found.

Signs/Symptoms

Bleeding is the most common sign of a coming miscarriage. You may have pain in your abdomen or back. A gush of warm liquid from your vagina is another sign, meaning your bag of water has broken early.

Care

• You may have an ultrasound test. It is done to check for your baby's heartbeat. Your doctor can tell if the miscarriage has happened or is about to happen.
• If your cervix (bottom part of the uterus) has opened and you are having painful cramps, a miscarriage is certain. Your doctor will watch you carefully if you start to bleed.
• After a miscarriage, you may have tissue left in your uterus. This tissue must be removed by a D & C (dilatation & curettage) because

it can cause infection. This can be done in your doctor's office or the emergency department. It is sometimes done in the operating room.
• You may need to go into the hospital if you are bleeding heavily or if you need more care.

Risks

Untreated bleeding or infection after a miscarriage could be fatal. But, the risks of serious illness or death are minimal if you follow your doctor's suggestions.

WHAT YOU SHOULD DO

Call Your Doctor If . . .

• You have heavy vaginal bleeding (soaking 1 pad each hour).
• You have fever or chills.
• You have severe abdominal pain.
• You have a bad odor coming from your vagina.
• Your have a high temperature.

IF YOU'RE HEADING FOR THE HOSPITAL . . .

What to Expect While You're There

You may encounter the following procedures and equipment during your stay.
• **Taking Vital Signs:** These include your temperature, blood pressure, pulse (counting your heartbeats), and respirations (counting your breaths). A stethoscope is used to listen to your heart and lungs. Your blood pressure is taken by wrapping a cuff around your arm.
• **D & C:** Any tissue left in the uterus could cause heavy bleeding, and must be removed by a D & C (dilatation & curettage) to prevent infection. You will get medicine to help you relax before and during the D & C. The procedure should not be painful.
• **Consent Form:** You or a close family member will be asked to sign this legal piece of paper. It will give your doctor permission to do tests and treatments. Be sure that all your questions have been answered before you sign this form.
• **Afterward:** You will return to your hospital room. Ask for medicine if you are having pain. You may want to have someone stay with you to give comfort and support. You will go home when you are eating, drinking, and able to care for yourself.
• **Activity:** You will be asked to rest in bed if you are bleeding heavily. Once the bleeding has slowed down you will be able to get out of bed.
• **IV:** A tube placed in your vein for giving medicine or liquids. It will be capped or have tubing connected to it.

- **Medicines:** You may get antibiotics and medicines to fight infection. They can be taken by mouth or put in your IV.
- **Blood:** Usually taken from a vein in your hand or from the bend in your elbow. Tests will be done on the blood.
- **Blood Transfusion:** May be necessary if you need more blood.
- **Abdominal and Vaginal Ultrasound:** This painless test is done while you are lying down. A dab of a jelly-like lotion is placed on your belly. The person doing the test will gently move a small handle through the lotion and across the skin. A TV-like screen is attached to the handle. To perform a vaginal ultrasound, a small tube is placed in your vagina. There is no pain.
- **Grief:** A miscarriage is frightening, confusing and depressing. You may feel sad or angry at the loss of your pregnancy, and may tend to blame yourself. These feelings are normal. To get past them, talk with your doctor or someone close to you.

After You Leave

- Your doctor will want to see you in 2 to 6 weeks.
- Take your medicine as directed by your doctor. If you feel it is not helping, call your doctor.
- You will have spotting from your vagina for 8 to 10 days. To keep from getting an infection, use sanitary pads rather than tampons.
- Rest and slowly begin normal activity. Eat healthy foods and drink liquids.
- Your doctor will tell you how soon you may resume sex.
- You should wait 2 or 3 normal periods before trying to get pregnant. If you do not want to get pregnant, use birth control. Ask your doctor about what is best for you.
- Exercise is good. Start slowly. Exercise more as you start to feel better. It will take your body 6 to 8 weeks to return to normal.
- Feelings of loss and grief are normal. After a miscarriage, you may have headaches, problems sleeping, little interest in eating, and feelings of fatigue. Talk about your feelings. This can help you accept your loss. Don't blame yourself for the miscarriage. In most cases, nothing could have prevented it.

Miscarriage, Threatened

See Threatened Miscarriage

Mitral Valve Prolapse

WHAT YOU SHOULD KNOW

The heart has 4 chambers in it. The upper chambers are called atria (A-tree-uh) and the lower chambers are called ventricles (VEN-trick-uls). When the heart "beats," the atria push blood into the ventricles and the ventricles push blood out of the heart.

Valves control the flow of blood between the atria and ventricles. The mitral (MY-tral) valve lies between the left atrium and the left ventricle. It is made up of two small doors or leaflets that come from each side of the valve and meet in the middle. Its job is to keep blood from moving back into the left atrium. The valve opens to let blood flow into the ventricle. It closes to keep blood in the ventricle until it is pushed out into the circulatory system.

Mitral valve prolapse occurs when one or both of the leaflets of the valve bulge backward into the atrium as the ventricle is pushing blood out of the heart. This is not normal.

This movement may cause a clicking noise that your doctor can hear while listening to the heart with a stethoscope. Also, some of the blood from the ventricle may be allowed back into the atrium, which causes a "whooshing" sound called a "murmur."

Signs/Symptoms
Most people with mitral valve prolapse do not have any symptoms. If your valve gets worse you may feel tired, dizzy, or faint; get headaches; have trouble breathing; or experience chest pain or an irregular heartbeat. If these symptoms occur, you should see your doctor.

Care
If you **do not** have signs/symptoms, you don't have to change the way you live. If you have a murmur, you may need to take antibiotics before dental check-ups and avoid sports in which you could be hurt. You should visit your doctor yearly or as directed.

If you **do** have signs/symptoms, you may not be able to exercise as much as before. You may also need medicine to control any symptoms and tests to find out how serious the prolapse is. One test is an echocardiogram (ek-oh-CARD-e-o-gram). This painless test allows the valves to be seen while the heart is beating. You may need surgery if the problems with the valve pose a real danger.

WHAT YOU SHOULD DO

- If you are prescribed medicine for this condition, be sure to take it as directed. If you feel it is not helping, call your doctor. Do not quit taking it on your own.
- If you take aspirin regularly, continue to take it. Aspirin helps thin the blood so blood clots don't form. Do not take acetaminophen or ibuprofen instead.
- Remind your doctor or dentist you have mitral valve prolapse. You may need to take an antibiotic before dental cleanings and before some kinds of surgery. These help kill any germs that may get into your blood and cause an infection in the valve.
- A diet low in fat, salt, and cholesterol is very important. It keeps your heart healthy and strong. Ask your doctor for guidelines on what to eat. It may take time getting used to a new diet. Special cookbooks may help you and the cook in your family find new recipes.
- Quit smoking. It harms the heart and lungs. If you are having trouble stopping, ask your doctor for help.
- If you have symptoms or a murmur, you may need to avoid heavy exercise or competitive sports. Ask your doctor about this. However, do exercise daily. It helps make the heart stronger, lowers blood pressure, and keeps you healthy. If your exercise plan seems too hard or too easy, talk to your doctor.
- Weighing too much can make the heart work harder. If you need to lose weight, ask your doctor for a weight-loss program.
- Wear your medic-alert bracelet every day especially if you have symptoms from your illness. Ask your doctor how to get one.
- For more information about the heart, call the **American Heart Association at 1-800-AHA-USA1 (1-800-242-8721)** or call your local **Red Cross**.

Call Your Doctor If . . .
- You have chest pain during exercise that doesn't go away with rest.
- You have new symptoms that you did not have when you last saw the doctor.
- You have worse headaches, are getting dizzier, or are more tired.

Seek Care Immediately If . . .
- You faint or have chest pain, trouble breathing, or an irregular heartbeat. **Call 911 or 0 (operator)** to get to the nearest hospital or clinic. **Do not drive yourself!**

Mittelschmerz

WHAT YOU SHOULD KNOW

Mittelschmerz (MITT-ul-shmurz) means "middle pain." It strikes some women when the ovary releases an egg into the tube leading to the uterus (womb). This occurs about 2 weeks before your period. It can cause pain and cramping; but it is not serious and usually goes away after about 6 to 8 hours.

Causes
An egg being released from an ovary.

Signs/Symptoms
Pain and sometimes cramps on one side of the lower abdomen. Some women feel sick to their stomach and note some spotting of blood from the vagina.

Care
Rest and try to drink plenty of fluids (about 8 glasses a day). To ease any pain, you can try a heating pad set on low or sit in a warm bath. If the pain is severe, your doctor may prescribe a pain medication.

WHAT YOU SHOULD DO

• Rest until you feel better.
• Take your temperature every 4 hours.
• Do not take any laxatives or pain killers unless ordered by your doctor.
• Drink plenty of fluids.

Call Your Doctor If . . .
• The pain does not go away in a few days.
• You have increased vaginal bleeding.
• You have any unusual vaginal discharge.

Seek Care Immediately If . . .
• The pain increases.
• You begin to vomit blood or find blood in your bowel movement.
• You are dizzy or faint.
• Your abdomen becomes swollen.
• You have a high temperature.
• You have difficulty passing urine.
• You have trouble breathing.

Mole Removal

Most moles are no threat to your health and need not be removed. Some, however, change over time and can lead to cancer. A mole usually is removed by shaving or cutting it from the skin. If it is large, you will need stitches. A small mole, or one that is shaved off, may require only a small bandage. Your doctor may send a piece of the mole to the laboratory to check for cancer.

WHAT YOU SHOULD DO

- After the removal, keep the wounded area raised above the level of your heart, if possible. This will ease pain and swelling and promote healing.
- Keep the wound and bandage clean and dry for 24 hours.
- If the bandage gets wet, unwrap it slowly and carefully. If it sticks, use warm water to gently loosen it. Pat the area dry with a clean towel before applying a new bandage.
- Clean the wound gently 2 to 3 times a day with a cotton swab dipped in a mixture of half water and half hydrogen peroxide.
- Do not go swimming or soak the wound. If the wound is on your arm, do not wash dishes.

Call Your Doctor If . . .
- You develop a high temperature.
- Blood soaks through the dressing.
- Pain and swelling in the injured area gets worse.
- You develop numbness or swelling below the area of the wound.
- You notice redness, swelling, pus, a bad smell, or red streaks coming from the wound. These are signs of infection.

Molluscum Contagiosum

WHAT YOU SHOULD KNOW

Molluscum (mo-LUS-kum) contagiosum (kun-TAGE-ee-O-sum) is a skin infection. It can appear anywhere on the body, and affects both children and adults.

Causes
The disease is caused by a virus. You can catch it by having sex or being in close contact with an infected person. It may take 2 weeks to 6 months after exposure for symptoms to appear.

Signs/Symptoms

The infection raises small, firm, smooth, skin-colored or white bumps on the skin. Adults may find them on their inner legs, belly, and genitals; children may get them on the face. The bumps do not hurt or itch.

Care

The bumps will disappear without treatment in 10 to 24 months. However, to prevent the infection from spreading, the bumps should be removed by freezing.

WHAT YOU SHOULD DO

- Do not scratch the bumps. Scratching may spread the infection to other parts of the body or to other people.
- Avoid all close contact (including sexual contact) with others until the bumps disappear.
- If you have liquid-nitrogen freezing treatment, blisters will form. Leave the blisters alone and cover with a bandage. The tops will come off by themselves in 7 to 14 days.

Call Your Doctor If . . .

- You develop a high temperature.
- You develop swelling, redness, pain, tenderness, or warmth in the areas of the bumps. They may be infected.

Mononucleosis

WHAT YOU SHOULD KNOW

Mononucleosis (mon-o-nu-klee-O-sis) is a viral infection that affects your lungs, liver, and lymphatic (lim-FA-tik) system or tissue fluids. The virus, known as Epstein-Barr, usually affects people between the ages of 12 and 40 years.

It can take from 10 days to 6 months to recover from mononucleosis. You may continue to feel tired for 3 to 6 weeks after your condition improves.

Causes

The virus is spread mainly by saliva and you can get it by close contact, such as kissing. You are more likely to catch the virus if you are tired, under stress, or have another illness.

Signs/Symptoms

Symptoms include fever, sore throat, swollen glands, headaches, body aches, fatigue, loss of appetite, swollen liver, swollen spleen, and occasionally yellow skin and eyes.

Care
There is no specific cure. Eating healthy foods and getting extra rest are important. Drink plenty of water or juice every day. While you still have this infection, remember to keep away from those who are most likely to catch it from you: infants and people who are already ill.

Risks
Without the proper care, you risk the loss of excessive amounts of body fluids and salts. You also may not get the vitamins and minerals your body needs. There is a slight chance that your spleen will rupture. Rarely, the heart, lungs, or brain and nervous system become affected. Deaths have occurred.

WHAT YOU SHOULD DO

- Anyone under 18 years of age should avoid taking aspirin or any medicines that contain aspirin. This could lead to brain and liver damage (Reye's syndrome). Be sure to read the label on any over-the-counter medicines you buy. For fever and pain, take acetaminophen instead.
- Gargling may help relieve your sore throat. Use warm salt water (1 teaspoon of salt in 1 cup of water) or double-strength tea. Sucking on hard candy also helps.
- Rest until your temperature returns to normal (98.6 F or 37 C). Get plenty of sleep. You may gradually resume your regular activity after your fever is gone, but be sure to rest when you are tired.
- Although you may not feel like eating while you are ill, try to eat a balanced diet. Drink at least 8 glasses of fluids each day, especially while you have a fever.
- Avoid physical activity such as heavy lifting, strenuous exercise, or sports for 4 to 5 weeks. Such activity may injure your spleen.
- Don't try to push yourself too hard. Most people recover in 2 to 4 weeks, but you may continue to feel tired for 3 to 6 weeks after the other symptoms are gone.

Call Your Doctor If . . .
- You develop a high temperature.
- Your fever isn't gone in a few days.
- You still have symptoms after several weeks.
- You have yellowing of the skin.

Seek Care Immediately If . . .
• You have severe pain in your abdomen or shoulder.
• You have trouble swallowing or breathing.
• You feel dizzy or confused.

IF YOU'RE HEADING FOR THE HOSPITAL . . .

What to Expect While You're There
You may encounter the following procedures and equipment during your stay.
• **CT Scan:** Also called a "CAT" scan. This is an x-ray using a computer. It will be used to take pictures of your liver and spleen.
• **Abdominal Ultrasound:** This painless test is done while you are lying down. A dab of a jelly-like lotion is placed on your stomach. The person doing the test will gently move a small handle through the lotion and across the skin. A TV-like screen attached to the handle shows pictures of the internal organs. This study helps the doctor examine your spleen and liver.
• **Chest X-ray:** This picture of your lungs and heart shows the doctor how well they are handling the illness.
• **Activity:** Rest in bed as much as possible. Do not get up by yourself if you are dizzy or light-headed.
• **Taking Vital Signs:** These include your temperature, blood pressure, pulse (counting your heartbeats), and respirations (counting your breaths). A stethoscope is used to listen to your heart and lungs. Your blood pressure is taken by wrapping a cuff around your arm.
• **Pulse Oximeter:** While you are getting oxygen, you may be hooked up to a pulse oximeter (ox-IM-uh-ter). It is placed on your ear, finger, or toe and is connected to a machine that measures the oxygen in your blood.
• **IV:** A tube placed in your vein for giving medicine or liquids. It will be capped or have tubing connected to it.
• **Blood:** Usually taken from a vein in your hand or from the bend in your elbow. Tests will be done on the blood.

Morning Sickness

WHAT YOU SHOULD KNOW

Morning sickness—the nausea and vomiting of pregnancy—is especially common the first half of pregnancy. Most pregnant women have some morning sickness. Although unpleasant, it is usually not serious. By the second half of pregnancy, it typically clears up.

Causes

Experts are unsure of the reason for morning sickness. Changes in your hormones and blood sugar may cause it. Stress and nerves can make the problem worse.

Signs/Symptoms

Excessive vomiting can cause dehydration. Dizziness, reduced urination, dry mouth, and cracked lips are signs of dehydration.

Care

Eating small, frequent meals will help ease nausea. Avoid greasy foods, alcohol, and caffeine drinks. Eating soda crackers or dry toast may help. Try to get plenty of rest.

WHAT YOU SHOULD DO

- Keep soda crackers by your bed. Eat a few of them or a slice of bread before you get up. Get out of bed slowly. Sudden movements could cause you to get dizzy and nauseated.
- Eat small amounts of food high in protein, such as cheese or peanut butter. Stay away from greasy, fried, or spicy foods. Try to eat every 2 to 3 hours even if you are not hungry. Sit straight up after eating. This will keep food from backing up and making you nauseous.
- Have a snack such as yogurt, milk, bread, dry cereal, or a small sandwich before going to bed. Try eating during the night. This may prevent nausea in the morning.
- Drink 8 to 10 glasses (soda-can size) of liquid each day. Clear broths, fruit juices, and water are the best choices. You may enjoy herbal teas such as spearmint, peppermint, or chamomile. Drink them slowly and between meals. This will keep you from eating large amounts during meals, which can be a cause of nausea.
- The smell of some foods may make you feel sick. Stay away from these foods.
- Do not brush your teeth right after eating as this can cause nausea.
- Keep your feet up and your head slightly raised on a pillow when resting.
- Getting fresh air may help you feel better. Take a short walk or try to sleep with the window open. When you are cooking, open windows to get rid of odors.
- Don't smoke cigarettes. Ask other people not to smoke around you.
- Do not take medicine or try home remedies without asking your doctor.

Call Your Doctor Immediately If . . .
• None of the above ideas help.
• You are vomiting more than 3 or 4 times daily.
• You are loosing weight.
• You are vomiting blood or liquid that looks like coffee grounds.

Motion Sickness

WHAT YOU SHOULD KNOW

Motion sickness—often called sea-, car-, or air-sickness—is an uncomfortable but minor problem that usually goes away without treatment in a day or two at most.

Causes
Travel in any type of vehicle can cause the problem. Motion disturbs the fluid in your inner ear, causing problems with your balance that can lead to stomach upset.

Signs/Symptoms
The usual symptoms include upset stomach, vomiting, headache, yawning, sweating, dizziness, fatigue, and loss of appetite.

Care
Usually, no special care is needed. Try resting with a cool towel over your eyes and forehead. It is all right to throw up if you have the urge.

WHAT YOU SHOULD DO

• Use over-the-counter or prescription medication to prevent motion sickness. If you feel it is not helping, call your doctor.
• To reduce the chance of an attack, the following steps may help:
  —Do not eat large meals or drink alcohol before or during travel.
  —Take frequent sips of liquids.
  —Sit in an area of the plane (near the wing) or boat with the least motion. Lie back in your seat, if possible.
  —Breathe slowly and deeply.
  —Do not read or watch the horizon, especially in rough weather.
  —Try to stay away from areas where people are smoking, if possible.

Call Your Doctor If . . .
• You are throwing up a lot and your medicine is not helping.
• You have been throwing up and feel dizzy or faint; cannot drink or are very thirsty; have not urinated in 8 hours or have dark yellow

urine; and have very dry skin. These are signs that your body has
lost too much water and has become dehydrated.

Mountain Sickness

WHAT YOU SHOULD KNOW

Mountain sickness, also called high altitude sickness, usually occurs
at heights of 8,500 feet or more, where the oxygen in the air is significantly reduced. You are especially likely to develop this problem
when you travel to the mountains after living in an area close to sea
level.

Young people have mountain sickness more frequently than older
adults, and you don't have to be out of shape to be affected. Although
it is not usually a serious illness, a really bad attack can make you
very ill.

Causes

You're most likely to have this problem when you experience a
sudden change in elevation. For example, if you rush right from Los
Angeles to Colorado's Rocky Mountains without stopping a while in
Denver to get used to the altitude, you may develop symptoms.

Signs/Symptoms

Typical signs of mountain sickness include headache, nausea, vomiting, loss of appetite, tiredness, dizziness, trouble walking, insomnia,
and trouble breathing.

Care

If your symptoms are mild, you may not need treatment. If you have
a headache, you may need medicine. If your symptoms are serious,
you may be given oxygen or hospitalized.

WHAT YOU SHOULD DO

- For the first 24 to 36 hours, restrict yourself to light exercise; heavy
  exercise will make you feel worse.
- Rest, drink plenty of fluids and eat small, light meals. Don't smoke
  or drink alcoholic beverages. Do not take sleeping pills or other
  sedatives.
- To prevent high altitude sickness during future trips:
  —Give your body a few days to adjust to the change in altitude before you start your activities.
  —Go to higher elevations as slowly as possible (no more than 1000
  feet per day).

—Visit higher elevations during the daytime and return to a lower altitude in the evening.
—Ask your family doctor about medicines that may help.

Call Your Doctor If . . .
• You do not feel better in a few days.
• You have headache, nausea, vomiting, tiredness, shortness of breath, dizziness, and difficulty sleeping and going to a lower elevation does not relieve these symptoms.

Seek Care Immediately If . . .
• You have a great deal of trouble breathing, chest pain, a dry cough or a cough that produces bloody sputum, increasingly severe headache, difficulty walking, fast heartbeat, difficulty concentrating, or a feeling of confusion.

Mumps

WHAT YOU SHOULD KNOW

Mumps usually affects children between 2 and 12 years old, but can occur in people of all ages. It's an infection that causes pain and swelling in glands in the neck located a little below the ear. These glands make saliva. It takes 2 to 3 weeks for symptoms to develop after you catch the disease from an infected individual. Most people who come down with mumps are completely well after about 10 days.

Causes
Mumps is caused by a virus that spreads through saliva. It is very contagious; you can get it simply by being near someone who has the disease. The chances of getting the disease are greater if you have never received the mumps vaccine (part of the MMR shot).

Signs/Symptoms
The first symptoms are fever, chills, headache, and loss of appetite. After 1 or 2 days, the saliva glands on one or both sides of the neck become swollen, hard, and painful. The ears may hurt, and it may become hard to chew or move the mouth. If the disease strikes a male after puberty, one or both testicles may also become red, swollen, and painful.

Care

Antibiotics won't help. Care consists of making the child as comfortable as possible.

WHAT YOU SHOULD DO

- Do NOT give aspirin to children with mumps who are under 18 years of age. This could lead to brain and liver damage (Reye's syndrome). Be sure to check for aspirin on the label of any over-the-counter medicines you buy.
- You MAY give acetaminophen for fever and pain.
- A warm towel or heating pad set on low may help ease the pain in the swollen glands. An ice pack also may help.
- Have the child rest as much as possible.
- The child may eat normally, but should not have foods that need lots of chewing. Give plenty of fluids such as ginger ale, cola, iced tea, or water (6 to 8 soda-can size glasses each day). Do not give fruit juices; they may make the pain worse.
- Call your child's school or day-care center and let them know the child has the mumps.
- Mumps is easily spread until the swelling is gone—usually about 1 week. Keep your child away from other children who have not had mumps or a mumps shot. Adults whose brothers or sisters had mumps when they were children can be considered protected. People who are not protected should call the doctor to see if they should get the mumps shot.

Call Your Doctor If . . .

- Your child gets a high temperature or fever lasts more than 5 days.
- Your child starts to vomit.
- Your child gets belly pain, pain or swelling of the testicles, or irritated or red eyes.
- The skin over the swollen area becomes red at any time.
- The swelling lasts for 8 days or more.

Seek Care Immediately If . . .

- Your child has a seizure, develops twitching of the face, seems drowsy, or can't be awakened.
- Your child gets a severe headache that is not relieved by pain medicine.

Muscle Strain

A muscle strain (also called a pulled muscle) occurs when a muscle is suddenly pulled or twisted, causing a tiny tear. Healing usually takes about 1 to 2 weeks.

Causes
The problem usually results from an accident, often during sports or exercise. The injury happens more easily when muscles are not stretched or warmed up before working out.

Signs/Symptoms
Symptoms typically include pain, tenderness, and swelling of the injured muscle. You may also not be able to move the area around the muscle very well because of the pain and swelling.

Care
Your doctor may order an x-ray to make sure you haven't broken a bone. If you have a bad strain, you may need a splint to keep the injured area from moving so it will heal. If you scratched or tore some skin, you may also get a tetanus shot.

Do's and Don'ts
To avoid strains and sprains, always warm up your muscles before you exercise. Stretching them gently is one good warm-up technique. Ask your doctor to show you some stretching exercises. Before heavy exercise, wrap weak joints with support bandages.

- Apply ice to the injury for 15 to 20 minutes each hour for the first 1 to 2 days. Put the ice in a plastic bag and place a towel between the bag of ice and your skin.
- After the first 1 to 2 days, you may put heat on the injury to help ease the pain. Use a heating pad (set on low), a whirlpool bath, or warm, moist towels for 15 to 20 minutes every hour for 48 hours.
- Do not use the pulled muscle for 2 to 3 days, or while you still have pain.
- Your doctor may suggest you wrap the injured area with an elastic (ace) bandage for a few days. Be careful not to wrap it too tightly because it may make the area numb or tingly. Loosen the wrap if you get these symptoms.

- If you need an air splint, your doctor can show you how to make it fit right. Wear the splint until the doctor says you may take it off.
- You can take off an air splint or ace wrap when showering or bathing.
- You may use over-the-counter medicines for pain. Always take medications exactly as directed.
- If you are given a tetanus shot, your arm may get swollen, red, and warm to the touch at the site of the shot. This is a normal reaction to the medicine.

Call Your Doctor If . . .
- The pain or swelling gets worse.

Myocardial Infarction

See Heart Attack

Myringotomy

See Pressure-Equalizing Ear Tubes

Nail Removal

WHAT YOU SHOULD KNOW

All or part of your finger or toenail may need to be removed because of injury, nail infection, or abnormal nail growth. After the procedure, your finger or toe will be tightly wrapped in a special nonstick bandage to prevent bleeding.

WHAT YOU SHOULD DO

- Keep your hand or foot elevated to reduce pain and swelling.
- Your doctor will tell you whether it is necessary to return to the hospital or the office to have your bandage changed or whether you can do it at home.
- Keep your bandage dry until after it is changed for the first time.
- After your bandage is changed for the first time, soak your hand or foot in warm water for 10 to 20 minutes 4 times a day to help reduce pain and swelling. If you wish, you may add Epsom salt to the water. After soaking your hand or foot, apply a clean, dry bandage. Change your bandage every time it gets wet or dirty.

Call Your Doctor If . . .
- You have increased pain, swelling, drainage or bleeding.

- You develop a temperature of greater than 101 degrees F (38.3 degrees C).

Narcotic Abuse

WHAT YOU SHOULD KNOW

Some narcotics, such as morphine and codeine, are routinely prescribed for severe pain. However, they have to be used with caution. If you take them steadily for several weeks, or take larger doses than prescribed, you can easily become addicted. Narcotic addicts constantly crave the drug and become physically ill if they stop taking it. The drug becomes the focus of their life, as they spend more and more of their time and money assuring a supply.

Using narcotics—particularly injecting heroin or morphine   puts your life in danger. Addicts are liable to develop infections; suffer serious problems with the lungs, liver, and brain; or die from an overdose. Injecting narcotics with dirty needles also can give you AIDS.

A narcotics habit is hard to kick, but there are medical treatments that will help.

Causes

Taking a narcotic drug regularly for several weeks, or taking large doses, almost always leads to addiction. Pregnant women who take these drugs can pass the addiction to their babies.

Signs/Symptoms

The initial "high" from the drug is followed by drowsiness and a slowdown in your breathing and heartbeat. Your skin may become red, warm, or itchy. The longer you keep taking the drug, the more you will need it. When you stop using it (go through withdrawal), you will go through a short period of physical illness.

The first signs of withdrawal are fast breathing, sweating, yawning, and runny nose. You may also shake and develop goose bumps on your skin, mood changes, and enlarged pupils. After 2 to 3 days, you may suffer insomnia, upset stomach, vomiting, diarrhea, stomach cramps, muscle pain, and a fast heart rate.

Care

To wean you from the drug, your doctor may prescribe another type of narcotic and slowly reduce the dose. You may need other drugs for a short time to help with the withdrawal symptoms. Joining a support group or getting counseling may help you stop taking the drug. Some people need to attend a special program for narcotic addicts.

WHAT YOU SHOULD DO

• If prescribed a narcotic medicine, be careful to follow your doctor's instructions. Do not increase the dose or take the drug any longer than absolutely necessary.

• Don't even experiment with "recreational" narcotics. Stay away from people who use drugs and who encourage others to use them.

• The first step to quitting is to admit you have a problem. Be honest and open with family and close friends. Ask for their help.

• Don't try to stop taking the drug all at once. You will need medical help to get you through a gradual withdrawal period.

• Tell your doctor exactly how much of the drug you have been taking. Also tell your doctor if you are taking any other medications. Don't hesitate to be honest. Doctors are familiar with the problem.

• Support-group meetings and counseling can help you quit. Take advantage of both.

• Eat a healthy diet, drink 6 to 8 glasses of water a day, and get plenty of rest.

• Don't smoke or drink coffee or alcohol. They can make you nervous and increase your withdrawal symptoms.

• Don't dwell on the problem. Find new things to do. Get out of the house every day. Go for walks outside.

Call Your Doctor If . . .

• You cannot fight the need to take more drugs. Call your doctor, a counselor, friend, or family member you trust RIGHT AWAY.

• You feel like your problems are getting the best of you and you can't deal with them on your own.

Seek Care Immediately If . . .

• You have chest pain, sweating, or trouble breathing.

• You get a severe headache; develop bad stomach pain; or notice pain, a numb or prickly feeling, or burning in your arms or legs.

Nasal Foreign Body

See Foreign Body in the Nose

Nasal Fracture

See Broken Nose

Nausea and Vomiting of Pregnancy

See Morning Sickness

Neck Sprain

See Whiplash

Needle Stick Injuries

WHAT YOU SHOULD KNOW

Anyone who works in health care is at risk of being stuck with a needle by accident. If the needle has blood or another body fluid on it, you can get an infection such as hepatitis or HIV (the AIDS virus). The same thing can happen any time you get cut with something that was used on a patient.

Causes

Any sharp object that comes in contact with a patient's body fluids may carry infection. Hepatitis is a greater danger than HIV. You are likely to get an HIV infection only if the stick is very deep, or if blood from the needle gets into your body.

Signs/Symptoms

At first, there will only be the pain and bleeding from the needle stick. Only later will you develop symptoms of infection.

Care

You'll need to be tested. You may be given shots to prevent you from getting hepatitis. If you have a positive test for HIV, the doctor may prescribe medicine to slow down the infection.

WHAT YOU SHOULD DO

- If you stick yourself with a needle used on a patient, report it immediately. Both you and the patient should be tested for hepatitis and HIV infection.
- See your doctor right away if the patient has AIDS or HIV infection or refuses to be tested.
- If you do not know which patient the needle came from, you and your doctor will need to decide what tests should be done and what treatment you should have.
- In case you've contracted hepatitis, wash your hands well before eating and after using the bathroom. Do not share food or drinks.
- Even if your first test shows you do not have HIV, you should get another test in 6 weeks and 3, 6, and 12 months after your needle stick injury. You should also take the steps necessary to avoid spreading

HIV: Use a condom when you have sex. Do not give blood. If you are breast feeding, use formula instead.
• To prevent needle stick injures:
   —Be careful when handling needles, scalpels, and any other sharp objects.
   —Do not put the cap back on a used needle; do not bend or break a needle by hand, and do not take the needle off a disposable syringe.
   —Put all sharp objects in a special holder that only contains sharp items.
• Always wear gloves when you touch anything that has blood or other body fluids on it.

Call Your Doctor If . . .
• You have not been given your test results.
• You can't drink fluids or you throw up after you eat.
• Your stomach or legs become swollen, itch, or break out in rash.
• You get a fever, rash, or muscle pain; feel tired; or can feel lumps in your neck or under your arms within a year of the injury.
• You vomit or have diarrhea or really bad abdominal pain for more than a few days.

Nephrolithiasis

See Kidney Stones

Nevus Removal

See Mole Removal

Newborn Jaundice

WHAT YOU SHOULD KNOW

Jaundice is a yellowing of the skin and whites of the eyes. In newborns, it often shows up in the first 2 to 4 days. Jaundice appears when there is too much bilirubin (bill-e-RUE-bin) in the body. Bilirubin is a normal breakdown product of red blood cells. It is taken out of the bloodstream by the liver.

Causes
Over half of all newborns have a liver that is not yet working normally, allowing bilirubin to build up in the baby's skin and blood. It is not a serious problem. It usually disappears after 1 to 2 weeks, when the liver is older and working better.

Care
With eyes covered, the baby is placed under lights. These "photo-therapy lights" help to lower the amount of bilirubin in the baby's body. Time spent under the lights depends on the baby's blood bilirubin level, which is checked daily.

Risks
The risks of serious problems with newborn jaundice are small if you follow your doctor's advice.

WHAT YOU SHOULD DO

• After you leave the hospital, it's important to observe your baby for signs of jaundice or worsening of any jaundice the baby had in the hospital. The amount of yellowishness is best determined by view-ing the baby undressed in natural sunlight by a window.
• You may give your baby a sun bath for 10 to 15 minutes twice a day inside a sunny window.

Call Your Doctor If . . .
• Your baby develops jaundice during the first 48 hours of life, the jaundice involves the arms or legs, the color gets deeper after 1 week, or the jaundice is not gone by day 14.

Seek Care Immediately If . . .
• Your baby starts to act sick or is difficult to awaken.

Nonspecific Urethritis in Men

WHAT YOU SHOULD KNOW

Urethritis (YOO-ree-THRI-tis) is a swelling and inflammation of the urethra, the duct that drains the bladder. "Nonspecific" is the medical way of saying that the exact cause may not be known. Once you begin treatment, the problem should begin to clear up in about a week.

Causes
Nonspecific urethritis is often an aftermath of unprotected sex. It is frequently the result of an infection with bacteria—most often chlamydia (clah-MID-ee-uh)—yeast, or other germs. Injury to the urethra by trauma, surgery, or chemicals can cause urethritis. It can also be triggered by bubble baths or bath oils.

Signs/Symptoms
Typical symptoms include pain or burning during urination; a cloudy,

white, or yellow-green mucous discharge from the penis; or pain during sex. In men older than 50, urinary dribbling may be a problem.

Care

If the doctor suspects an infection, you will be given antibiotic medicine.

WHAT YOU SHOULD DO

• If you are taking antibiotics, finish the entire prescription, even if you feel better. If you stop taking the drug too soon, some germs may survive and re-infect you.

• Do not have sex until the infection is gone. If you do have sex, use a condom to prevent the spread of infection.

• To help ease the pain, sit in a hot bath for about 15 minutes at least 2 times a day.

• Do not squeeze or otherwise irritate the penis. If you are not circumcised, leave the foreskin alone. Do not pull it back to see if discharge is still present.

• Keep the penis clean. Use plain, unscented soap.

• Drink at least 8 soda-can size glasses of water every day. Also, drink cranberry juice to make your urine more acidic. This may increase the effectiveness of your medication.

• During treatment, don't drink liquids that contain alcohol or caffeine.

• Tell all partners with whom you had sex before treatment that you have this infection so that they can get treatment, too.

Call Your Doctor If . . .

• You get a high temperature.

• You start bleeding from the urethra or have blood in your urine.

• Your symptoms last longer than 1 week or get worse during treatment.

• You develop any new or unexplained symptoms.

• You have any problems that may be related to the medicine you are taking (for example, a rash, swelling, or trouble breathing).

Nonspecific Vaginitis

See Bacterial Vaginosis

Nosebleeds

WHAT YOU SHOULD KNOW

Nosebleeds, known medically as epistaxis (epi-STAX-sis), are more common in children than in adults.

Causes
The problem can result from excessive dryness of the inside of the nose, an infection, or an injury. Other causes include high blood pressure, kidney or liver disease, or generalized bleeding problems.

Signs/Symptoms
Blood from the nose can be either dark or bright in color. If you lose a large amount of blood, you may become dizzy. If you swallow blood, your stools may turn black.

Care
To stop severe nosebleeds, the doctor will insert gauze packing high in the nose. If the bleeding won't stop, you may need to be hospitalized for tests and care.

WHAT YOU SHOULD DO

• You will need to return to the doctor to have the gauze packing removed. If part of the packing starts to come out of the nostril, either cut it off or gently tuck it back in. Do not pull it out.
• If there is no packing in your nose, apply a small amount of petroleum jelly inside the nostril 2 times a day for 4 or 5 days. This will help relieve dryness and irritation.
• To avoid loosening any blood clots, do not blow your nose for 12 hours after the bleeding stops. Do not pick your nose or put anything into it.
• If the bleeding starts again, sit up and lean forward. Breathe through your mouth. Pinch the soft part of your nose tightly and for 10 minutes without letting go.
• Use a cool-mist humidifier or vaporizer in your home; the increased moisture will help prevent nosebleeds.
• For a few days, keep your head on several pillows when lying down.
• To prevent the bleeding from starting again, do not use aspirin or drink alcohol for 2 or 3 days. You should also avoid hot drinks for several days.
• Avoid heavy lifting and straining for several days.
• You may resume your normal activities as soon as you feel better.

Call Your Doctor If . . .
- You have unexplained bruises on other parts of the body.
- You develop a high temperature.
- You continue to have frequent nosebleeds.
- You become nauseated or vomit.

Seek Care Immediately If . . .
- You cannot stop the bleeding after applying pressure to your nose for 10 minutes.
- You lose large amounts of blood.

Nose Fracture

See Broken Nose

Nursemaid's Elbow

See Pulled Elbow

Opiate Withdrawal

See Narcotic Abuse

Oral Candidiasis

See Thrush

Oral Herpes

See Cold Sores

Orbital Fracture

See Facial Fracture

Orchitis

WHAT YOU SHOULD KNOW

Orchitis (or-KITE-iss) is an inflammation of one or both testicles, usually resulting from an infection. The inflammation doesn't affect the production of male hormones, and very rarely results in sterility.

Causes
The most common causes are urinary tract infections, sexually transmitted infections such as gonorrhea, and cases of mumps contracted after puberty.

Signs/Symptoms
Pain, swelling, or redness of the testicle is often accompanied by fever. You may feel a lump in the testicle.

Care
For many types of infection, the doctor can prescribe an antibiotic. If the problem is caused by mumps, however, there are no drugs to speed recovery. Simply follow the instructions below to make the area as comfortable as possible.

WHAT YOU SHOULD DO

- Rest in bed until fever, pain, and swelling go down. Your testicle may stay swollen and hard for several days or even a few weeks.
- If your doctor prescribes an antibiotic to fight infection, take it exactly as prescribed and be sure to finish the entire prescription. If you stop taking the drug too soon, some germs may survive and re-infect you.
- To help relieve pain and swelling, place a rolled-up towel between your legs under the scrotum. This helps support the weight of the scrotum and tender testicles. Wearing briefs (jockey shorts) also provides support.
- Apply either cold or heat to the swollen area, whichever relieves the pain best. You may use warm or cold compresses, ice packs, an electric heating pad set on low, or a hot water bottle filled with warm water. Sitting in a warm bath for 15 minutes twice a day will help reduce the swelling more quickly. You may also use acetaminophen, aspirin, or ibuprofen
- Don't drink alcohol, tea, coffee, or carbonated beverages; they irritate the urinary system. Eat foods such as prunes, fresh fruit, whole-grain cereals, and nuts to prevent constipation.
- If the problem is caused by a sexually transmitted disease, remember that you can pass the infection to a partner; wait at least 1 month after all symptoms disappear before having sex. Using a condom will help to prevent the spread of infection.
- Be careful not to injure the inflamed testicle for 2 or 3 months. When you resume normal activities, wear an athletic supporter (jock strap) or two pairs of briefs.

Call Your Doctor If . . .
- You have a high temperature.
- Your pain is not relieved by bed rest, applying heat or cold, or scrotal support.
- You become constipated.

- Your symptoms do not improve in 3 to 4 days after treatment starts.
- You have any problems that may be related to the medicine you are taking.

Osteoarthritis

WHAT YOU SHOULD KNOW

Osteoarthritis, a form of arthritis or degenerative joint disease, occurs when the cartilage that normally cushions a joint becomes soft and breaks down. A bone "spur" (a pointed growth) that causes swelling and redness around the tissue may develop. The problem is most common in the fingers, feet, knees, hips, and the back and neck regions of the spine. It usually affects those over 50 years of age. The changes in the joints are long-term.

Causes
The exact cause of osteoarthritis is unknown.

Signs/Symptoms
The hallmarks of this disease are joint stiffness and pain. Joints may also swell. Cold and damp weather may make the aching worse. You may have trouble moving the affected joints; and when you do move them, you may hear a cracking sound. Usually, there is no fever, redness, or heat in the joints.

Care
Heat and medicine can help relieve the pain.

WHAT YOU SHOULD DO

- Applying heat to the affected area may ease the pain. Put a warm heating pad or warm, moist towels on the painful joint, or soak it in a whirlpool bath for 10 to 20 minutes every hour for 48 hours.
- Massaging the muscles around the joint also may relieve pain and stiffness, although massaging the joint itself is not helpful.
- If your back is affected:
  —You may be more comfortable at night if you sleep on a firm mattress or place a piece of 3/4-inch plywood between your mattress and the box springs.
  —Sleeping on a waterbed is helpful for some people.
- If your neck is affected and you have pain in your arms:
  —Wearing a soft neck collar may help relieve the pain.
  —If this is not helpful, ask your doctor if you can buy or rent a neck traction device to use at home.

• Activity:
  —Rest is important when the joint becomes very painful.
  —Resume normal activity when you feel better.
  —Regular exercise will strengthen your muscles and reduce your symptoms.
  —Cold may increase the pain in the affected joint. You may want to wear thermal underwear or avoid outdoor activity during cold weather.
• If you are overweight, it is important to lose weight.
• You may use over-the-counter medicines such as deep-heating ointments or lotions to relieve pain.

Call Your Doctor If . . .
• You have any problems that may be related to the medicine you are taking.

Seek Care Immediately If . . .
• You develop chills, fever, or redness and tenderness of the affected joint.

Osteoporosis

WHAT YOU SHOULD KNOW

Osteoporosis (AHS-tee-oh-pour-O-sis) is a thinning of the bones that can eventually lead to fractures and deformity. It is most common in women who have gone through menopause. Although osteoporosis is a life-long condition, exercise, diet, and hormone replacement therapy can slow its progress. There are also prescription drugs available that can reverse the disease.

Causes
Bones tend to lose strength with advancing age; and when estrogen levels decline after menopause, the process may pick up speed. Insufficient calcium in your diet will make the problem worse, as will a deficiency of vitamin D. Because weight-bearing exercise strengthens the bones, lack of exercise is an important contributing factor. Certain diseases and medicines may also lead to osteoporosis.

Signs/Symptoms
One early sign is a backache. Later, as bones in the spine begin to crumble, people with osteoporosis may lose height and develop a hump in the back. Falls are more likely to result in a broken arm or hip.

Care

Get plenty of exercise and make sure you have enough calcium in your diet. Ask your doctor about hormone replacement therapy and medicines such as calcitonin and Fosamax.

WHAT YOU SHOULD DO

- Falls are especially dangerous if you have osteoporosis. To avoid them:
  —If you are unsteady on your feet, use a cane or have someone help you walk.
  —Remove loose rugs and long electrical cords from your home.
  —Keep your home well lighted at night.
  —Avoid icy streets and wet or waxed floors. Hold the railing when using stairs.
- If your back is affected, a firm mattress may help you sleep better.
- To pick up objects, bend at the knees rather than from the waist.
- Eat a balanced diet that is high in calcium and vitamin D and contains lots of green vegetables and milk.
- Ask your doctor to suggest a good exercise program.
- To relieve pain, you may use over-the-counter pain-killers such as aspirin, acetaminophen, and ibuprofen.

Call Your Doctor If . . .

- You develop new, unexplained symptoms. They may be related to a medicine you are taking.

Seek Care Immediately If . . .

- You develop sudden, severe pain in your back.
- You have pain after an injury or fall.

Otitis Externa

WHAT YOU SHOULD KNOW

Otitis (o-TIE-tis) externa (ex-TER-na), also called swimmer's ear, is a skin infection of the outer ear canal (the area that extends from the eardrum to the outside of the ear). With treatment, the infection should be gone in 7 to 10 days.

Causes

The condition may be caused by either bacteria or a fungus. Swimming in dirty water or swimming frequently in pools with chlorine increase your chances of infection. You're also more likely to contract the problem if you have excess moisture in the ear, have had previous ear infections, or suffer from skin allergies.

Signs/Symptoms
This condition is marked by plugged ears or ear pain that becomes worse when your ear lobe is pulled. Other possible symptoms are itching, a discharge of pus, short-term hearing loss, and fever.

Care
Your doctor may gently clean your ear. You may need antibiotic ear medicine to fight the infection.

WHAT YOU SHOULD DO

• Over-the-counter pain medicine and warm packs placed over the ear will help relieve your pain.
• Sleeping with your head raised may help relieve pain.
• It is important to keep your ear dry. For three weeks after the infection is gone, do not swim or get water in your ear. Use ear plugs or a shower cap when showering.
• Use a cotton tipped applicator to apply medication.

Call Your Doctor If . . .
• Your pain is not relieved by ear drops or heat.
• You develop a high temperature.
• There is any discharge from the ear, the outer ear becomes red or swollen, or you notice swelling behind your earlobe.
• Your ear is still painful after 3 days.

Otitis Media in Adults

WHAT YOU SHOULD KNOW

Otitis (o-TIE-tis) media (me-DEE-uh) is an infection of the middle ear (the area behind the eardrum). With treatment, you will feel better in a few days. However, if you are not treated, your eardrum could break or the infection could spread. You might also develop a permanent hearing loss.

Causes
Middle ear infections can be caused by a variety of viruses and bacteria. They often follow a cold. People who have allergy attacks and those with broken eardrums are especially prone to this type of infection. The ear infection is not contagious.

Signs/Symptoms
Likely symptoms include ear pain, plugged ears, diminished hearing, ringing in the ear, headache, and fever. You may feel dizzy and have trouble walking. Some people get an upset stomach and vomit or have diarrhea. If the eardrum breaks, you may notice fluid leaking from the ear.

Care
Antibiotics are often prescribed to treat a middle ear infection. You may also need medicine to reduce pain and fever. For severe infections, the doctor may recommend insertion of a pressure-equalizing tube through the eardrum.

WHAT YOU SHOULD DO

- If your doctor has prescribed antibiotics, be sure to finish all the medication. If you stop treatment too soon, some bacteria may survive and cause a second infection.
- A heating pad (set on low) or a warm water bottle on the ear may provide some relief. Do not lie on the heating pad.
- You may also put an icebag or ice in a wet washcloth over the ear to ease the pain.
- Do not put anything in your ear unless your doctor tells you to.
- Over-the-counter drugs, such as acetaminophen and ibuprofen, are effective in relieving pain. Your doctor may also give you ear drops to ease your discomfort. Always take medicine exactly as directed.
- You may return to school or work when your temperature is normal (98.6 degrees F or 37 degrees C).
- Do not smoke or go swimming as long as you are taking antibiotics.
- Cover your ears in cold weather.
- Try to stay away from people with colds, and wash your hands if you touch someone who has this kind of infection.

Call Your Doctor If . . .
- You do not feel better in a few hours.
- You develop a high temperature, start vomiting, or have diarrhea.
- Your ear pain gets worse or you develop swelling around the ear.
- You develop a rash, itching, or swelling after taking your medicine.
- You get a really bad headache or pain near your ear.

Seek Care Immediately If . . .
- You have a seizure, your facial muscles begin to twitch, or you pass out.
- You become dizzy, develop a stiff neck, or cannot walk normally.

Otitis Media in Children

See Earache in Children

Ovarian Cyst

WHAT YOU SHOULD KNOW

Ovarian cysts are growths, like blisters, that sometimes appear on the ovaries (the two small organs in the lower abdomen that hold eggs). Ovarian cysts are common in young women. They are usually small and go away by themselves. However, they sometimes grow large and cause problems. Ovarian cysts are usually NOT a form of cancer.

Cause

The cysts tend to appear when too much of a hormone called estrogen is put out by the ovary.

Signs/Symptoms

Many cysts cause no symptoms—you may not feel anything or even know that you have a cyst. Larger cysts can cause a dull ache or a feeling of fullness (bloating) in the lower belly or back. Sometimes the cysts make sex painful, or disrupt your regular periods. Cysts also may make your periods very painful.

    If a cyst breaks open, it can cause severe pain and swelling of your lower abdomen.

Care

The doctor may take a blood sample for testing. Often no treatment is needed. However, your doctor may give you hormone medicine (such as birth control pills) to shrink the cyst. In severe cases, surgery may be needed.

WHAT YOU SHOULD DO

- You may continue your normal activities.
- You may need to go back to the doctor later or make an appointment with another doctor to find the exact cause of your cyst.

Call Your Doctor If . . .

- Your periods are late, irregular, or painful.
- Your abdominal pain doesn't go away.
- Your abdomen becomes enlarged or swollen.
- You have trouble emptying your bladder completely.
- You have pain during sexual intercourse.

- You have feelings of fullness, pressure, or discomfort in your abdomen.
- You lose weight for no apparent reason.
- You feel generally ill.

Seek Care Immediately If . . .
- You have severe abdominal pain, nausea and vomiting, and fever that comes on suddenly.

Oxyuriasis

See Pinworms

Pain After Surgery

WHAT YOU SHOULD DO

There's no way around it: Even minor surgery will leave you with some degree of pain. However, keeping this pain to a minimum will not only increase your comfort, but actually speed healing. Your doctor will prescribe strong pain-killers to achieve this.

Causes
Pain after surgery is an inevitable result of injury to your skin, muscles, and nerves during the operation. The amount of discomfort may be affected by the length of the operation. Other causes of postsurgical pain include the type of anesthetic used during the operation, gas in your bowels, and anxiety.

Signs/Symptoms
Pain in the area of the surgery may be accompanied by anxiety, restlessness, sweating, and an inability to move. If you have too much pain to walk, talk, or breathe normally, you need more medication to ease your suffering.

Care
While you are still in the hospital, you will get pain medicine in your IV, as a shot, or by mouth. When you return home, you'll be prescribed pain medication you can take by mouth.

WHAT YOU SHOULD DO

- To stay comfortable and heal more quickly, be sure to take your pain medication exactly as directed. If the pain does not go away or comes back, tell a doctor right away.

- Check with your doctor before taking any other medications. Do not drink alcohol or drive while you are taking narcotic pain medication.
- If the operation was on your arm or leg, keep it elevated. This will help relieve the pain and swelling, and will reduce the amount of blood flowing toward the wound.
- If the incision is on your chest or abdomen, hold a pillow firmly over that area while coughing and breathing deeply. This "splinting" will reduce the pain of deep coughing and breathing, which are needed to help prevent lung infections.
- Your doctor may suggest you try to reduce the pain by applying warm compresses, a heating pad set on low, or cold packs to the incision. (Be sure to place a washcloth between your skin and the cold pack.)
- Changing positions in bed or having your back rubbed may help your pain. You may feel better if you put a cool cloth on your hands or face. Try to take your mind off your pain by watching TV or listening to the radio.
- Constipation is a common side effect with many narcotic pain medications, so increase the fluids and fiber in your diet. A high fiber diet includes whole grain foods such as wheat bread and brown rice, raw fruit and vegetables, and legumes (beans).
- Get plenty of rest so your body can repair itself.
- Try to get up and around and take care of your personal needs as much as possible.

Call Your Doctor If . . .
- You have pain an hour after taking your pain medication (it may not be strong enough).
- You feel very sleepy or groggy (your pain medication may be too strong).
- You have side effects such as nausea, vomiting, or a rash.
- You have increased redness, swelling, bleeding, or pus-like drainage coming from the wound.
- You have tingling, numbness, swelling, or bluish fingers or toes.
- Your incision opens up.
- You have significant pain or discomfort after routine activity.
- You develop a temperature of over 100 degrees F (37.8 degrees C).

Palpitations

WHAT YOU SHOULD KNOW

Palpitations (pal-pih-TAY-shuns) are the feeling that your heart has a change in rate, rhythm, or strength of the beat. Although this can be frightening, it usually isn't serious.

Causes
Palpitations can be caused by anxiety, lack of sleep, certain medicines, caffeine, or too much heavy exercise. They also may be a sign of heart disease or other diseases.

Signs/Symptoms
Palpitations often feel like your heart is "skipping beats," "fluttering in your chest," or "racing." If you also feel dizzy, light-headed, short of breath, or have chest pain along with palpitations, it could be a sign of a life-threatening problem.

Care
Depends on the cause. If the palpitations are due to a serious problem, you'll need to have it treated. If a medicine is causing your heart to skip beats or race, your doctor may stop or change the prescription. Otherwise, you will need to stop eating or drinking foods with caffeine in them. You will also need to make sure you get enough rest. Remember, also, to avoid over-exercising, and try not to get too stressed-out.

Risks
If you do not go for treatment, the cause of the palpitations will remain unknown. Since palpitations sometimes signal a dangerous problem, you could be at risk for your life.

WHAT YOU SHOULD DO

- If you are prescribed a medication, be sure to take it as directed. If you feel it is not helping, call your doctor. Do not quit taking it on your own.
- To help keep the palpitations from coming back:
  —Drink decaffeinated coffee, tea, and soda pop. Do not eat chocolate.
  —If you smoke, quit or cut down as much as you can.
  —Try not to get too stressed-out or upset. Biofeedback, yoga, or meditation will help you relax. Exercise such as swimming, jogging, or walking also may help reduce stress.
  —Excess weight can make the heart work harder. If you need to lose weight, ask your doctor about the best plan for you.

Call Your Doctor If . . .
- You continue to have a fast heartbeat.
- Your palpitations occur more often.

Seek Care Immediately If . . .

• You get a really bad headache, dizziness, or fainting.
• You have chest pain that spreads to your arms, jaw, or back, and you are sweating, feel sick to your stomach (nauseated), and have trouble breathing. These are signs of a heart attack. **THIS IS AN EMERGENCY. Call 911 or 0 (operator)** to get to the nearest hospital or clinic. **Do not drive yourself!**

IF YOU'RE HEADING FOR THE HOSPITAL . . .

What to Expect While You're There

You may encounter the following procedures and equipment during your stay.

• **Taking Vital Signs:** These include your temperature, blood pressure, pulse (counting your heartbeats), and respirations (counting your breaths). A stethoscope is used to listen to your heart and lungs. Your blood pressure is taken by wrapping a cuff around your arm.

• **Pulse Oximeter:** You may be hooked up to a pulse oximeter (ox-IM-uh-ter). It is placed on your ear, finger, or toe and is connected to a machine. It measures the oxygen in your blood.

• **Oxygen:** Your body may need extra oxygen at this time. It is given either by a mask or nasal prongs. Tell your doctor if the oxygen is drying out your nose or if the nasal prongs bother you.

• **Blood:** Usually taken from a vein in your hand or from the bend in your elbow. Tests will be done on the blood.

• **Blood Gases:** Blood is taken from an artery in your wrist, elbow, or groin. It is tested for the amount of oxygen in your blood.

• **ECG:** Also called a heart monitor, an electrocardiograph (e-lek-tro-CAR-dee-o-graf), or EKG. The patches on your chest are hooked up to a TV-type screen or a small portable box (telemetry unit). This screen shows a tracing of each heartbeat. The ECG helps to detect the source of the problem.

• **IV:** A tube placed in your vein for giving medicine or liquids. It will be capped or have tubing connected to it.

Pancreatitis

WHAT YOU SHOULD KNOW

Pancreatitis (pan-cree-uh-TIE-tis) is an irritation of the pancreas that may begin quickly, then disappear after treatment. It may come and go repeatedly. This disease can make you very sick.

Causes

Pancreatitis runs in families. You can trigger it by drinking too much alcohol or eating foods high in fat. It can also be a result of gall-bladder disease or injury to your abdomen (the area around your stomach). Other causes are heavy smoking, surgery, infection, and some medicines.

Signs/Symptoms

Typical symptoms include fever, nausea, vomiting, severe abdominal pain, gas, and muscle aches. You also may lose weight, get dizzy, and have jaundice (a yellow tint to your skin or eyes).

Care

Your doctor may have you rest at home until you feel better. If the attacks are serious, you may need to check into the hospital for more tests and treatment.

Risks

Although you can die from pancreatitis, the risks of serious illness or death are decreased if you follow your doctor's suggestions.

WHAT YOU SHOULD DO

- You should drink clear liquids for the first few hours. Then return to a normal diet as your stomach allows.
- To ease the pain, you may use a warm washcloth or a heating pad set on *low*.
- Take your medicines exactly as directed by the doctor.
- You may return to your normal activities when you feel better. Avoid alcohol, and eat a normal, well-balanced diet.

Call Your Doctor If . . .

- You have severe stomach pain, vomiting, swelling and gas in your abdomen, or muscle aches.
- You have a high fever.
- You have continual weight loss.
- You have muscle cramps or spasms.
- Your skin or the whites of your eyes turn yellow.

Seek Care Immediately If . . .

- You have increasing pain or nausea and vomiting.
- You have cold hands and feet; pale, moist and sweaty skin; difficulty breathing; or fast breathing. These are symptoms of shock. Dial **911**

or **0 (operator)** and get to the hospital immediately. **THIS IS A LIFE-THREATENING EMERGENCY!**

IF YOU'RE HEADING FOR THE HOSPITAL . . .

What to Expect While You're There

You may encounter the following procedures and equipment during your stay.

- **Pancreas Ultrasound:** This painless test gives the doctor a view of the pancreas. It's done while you're lying down. A dab of a jelly-like lotion is placed on your stomach. The person doing the test will gently move a small handle through the lotion and across the skin. A TV-like screen is attached to the handle.

- **CT Scan:** Also called a "CAT" scan, this computer x-ray makes pictures of the pancreas that the doctor examines for problems.

- **Endoscopy** (end-OS-ko-pee): Your doctor will run a tube through your mouth and down into your stomach. A light and camera at the end allows the doctor to inspect the upper digestive tract.

- **Medicines:**
  —**Antibiotics** may be given to fight infection.
  —**Pain Medicine** may be given in your IV, as a shot, or by mouth. If the pain does not go away, tell a nurse right away.

- **Nasogastric Tube:** This tube may be threaded through your nose or mouth and down into your stomach. The tube is then attached to suction that will keep the stomach empty.

- **IV:** A tube placed in your vein for giving medicine or liquids. It will be capped or have tubing connected to it.

- **Eating:** If you have been vomiting, your stomach will need rest. You will not be able to eat until the vomiting has stopped. The IV will give you all the vitamins and liquids you need until you can eat again.

- **Taking Vital Signs:** These include your temperature, blood pressure, pulse (counting your heartbeats), and respirations (counting your breaths). A stethoscope is used to listen to your heart and lungs. Your blood pressure is taken by wrapping a cuff around your arm.

- **Blood:** Usually taken from a vein in your hand or from the bend in your elbow. Tests will be done on the blood.

- **Chest X-ray:** This picture of your lungs and heart will show how they are handling the illness.

- **ECG:** Also called a heart monitor, an electrocardiograph (e-lec-tro-CAR-dee-o-graf), or EKG. Patches on your chest are hooked up to a TV-type screen or a small portable box (telemetry unit). This screen shows a tracing of each heartbeat. Your heart will be watched for signs of injury or damage that could be related to your illness.

• **Other Care:** The doctor may have to operate to remove your gall-bladder or drain pockets of infection in your abdomen.

Panic Attack

WHAT YOU SHOULD KNOW

Panic attacks are a type of anxiety disorder. They are marked by overwhelming feelings of fear that last anywhere from a few minutes to an hour or two. They may strike for no apparent reason. The problem can usually be treated with a combination of counseling and medicine. If not treated, the attacks can lead to more severe problems.

Causes

Illness, stress, or certain medicines may trigger the first attack. Past injuries and dangers may also be a factor. Fear of additional attacks can actually set them off.

Signs/Symptoms

Adrenaline (uh-DREN-uh-lin), a chemical made by your system in response to danger (real or imagined), causes many of the body changes typically felt during a panic attack. Among these symptoms are a feeling of dread, fear, or danger; a fast heart rate and breathing; trembling; upset stomach; dry mouth; sweating; dizziness or fainting; and sometimes diarrhea. You may also feel detached from the people or things around you.

Care

The doctor may run tests for underlying physical disorders. Certain tranquilizers and antidepressant medications can relieve the attacks. Counseling may help you understand the cause of the panic and prepare you to deal effectively with the attacks. Learning to relax through muscle relaxation or biofeedback techniques can reduce your overall level of anxiety.

WHAT YOU SHOULD DO

• Don't smoke, use drugs, drink alcohol, or take high-caffeine foods and beverages such as coffee, tea, soda, and chocolate. They can either cause anxiety or make your symptoms worse.
• Try to spend time outdoors.
• Get plenty of rest.
• Muscle relaxation or aerobic exercise (such as walking) can help

you relax. Ask your doctor to recommend the best exercise program
for you.
- Take any medications exactly as prescribed. Do not change the
  dosage. If you feel the medicine is not helping, let your doctor
  know; but don't stop taking it on your own. It is important to stick
  with a regular program of therapy.
- For more information, get in touch with the following associations:
  —Anxiety Disorders Association of America, 6000 Executive
    Blvd., Suite 200, Rockville, MD 20852
  —National Institute of Mental Health Panic Campaign, Room
    15C-05, 5600 Fishers Lane, Rockville, MD 20857

Call Your Doctor If . . .
- Your feelings of anxiety become worse.
- You develop new, unexplained symptoms.
- You have problems that may be related to medication you are
  taking.

Seek Care Immediately If . . .
- You have a sudden feeling of panic that you can't control.
- You develop chest pain, sweating, trouble breathing, or pain in your
  jaw, neck, and arm during an anxiety attack.

Paraphimosis

WHAT YOU SHOULD KNOW

If the foreskin of the penis is tight and gets stuck behind the head, the
condition is known as paraphimosis (PAIR-uh-fim-OH-sis).

Causes
The problem may occur during sex, result from an infection, or
happen when the foreskin is pulled back so the tip of the penis can be
washed.

Signs/Symptoms
The condition can cause pain and swelling at the tip of the penis and
lead to problems with urination. The tip of the penis may turn red
or blue.

Care
Sometimes the foreskin can be worked back into place manually.
However, the doctor may need to make a slit in the foreskin to relieve

the pressure. Removal of the foreskin (circumcision) is often recommended.

WHAT YOU SHOULD DO

- If the doctor slits the foreskin, keep the dressing clean and dry and leave it in place until you return to the doctor.
- Apply ice packs to the penis to reduce swelling.
- You may take over-the-counter pain medicines such as aspirin, acetaminophen, or ibuprofen. Your doctor may prescribe additional medication.
- Do not try to pull back the foreskin until after your follow-up visit.
- Avoid sexual intercourse for 7 to 10 days.
- In uncircumcised babies, the foreskin is normally tight. It usually doesn't start to loosen enough to be pulled back until the baby is at least 18 months old. Until then, leave the foreskin alone. Later, you may gently pull back the foreskin during bathing.

Call Your Doctor If . . .
- The pain gets worse.
- The foreskin stays swollen for 24 hours, or the swelling gets worse.
- You have increasing redness, swelling, or drainage from the area. These are signs of infection.

Seek Care Immediately If . . .
- You are unable to urinate.
- You develop severe pain.
- You have bleeding from the area that will not stop with gentle pressure.
- You have a high temperature.

Paronychia

WHAT YOU SHOULD KNOW

A paronychia (PAIR-uh-NIK-ee-uh) is an infection of the skin around a fingernail or toenail. With treatment, the disease will be gone in 2 weeks to 6 months. However, these infections sometimes return.

Causes
The infection can be caused by either bacteria or a fungus. A bacterial paronychia may follow an injury, such as a torn hangnail. A fungal paronychia results from growth of fungus or yeast.

Signs/Symptoms

Signs of a bacterial paronychia include pain, tenderness, redness, swelling, warmth, and itching of the skin around the nail. Some of the skin may be pus-filled. A fungal paronychia is also accompanied by swelling and redness around the fingernail, but does not produce warmth, pain, pus, or itching.

Care

If there is pus around the nail, you may need an antibiotic to treat the infection. If the infection is severe, your doctor may need to make a cut in the area to let it drain.

WHAT YOU SHOULD DO

- If your doctor prescribes an antibiotic, take it exactly as directed. For pain or fever, you may use over-the-counter medicines such as acetaminophen or ibuprofen.
- Soak the nail in warm water for 10 to 20 minutes, 5 or 6 times a day, for several days.
- If the nail has been bandaged, keep the bandage dry until it is changed for the first time. Then start soaking the nail before applying each new bandage.
- To decrease swelling, elevate your hand or foot on a pillow whenever possible.
- To prevent further infections, protect your hands. Wear gloves when your hands are in water, when you are using irritating chemicals, or when you might injure your fingertips.
- Leave hangnails alone. Carefully trim your nails, but avoid cutting them too short.

Call Your Doctor If . . .

- You develop a high temperature.
- The pain gets worse.
- The swelling increases—especially if it affects the whole tip of the finger or toe.
- You notice red streaks coming from the infected area.

Pelvic Inflammatory Disease

WHAT YOU SHOULD KNOW

Pelvic inflammatory (in-FLAM-uh-tory) disease (PID) is an infection of the female organs. It is most common in women in their late teens or early 20's who have more than one sexual partner.

The disease starts in the vagina and moves into the uterus, up the tubes, and into the ovaries. Sometimes it spreads to other areas in the abdomen.

PID can make it difficult to become pregnant in the future, and can cause chronic (long-term) abdominal pain. The disease can also lead to a tubal pregnancy, which can be a serious problem.

Causes

PID can be caused by either bacteria or viruses. You can get it by having sex with an infected partner. The more sexual partners you have, the higher the risk of getting PID. Childbirth, abortion, or abdominal surgery can also cause PID.

Signs/Symptoms

Fever, painful periods, pain during sex, abdominal pain, and bad-smelling vaginal discharge are typical symptoms.

You also may have pain when you urinate and you may urinate more often. And you may have vaginal bleeding.

Your symptoms will depend on where the infection is and which germ has caused it. You may feel worse if you have had the infection longer than a week.

Care

Your doctor will do a pelvic exam (also called an "internal"). Samples of discharge from your vagina will be sent to the lab for tests. Blood samples will be taken.

You may be prescribed an antibiotic to treat your infection. Take it until it is all gone, even if you feel better. Your sexual partner (or partners) will also need antibiotic treatment.

You may need to be put in the hospital if your infection is serious.

Risks

Without treatment the infection can get worse and possibly even fatal.

WHAT YOU SHOULD DO

Call Your Doctor If . . .

• Your symptoms come back after you have finished your medicine.
• You get any new symptoms. They could be caused by your medicine.

Seek Care Immediately If . . .

• Your abdominal pain gets worse.
• You get chills, fever, nausea or vomiting.

What to Expect While You're There

You may encounter the following procedures and equipment during your stay.

- **Taking Vital Signs:** These include your temperature, blood pressure, pulse (counting your heartbeats), and respirations (counting your breaths). A stethoscope is used to listen to your heart and lungs. Your blood pressure is taken by wrapping a cuff around your arm.
- **IV:** A tube placed in your vein for giving medicine or liquids. It will be capped or have tubing connected to it.
- **Medicines:** You will probably be given antibiotics to fight the infection. Your doctor may also give you medicines to help your pain. Either can be taken by mouth or put in your IV.
- **Blood:** Usually taken from a vein in your hand or from the bend in your elbow. Tests will be done on the blood.

After You Leave

- Take all your medicine. Call your doctor if you do not feel it is working. Do not stop taking it on your own.
- Warm baths or a heating pad on "low" may help relieve your pain.
- Do not put anything in your vagina until your infection is gone. You should not douche.
- Use sanitary pads if you have a period while taking your medicines.
- Your doctor will tell you how soon you can have sex.
- Make sure your partner(s) have finished their antibiotic treatment before having sex with them.
- Have your male partner(s) use condoms. This will help protect you from being infected again.
- Remember, if you have sex with only one partner, you have less of a chance of getting PID.

Peptic Ulcers

See Ulcers

Perforated Eardrum

WHAT YOU SHOULD KNOW

The eardrum—also known as the tympanic (tim-PAN-ik) membrane—is a thin, round sheet of tissue that divides the ear canal from the middle ear. This fragile membrane is easily torn or perforated. The injury usually heals in 2 months without treatment. Your hearing should not be affected.

Causes

The culprit is often a sharp object jammed into the ear. The membrane can also rupture under the sudden increase in pressure that occurs during an explosion or while diving. A blow to the outer ear sometimes damages the eardrum; and a middle ear infection also can lead to perforation.

Signs/Symptoms

Typical symptoms include sudden ear pain, hearing loss, dizziness, ringing in the ear, and bleeding or discharge from the ear. Signs of a serious problem are hearing loss in both ears, severe dizziness, or feeling as though you are spinning.

Care

If you develop an infection, your doctor may prescribe an antibiotic. Surgery may be needed if the eardrum does not heal on its own.

WHAT YOU SHOULD DO

- Keep your ear dry. Water inside the ear may delay or prevent healing.
  - —Do not swim or take showers until the eardrum is healed.
  - —When taking a bath, place a piece of cotton covered with petroleum jelly in the outer ear canal to prevent water from entering the ear.
- To help relieve pain, apply heat to the ear with a warm water bottle or a heating pad set on low. Avoid high temperatures that could burn your ear or face.
- You may use over-the-counter medicines such as acetaminophen or ibuprofen to relieve pain. Be sure to use them exactly as directed.
- Blow your nose gently to avoid changes in pressure that could further damage the ear.
- You may resume normal activities when you feel better.

Call Your Doctor If . . .

- You have increased bleeding or a pus-like discharge from the ear.
- You still feel dizzy after 12 to 24 hours.
- You feel nauseated or start to vomit.
- You develop a high temperature.
- You continue to have pain in your ear despite treatment.

Periorbital Hematoma

See Black Eye

Perirectal Abscess

WHAT YOU SHOULD KNOW

A perirectal (pair-ee-REK-tuhl) abscess (AB-sess) is a pocket of pus in the tissues around the rectum, the last part of the bowel that ends at the anus.

Causes
Bacteria invade the tissue around the rectum through a cut or tear.

Signs/Symptoms
The primary symptom is a lump that is tender, firm, or moves about when you push on it. You may also have pain and a fever. If you can see the abscess on the skin, it will probably look red and swollen.

Care
You will probably need surgery to open the abscess and drain the pus. You may need to take antibiotics or other medicines. You'll also need to take a stool softener to make bowel movements easier.

Do's and Don'ts
To keep from getting more tears in your rectum that could lead to another abscess, try to keep your stool soft by eating foods that are high in fiber. Do not use enemas, and avoid anal sex.

Risks
Without treatment, the abscess can develop into a tear or hole where stool can get caught. The infection can spread to other parts of your body and cause severe illness. At the very least, if the cause of the abscess is not found and fixed, it can keep coming back.

IF YOU'RE HEADING FOR THE HOSPITAL . . .

What to Expect While You're There
You may encounter the following procedures and equipment during your stay.
- **Taking Vital Signs:** These include your temperature, blood pressure, pulse (counting your heartbeats), and respirations (counting your breaths). A stethoscope is used to listen to your heart and lungs. Your blood pressure is taken by wrapping a cuff around your arm.
- **Pulse Oximeter:** You may be hooked up to a pulse oximeter (ox-IM-uh-ter). It is placed on your ear, finger, or toe and is connected to a machine that measures the oxygen in your blood.

- **Blood:** Usually taken from a vein in your hand or from the bend in your elbow. Tests will be done on the blood.
- **IV:** A tube placed in your vein for giving medicine or liquids. It will be capped or have tubing connected to it.
- **ECG:** Also called a heart monitor, an electrocardiograph (e-lec-tro-CAR-dee-o-graf), or EKG. The patches on your chest are hooked up to a TV-type screen or a small portable box (telemetry unit). This screen shows a tracing of each heartbeat. Your heart will be watched for signs of injury or damage that could be related to your illness.
- **Oxygen:** Your body may need extra oxygen at this time. It is given either by a mask or nasal prongs. Tell your doctor if the oxygen is drying out your nose or if the nasal prongs bother you.
- **Foley Catheter:** This tube may be inserted to drain the bladder until you are able to urinate on your own.
- **Strict Intake/Output:** Nurses will carefully watch how much liquid you are getting by mouth and in your IV. They will also measure how much you are urinating.
- **Activity:** You may need to rest in bed. Once you are feeling better, you will be allowed to get up.
- **Cold/Heat:** Placing a cool towel or heating pad (set on low) on the area may help ease the pain.
- **Medicines:** You may receive several drugs by IV, in a shot, or by mouth.
  —**Antibiotics** may be prescribed if the abscess is infected with bacteria.
  —**Antifungal medicine** may be prescribed if the infection is caused by a fungus.
  —**Pain medicine** may also be needed. If the pain does not go away or comes back, tell a nurse right away.

After You Leave
- A small piece of gauze will be left at the abscess so it can drain. Do not remove the gauze until your doctor says it's okay.
- You may put a loose dressing over the site of the abscess. Keep the dressing clean and dry. You may need to change it several times a day.
- After the gauze drain is removed, you may wash the area gently with mild soap before putting the dressing back on.
- To ease the pain and discomfort, put warm wet washcloths on the area or use a heating pad set on low. After the drain is removed, it may help to sit in a tub of warm water for 10 to 20 minutes, 3 or 4 times a day.
- A special plastic cushion that's shaped like a doughnut may make

sitting more comfortable. These cushions can often be found in drugstores.
• To reduce pain and straining during bowel movements:
    —Eat a diet high in fiber (vegetables, fruits, and whole grains).
    —Take stool softeners as suggested by your doctor.

Call Your Doctor If . . .
• You have increasing pain, redness, swelling, drainage, or bleeding in the area.
• You develop any new symptoms.
• You develop chills or a high temperature.

Peritonsillar Abscess

WHAT YOU SHOULD KNOW

A peritonsillar (PAIR-ee-TON-sill-er) abscess (AB-sess), also called quinsy (kwin-z) sore throat, is a pus-filled cavity in back of the throat near the tonsils. If you don't get treatment, the abscess may spread into your head and neck. An abscess that grows very large can even interfere with breathing. With care, however, the problem will begin to clear up in a few days.

Causes
The abscess is usually caused by bacteria that produce an infection in your tonsils, throat, or mouth which then spreads deep into the neck.

Signs/Symptoms
The abscess is accompanied by severe pain, swelling, and redness in the throat; ear pain; trouble swallowing and talking; drooling; and bad breath. You may also have a fever and headache.

Care
The abscess must be broken to drain out the pus. The doctor may prick it with a special needle or make a cut in it. If the condition is severe, you may need to have your tonsils removed.

WHAT YOU SHOULD DO

• Rinse your throat with warm salt water or hydrogen peroxide: Mix 1 teaspoon of salt in 1 cup of warm water or 1/2 cup of hydrogen peroxide in 1/2 cup of warm water. After you finish rinsing, spit out the water; DO NOT SWALLOW IT. Rinse every 2 to 4 hours for several days.

- To help ease the pain, fill a plastic bag with ice and wrap it in a towel. Hold the ice on your neck for 20 minutes, 3 or 4 times a day.
- Over-the-counter medications, such as acetaminophen and ibuprofen, will also ease pain and fever. Take these and other medicines exactly as directed.
- If your doctor prescribes antibiotics, finish all the medication even if you begin to feel better. If you stop treatment too soon, some bacteria in the abscess may survive and cause a second infection.
- Rest in bed for 1 or 2 days, then slowly resume your regular activities.
- Eat soft or liquid foods for several days until your throat feels better. Milk, milk shakes, ice cream, gelatin, soups, and instant breakfast drinks are good choices. Slowly return to your normal diet.
- Drink 8 to 10 (soda-can size) glasses of water each day. For the first 1 or 2 days, it may feel better to sip the fluids.
- While your throat is sore, try not to cough, clear your throat, sing, talk loudly, or shout.
- Do not smoke until your throat feels better.

Call Your Doctor If . . .
- You have more pain, swelling, redness, or pus draining in your throat.
- You develop a high temperature.
- You get dizzy, have a really bad headache, or feel very sick all over.

Seek Care Immediately If . . .
- You cough or throw up blood.
- Your throat pain gets worse and you begin to drool.
- You have trouble breathing, or there is a change in your voice.

Pertussis in Children

See Whooping Cough

Pharyngitis

See Strep Throat

Phimosis

WHAT YOU SHOULD KNOW

If the foreskin of the penis is so tight that it can't be pulled back, the condition is known as phimosis (fim-O-sis). It is seen most frequently in children.

Causes
The problem may be present from birth. It also can be caused by an infection or scar tissue from an injury.

Care
If the boy is unable to urinate, seek medical attention at once. The doctor may need to thread a tube (catheter) into the tip of the penis, through the urinary canal (urethra), and into the bladder to drain the urine. If the boy can urinate, he may not need treatment right away. The usual remedy is circumcision to remove the foreskin.

WHAT YOU SHOULD DO

- Do NOT use force to pull the foreskin back. This can cause scarring and make the condition worse. Clean under the foreskin regularly if possible.
- In uncircumcised babies, the foreskin is normally tight. It usually doesn't start to loosen enough to be pulled back until the baby is at least 18 months old. Until then, leave the foreskin alone. Later, you may gently pull back the foreskin during bathing.

Call Your Doctor If . . .
- There is redness, swelling, or drainage from the foreskin. These are signs of infection.
- The boy has pain when urinating.
- The boy gets a high temperature.

Seek Care Immediately If . . .
- The boy has not urinated in 24 hours.

Phlebitis

See Deep Vein Thrombophlebitis

PID

See Pelvic Inflammatory Disease

Piles

See Hemorrhoids

Pilonidal Cyst

WHAT YOU SHOULD KNOW

A pilonidal (PIE-low-NI-dal) cyst is a sac under the skin at the base of the spine. It looks like a small hole, often with a few hairs coming out. The cyst may become infected. Pilonidal cysts are most common in young men.

Causes
The cysts form before birth, but present no problem until bacteria cause them to become infected.

Signs/Symptoms
Typically, there will be pain, redness, and swelling in the area of the cyst. A pus-like discharge may come from the cyst, and you may have fever and chills.

Care
You may need an antibiotic to fight the infection. Your doctor may have to open the cyst to drain the pus, and may need to remove the cyst surgically.

WHAT YOU SHOULD DO

- If the cyst is not infected, keep the area clean and dry. Bathe or shower daily and wash the area well with a germ-killing soap. Taking hot tub baths helps prevent infection. Dry the area well with a towel.
- Avoid tight clothing.
- If the cyst is infected and needs to be cut open and drained, your doctor will pack the wound with gauze. This allows the wound to heal from the inside outwards. You should return to the doctor's office in a few days for a follow-up wound check.
- Do not take tub baths or showers until the gauze is removed. You may wash at the sink.
- After the gauze is removed, apply a warm, wet wash cloth to the area or sit in a tub of warm water for 15 to 20 minutes several times a day to relieve the pain. Then clean the wound gently with mild, unscented soap.
- If your doctor prescribes an antibiotic to fight the infection, take all of the medication exactly as directed, even if you are feeling better. If you stop treatment too soon, some bacteria may survive and re-infect you. If you are using a pain reliever, take it exactly as directed.

Call Your Doctor If . . .
- You have increased pain, swelling, redness, drainage, or bleeding from the area.
- You develop a high temperature.
- You develop muscle aches, dizziness, or a general ill feeling.

Pinkeye

WHAT YOU SHOULD KNOW

Pinkeye, known medically as conjunctivitis (cun-JUNK-tuh-VI-tis), is an irritation of the inner eyelid and the surface of the white part of the eye. If caused by an infection, the disease spreads easily from person to person. With care, the problem should clear up in 7 days.

Causes
Infections and allergies are the most common causes. Air pollution, smoke, dust, and pollen may also be at fault.

Signs/Symptoms
Typically, you'll have painful red eyes, puffy eyelids, or a gritty feeling in the eyes. You may have clear, yellow, or green-colored eye discharge that may form crusts and cause the eyelids to stick together, especially in the morning.

Care
Your doctor will order tests to find the cause. If a bacterial infection is the culprit, the doctor may prescribe antibiotic medication.

WHAT YOU SHOULD DO

- To ease discomfort, apply a clean, warm or cool washcloth to your eye several times a day for 10 to 20 minutes.
- Do not touch or rub your eyes with your hands.
- Gently wipe away any discharge from the eyes with tissues.
- To keep from spreading infection, wash your hands often with soap and use paper towels to dry.
- Do not share towels or washcloths.
- Sunglasses may be helpful if light bothers your eyes.
- Do not use eye makeup. Keep contact lenses out of eyes until the irritation is gone.
- Do not drive or operate machinery if your vision is blurred.
- Keep children home from school or daycare until the eye is no longer pink.
- Your doctor may give you antibiotic medicine to treat your eye

infection. You may also use nonprescription eyedrops to help your pain.

Call Your Doctor If . . .
- The eye is still pink 3 days after starting treatment with medicine.
- Pain in the eye increases, the redness spreads, or your vision becomes blurred.
- You develop a high temperature.
- You have any problems that may be related to the medicine you are taking.

Pinworms

WHAT YOU SHOULD KNOW

Pinworm is also known as seatworm or threadworm. Medically, it is called enterobiasis (en-ter-o-BI-uh-sis) or oxyuriasis (ox-e-yur-EYE-uh-sis). It is an infection of the end of the bowel and anal area with tiny, white, thread-like worms that you can barely see. Because the worms live by getting their food from the person they have infected, they are called parasites. Infection with the worms is more common in warm climates.

Causes
Pinworm eggs can move from toilet seats to the body. They also spread through hand-to-hand or hand-to-mouth contact, and they can float in the air and be breathed in or swallowed. Once inside the body, the eggs travel to the small intestine and hatch.

Signs/Symptoms
The chief symptom is irritated skin and painful itching around the anus. The itching is worse at night and may keep you awake. If pinworms move to the opening of the vagina, they may cause itching, soreness, or a discharge. Other symptoms include loss of appetite and stomach pain, though this is rare. The skin may become pale and colorless.

Care
Your whole family may need treatment, which consists of medication to kill the worms. It usually only takes 1 or 2 treatments before the problem is under control or cured, but it is common for pinworms to come back.

WHAT YOU SHOULD DO

- Your doctor will prescribe medicine to kill the pinworms. The medicine may cause upset stomach, vomiting, or diarrhea, but must be used exactly as directed.
- On the day of treatment, do the following:
  —Thoroughly clean your house.
  —Machine wash sheets, clothing, and dishes at the hottest water setting.
  —Change all towels.
  —Cut and clean the fingernails of those who are infected.
- Everyone in your household—especially those who are infected— should wash hands well after using the toilet and before touching food.
- At least once a day, wash the anal area. Do this under a shower, if possible.
- When using public toilet seats, cover them with clean paper first.
- Try to keep children from scratching the anus. Have them keep their fingers away from the nose and mouth.
- Change sheets, pillowcases, towels, and nightwear often. Machine wash them on the hottest water setting. Change underwear daily.
- Have children wear snug cotton underpants.
- After the treatment, stools may look like the color of the medicine used to kill the worms.
- Be sure to keep any follow-up appointment the doctor may schedule.

Call Your Doctor If . . .
- The skin around the anus becomes sore and red.
- Itching still continues one week after treatment.
- Another family member has symptoms of pinworms after treatment.
- The medicine causes severe problems (a lot of throwing up or diarrhea, or really bad stomach pain).

Plantar Warts

WHAT YOU SHOULD KNOW

A plantar wart is a flat, hard lump on the bottom of your foot. The warts are most common in people 12 to 16 years of age, and may last for many years.

Causes

The warts are caused by a virus called the human papillomavirus (PAP-ih-LOW-muh-VI-russ), or HPV.

Signs/Symptoms

Plantar warts occur only on the sole of the foot. They form a lump that consists of a main circle or oval area surrounded by a build-up of skin layers. They can cause a great deal of pain when you stand or walk.

Care

The warts may go away without treatment. If over-the-counter medicine does not get rid of the wart, your doctor may need to remove it.

Risks

If the wart is surgically removed, you could develop an infection. Following your doctor's instructions carefully will usually prevent this from happening.

IF YOU'RE HEADING FOR THE HOSPITAL . . .

What to Expect While You're There

Professional wart removal usually involves the following steps.

- The wart and the area around it will be cleaned. Your doctor may be able to cut or shave off some of the dead skin.
- The doctor will put an acid chemical on the wart. He or she may use liquid acid called "paint," or may apply a "plaster" that contains the acid. The plaster is cut to the size and shape of the wart and held on with tape.
- When your doctor says it is all right to take off the acid paint or plaster, you should soak your foot in water and then rub, file, or cut off the dead skin.
- To keep pressure off the bottom of your foot, you can apply a donut-like pad over the wart.
- The treatment will take about 15 to 20 minutes. You may need more than one treatment to get rid of the wart.

After You Leave

- Follow your doctor's directions carefully.
- Keep the area clean and dry between treatments.
- DO NOT cut or shave the area being treated unless instructed to do so.
- It is important to return for additional treatments if instructed to do so.

Call Your Doctor If . . .
- You experience increasing pain or bleeding that won't stop after a treatment.
- You notice increasing redness, swelling, or drainage from the treated area. These are signs of infection.
- Your foot becomes painful, red, or swollen.
- You develop a high temperature.

Pleurisy

WHAT YOU SHOULD KNOW

Pleurisy (PLOOR-iss-ee) is caused by swelling and irritation of the membrane that surrounds the lungs. It is usually a symptom of another illness. It is also called Pleuritic Chest Pain.

Causes
Pleurisy can develop from many things, including bacterial or viral infections of the lungs (such as pneumonia), TB, lupus, chest injury or trauma, a blood clot in the lung, or cancer.

Sometimes a cause cannot be found. Doctors call this ideopathic (id-e-o-PATH-ik) pleurisy. Even though the cause isn't known, the problem can still be treated.

Signs/Symptoms
The hallmark of pleurisy is severe chest pain that starts suddenly. The pain is often strong or stabbing when you take a deep breath. It usually subsides or disappears between breaths. It's usually felt on one side of the stomach area or lower chest. Deep breathing and coughing often make it worse.

You may also have a fever, pain when moving, or fast, shallow breathing. Typically, you will be able to point to the exact location of the pain. In some people, the pain spreads to the neck, shoulder, or abdomen.

Care
While your doctor looks for the cause, you will get medicine to ease the pain. This will help you breathe more easily too.

Risks
Some cases of pleurisy clear up by themselves, but it's more likely that your lung problems will get worse. Possible problems include pneumonia or fluid build-up in the lining of the lungs. Some problems can cause damage to the lungs and affect your ability to breathe.

WHAT YOU SHOULD DO

• Always take your medicine as directed. If you feel it is not helping, call your doctor. Do not quit taking it on your own.
• If you are taking antibiotics, continue to take them until they are all gone—even if you feel well.
• If you are taking medicine that makes you drowsy, do not drive or use heavy equipment.
• Quit smoking. It harms the lungs. If you are having trouble quitting, ask your doctor for help.
• To ease the pain:
  —When you cough, hold a pillow tightly against your chest.
  —Lie on the side that hurts.
  —You may need to loosely wrap a 6 inch elastic ace bandage around your chest. You should unwrap it several times a day.
• To help keep your lungs free of infection, take 2 or 3 deep breaths and then cough. Do this often during the day.
• If you are coughing up sputum and milk seems to make the sputum thicker, do not eat or drink foods that contain milk.
• If you do not have to limit the amount of liquids you drink, drink 8 to 10 (soda-can size) glasses of water each day. This helps thin the sputum so it can be coughed up more easily.
• Use a humidifier to help keep the air moist and your sputum thin. This makes it easier to cough up the sputum. You must keep the humidifier free of fungus. Clean it every day.
• Rest until you feel better. You may return to work or school when your temperature is around 98.6 degrees F (37 degrees C).

Call Your Doctor If . . .
• You have a high temperature.
• You cough up yellow, green, gray, or bloody sputum.
• Your pain gets worse.

Seek Care Immediately If . . .
• You have blue or pale lips, fingernails, or toenails.
• You have increased trouble breathing even if the pain is less.

IF YOU'RE HEADING FOR THE HOSPITAL . . .

What to Expect While You're There
You may encounter the following procedures and equipment during your stay.
• **Activity:** At first you will need to rest in bed, with a few pillows to keep you sitting up a little. This will help your breathing. Do not lie

flat. Once you are breathing more easily, you will be allowed to increase your exercise.

- **Taking Vital Signs:** These include your temperature, blood pressure, pulse (counting your heartbeats), and respirations (counting your breaths). A stethoscope is used to listen to your heart and lungs. Your blood pressure is taken by wrapping a cuff around your arm.

- **Oxygen:** Your body may need extra oxygen at this time. It is given either by a mask or nasal prongs. Tell your doctor if the oxygen is drying out your nose or if the nasal prongs bother you.

- **Pulse Oximeter:** While you are getting oxygen, you may be hooked up to a pulse oximeter (ox-IM-uh-ter). It is placed on your ear, finger, or toe and is connected to a machine. It tells how much oxygen is in your blood.

- **ECG:** Also called a heart monitor, an electrocardiograph (e-lec-tro-CAR-dee-o-graf), or EKG. The patches on your chest are hooked up to a TV-type screen or a small portable box (telemetry unit). This screen shows a tracing of each heartbeat. Your heart will be watched for signs of injury or damage that could be related to your illness.

- **12 Lead ECG:** This test makes tracings from different parts of your heart. It can help your doctor decide whether there is a heart problem.

- **Chest X-ray:** This picture of your lungs and heart shows how they are handling the illness.

- **Blood:** Usually taken from a vein in your hand or from the bend in your elbow. Tests will be done on the blood.

- **IV:** A tube placed in your vein for giving medicine or liquids. It will be capped or have tubing connected to it.

- **Medicines:** You will be given medicine to ease the pain. This will help you breathe more easily also. You may also need antibiotics to fight infection.

- **Coughing and Deep Breathing:** It is important to do this often because it helps prevent infections in your lungs.
  - —To ease your pain during breathing, you may need to loosely wrap your rib cage with a 6 inch elastic bandage.
  - —Holding a pillow tightly against your chest when you cough can help reduce the pain. Lying on the side that is hurting, may also help ease the pain.

- **Cold/Heat:** A cool towel or heating pad (set on low) placed on the area that hurts may help ease the pain.

- **Sputum Sample:** If you are coughing up sputum, your doctor may need to send a sample to the lab. This sample may show what is causing your illness. It will also help the doctor choose the medicine you need.

- **Other Care:**
  - **Nerve Block:** You may need this if your pain gets worse. This is a shot of pain-killers in the nerves serving the chest (intercostal) muscles.
  - **Thoracentesis** (thor-uh-cent-E-sis): In this procedure, a needle is pushed through the chest wall to drain fluid from the chest. You will be given medicine to numb the area. Removing this fluid will allow you to breathe more easily.

After You Leave

Follow the directions listed under "What You Should Do."

PMS

See Premenstrual Syndrome

Pneumonia, Bacterial

See Bacterial Pneumonia

Pneumothorax

See Collapsed Lung

Poison Ivy

WHAT YOU SHOULD KNOW

Poison ivy causes a severe rash in sensitive individuals. The plant has three large, shiny leaves on each stem, and grows wild in woods and fields. Poison oak, poison sumac, and ragweed can cause a similar rash.

Causes

The rash is caused by an oil on the plant's leaves.

Signs/Symptoms

The rash is typically red, itchy, and swollen, with blisters on the part of the skin that touched the poison ivy. It usually oozes at first, then gets crusty and scaly. The liquid inside the blisters will not cause the rash to spread.

Care

Your doctor can prescribe medicine to relieve the itching and swelling. In addition, follow the directions listed below.

WHAT YOU SHOULD DO

• Do not scratch the rash or it may spread to other parts of your body. Fluid from the blisters will not cause the rash to spread, but any oil from the plant that remains on the skin can cause new problems.

• Wash the area with soap and water as soon as possible. Put calamine lotion on the rash to help dry the blisters.

• Wash the clothes you were wearing when you touched the plant. Wash anything else that may have picked up oil from the plant, including shoes, hunting and sports equipment, and tools.

• If your dog was with you, give him a bath in soap and water to wash off any oil from his fur.

• Put cool wet cloths on the rash to reduce the itching.
  —Use plain water or Burow's solution (Domeboro® powder), which you can buy over-the-counter. Dissolve 1 packet in 2 cups of cool water. Soak a clean towel in the solution, wring it out, and apply it to the rash.
  —Resoak the towel every few minutes. Apply the solution to the rash for about an hour several times a day.

• If the area is too large to cover with wet cloths, take 3 or 4 cornstarch baths daily. Mix 1 pound of cornstarch with a little water to make a paste and add it to a tub full of water.

• Taking hot, soapless showers may also be helpful.

• To keep from getting poison ivy, watch out for the plant and wear pants and long sleeved shirts when hiking in woods or fields.

• If you touch poison ivy again, try to prevent the rash by:
  —Removing your clothes as soon as possible and washing your entire body with soap and water.
  —Cleaning your fingernails to remove the plant oil.

Call Your Doctor If . . .

• You have a high temperature.

• The rash gets tender, exudes pus, or has soft yellow scabs.

• The itching gets worse or keeps you awake at night.

• The rash spreads to your eyes, mouth, or genital area, or covers more than a quarter of your skin.

• The rash is not better within a few days.

Poison-Proofing Your Home

WHAT YOU SHOULD KNOW

Children are extremely curious; they want to climb, touch, taste, and chew everything in sight. Unfortunately, each year about 6 million children—most of them less than five years old—swallow something harmful. That's why it is so important to keep all poisons out of their reach.

WHAT YOU SHOULD DO

- Keep all drugs and chemicals locked up or out of reach. Store them in childproof containers. Place child safety latches on cabinets and drawers that contain dangerous products.
- Keep all drugs and household products in their original containers. Don't store dangerous liquids in soft drink bottles.
- Don't leave medicines or household products sitting out, especially when you are called to the telephone or door.
- Don't leave medicine in a purse. Keep your guests' purses out of reach.
- Never call a medicine "candy."
- Put alcoholic beverages away after a party. Keep them out of reach of children. Don't leave partly filled glasses or open bottles or cans sitting out.
- Keep cigarettes and ashtrays out of reach.
- Check your house plants. Some varieties can make children sick. Teach your children not to put anything from a plant in their mouths.
- Keep a bottle of the poison remedy called syrup of ipecac in your medicine cabinet. (Check with your doctor or a poison control center before using this remedy. For certain types of poisoning, it MUST NOT be used.)
- Keep the telephone number of the nearest Poison Control Center next to each phone in your home.
- Go through each room in your house and look for anything that could harm a child. If you find any potentially dangerous items, remove them or put them in a safe location.
- In the **KITCHEN:**
  —Keep dishwashing soaps, drain cleaner, scouring pads, and oven cleaners out of reach. Don't store them under the sink.
- In the **BATHROOM:**
  —Keep toilet cleaner, medicines, sprays, powders, makeup, fingernail polish and remover, hair care products, aftershave lotions, and mouthwash out of reach.
  —Both prescription and nonprescription medicines can be dangerous. The most dangerous nonprescription medicines are aspirin and iron pills.
  —Keep the safety cap on all medicines. Flush old medicine down the toilet.

• In the **BEDROOM:**
—Don't leave medicine on your dresser or nightstand.
—Keep all perfume and makeup out of reach.
• In the **LAUNDRY AREA:**
—Keep detergents, soaps, bleach, fabric softener, and sprays out of reach.
• In the **GARAGE AND BASEMENT:**
—Keep gasoline and car care products, insect sprays, weed killers, turpentine, paint, paint thinner, antifreeze, and grease remover locked up or out of reach.

Postpartum Depression

WHAT YOU SHOULD KNOW

Many women feel sad, afraid, and unable to cope in the first few days after having a baby. This feeling is called postpartum (post-PAR-tum) blues, or baby blues. It usually goes away within two weeks.

When it doesn't go away or gets worse, you may find yourself unable to care for the baby or yourself. This is called postpartum depression. Treatment can relieve even the worst of such depressions. Without treatment, however, the condition could get worse and lead to dangerous thoughts about hurting yourself or your baby.

Causes
Fast changes in the body's hormone levels are partially to blame. Stress, lack of sleep, poor diet, and lack of help from family and friends also can bring on depression. Women who have emotional problems before the baby is born are more likely to develop the problem.

Signs/Symptoms
You may feel sad, nervous, irritated, or moody. Sometimes women feel angry at their baby, their partner, or their other children. Trouble sleeping, eating, or making decisions is common. In very bad cases, self-destructive thoughts may emerge.

Care
Many cases of postpartum blues will go away if a woman can get rest and help from family and friends. However, if the depression continues, medications and counseling may be needed.

WHAT YOU SHOULD DO

- Remember that it's normal to feel sad or worried right after your baby is born. This is a very big change in your life. Don't feel guilty.
- Rest is important. Don't try to do everything. Do only what is needed and let everything else go. Ask your partner, family, or friends to help, especially if you have other children.
- Try to nap when the baby naps. Ask your partner's help with night feedings or other baby care.
- Share your feelings with your partner, a friend, or another mother. Often just talking things out with someone you trust can be a big help.
- Take good care of yourself. Shower and dress each day. Don't forget to eat. Try to get out of the house a little each day. Go for a walk or meet with a friend. Get a baby-sitter or take the baby with you.
- Call your doctor, a hospital emergency department, or a mental health center if you need to talk about your problems. They will help you sort through your feelings. They also may be able to help you find a support group.

Call Your doctor If . . .
- You feel you are getting worse, or your depression does not go away.

Seek Care Immediately If . . .
- You feel like hurting yourself, your baby, or others.

Postpartum Perineal Care

WHAT YOU SHOULD KNOW

The perineum (PEAR-i-NEE-um) is the part of your body between your legs, including the vagina (birth canal) and rectum. After having a baby, you need to give this area special attention. Postpartum perineal care includes all the things you need to do to make the area feel better, heal properly, and avoid infection. You will need to do this for 1 to 3 weeks.

Causes
The perineum is severely stressed as a baby is pushed through the vagina (birth canal). Also, the doctor may have made a small opening called an episiotomy (eh-pee-z-AH-toe-mee) so that the vagina wouldn't tear when the baby was coming out. Although this is sewn back together, it will take time to heal.

Signs/Symptoms

There will be pain and swelling around the vagina because of stretching when the baby was born. You will also notice a discharge from the vagina. At first it will be bloody, then it will turn pink. Later it will turn yellow and then go away. You may have a tear in your vagina. You may also have stitches in your vagina.

Sometimes because of pushing and straining, hemorrhoids (HEM-uh-roids) may occur around the rectum. A hemorrhoid is a bulge in a blood vessel that can be very sore. Hemorrhoids feel worse when you are sitting up.

Care

You may need ice packs, or an ice sitz bath, to relieve the pain right after you give birth. You may be given pain medicine; and you also may get sprays or wipes that contain a numbing agent to help ease the pain. In addition, your doctor may give you medicine to help soften your stools so that it doesn't hurt as much when you go to the bathroom.

Keeping the area clean with a peri-bottle (a hand-held squirt bottle) can be soothing and help prevent infection. You will also need to use peri-pads in your underwear to catch the blood and discharge from the vagina.

WHAT YOU SHOULD DO

- Keep a supply of the following items at home: peri-pads, peri-bottle, toilet paper or cotton wipes, pain medicine such as acetaminophen, and other medicines your doctor asks you to take. Let your doctor know if you have any problems or questions.
- Check the amount and color of the discharge from your vagina. This shows how fast you are healing.
  - —For the first 2 to 3 days after you have had your baby, the blood will be a heavy flow and dark red. Some women pass clots and blood for 3 to 5 days.
  - —From the 3rd to the 10th day, the discharge gradually becomes pink, and the flow is lighter. After that, you will have a creamy or yellowish discharge for another 1 or 2 weeks.
- Clean the perineal area each time you use the toilet or change your perineal pads. Proceed as follows:
  - —Use a hand-held squirt bottle (peri-bottle) filled with warm tap water.
  - —While sitting on the toilet, rinse your perineum for at least 2 minutes. Aim the water from front to back.

—Pat the area dry with toilet paper or cotton wipes, again from front to back.

—Put on a fresh perineal pad.

—Stand up before flushing the toilet to avoid being sprayed with the water.

• Sitz baths during the first week may help you feel better. Fill the bathtub with warm water. Sit for 10 minutes twice a day. Put on a fresh perineal pad after the bath.

Call Your Doctor If . . .
• Your vaginal discharge:

—Gets heavier (soaking 1 pad every 1 to 2 hours).

—Turns bright red.

—Develops a bad smell.

• You start having a high temperature.

• You have pain in the abdomen.

Pregnancy

WHAT YOU SHOULD KNOW

During the 40 weeks of pregnancy, as your baby is growing inside the uterus (womb), there are many things you can do to ensure good health for both you and the baby.

Prenatal Care
This includes checkups with your doctor and any necessary medical care before your baby is born. Getting good prenatal care is very important. It helps prevent problems during pregnancy and childbirth.

You will probably have a pelvic exam (also called an "internal") during your first visit. Your doctor will check the size and shape of your uterus. A Pap smear to check for cancer of the cervix (the opening of the uterus) also may be done on the first visit, along with blood and urine tests.

Your doctor will want to see you monthly during most of your pregnancy. During the last 8 weeks, your visits will be more frequent. At each visit, you will be weighed and have your blood pressure checked. Your urine will be tested and the baby's growth will be checked. At some visits you may get an ultrasound, a painless test that shows the baby's growth and helps determine the due date. You may also need additional blood tests during the pregnancy.

Signs/Symptoms
As the baby grows, your body will go through many changes.

- You may have nausea and vomiting during early pregnancy.
- Your breasts will get larger and can make you uncomfortable.
- Red marks called stretch marks may show up on your skin.
- You may have back and leg aches from the weight of the growing baby.
- You may have mood changes going from joy to mild depression. These changes are normal; but talk to your doctor if you are depressed all the time.

Care

Pregnancy is a time to "listen" to your body. You can probably tell what you should and shouldn't do by the way you feel. For example, if you are tired, rest. If you are nauseated, eat a few soda crackers.

WHAT YOU SHOULD DO

Eating

- Focus on healthy foods. What you eat feeds both you and the baby. Choose from each of these food groups every day:
  —Fruits and vegetables.
  —Whole-grain breads and cereals.
  —Meat, fish, poultry, eggs, nuts, and beans.
  —Milk and milk products and cheese.
- Drink at least 6 to 8 glasses (soda-can size) of liquids such as milk, water, or juice. Cut down on drinks that have caffeine in them such as coffee, tea, and cola.
- Although you should get as many vitamins as possible from what you eat, your doctor may still want you to take daily vitamins and iron pills. The iron pills can cause constipation, so remember to drink liquids, eat good foods, and exercise.
- Your doctor will tell you about how much weight you should gain. Too much or too little weight gain can harm your baby. This is not the time to go on a diet.

Relieving Common Symptoms

- Here are some tips for controlling the many symptoms that accompany pregnancy:
  —**Morning Sickness:** You may have nausea and vomiting any time during the day. Eating small, frequent meals and avoiding greasy or spicy foods should help. Try eating a few soda crackers or a piece of dry toast before getting out of bed in the morning.

  Talk to your doctor if the nausea and vomiting lasts past the first 3 months of pregnancy or if you are losing weight. Do **not** take medicine for nausea and vomiting without asking your doctor.

—**Tiredness:** You may need more sleep to feel your best. Taking a few 10 or 15 minute rest breaks during the day may help you feel better. Try to stay well-rested. This will help you deal with the physical and emotional changes of pregnancy.

—**Back Pain:** You are likely to have back pain as your baby grows. When you need to bend down, try squatting instead. When squatting, use your leg muscles rather than your back muscles.

Try to maintain good posture by standing straight. Wear shoes with good support. Back rubs also may help.

—**Leg Cramps ("Charley Horse"):** As your baby grows and puts pressure on your lower body, your legs may not get enough blood. Leg cramps can develop when you are tired or not getting enough calcium in your diet.

Try to rest often with your legs higher than your heart. Drink milk and eat yogurt and cheeses. Talk to your doctor about your diet. You may need to take daily calcium pills.

—**Varicose (VARE-ih-koz) Veins:** These are swollen veins in your lower body, often the legs, where blood moves slowly. You are more likely to get varicose veins if other members of your family have them. The growing baby and long periods of standing can both put pressure on these veins.

If you have varicose veins in your legs, you should rest often with legs raised higher than your heart. Wearing support panty hose also helps. If you have varicose veins in the genital area, rest often with a small pillow under your bottom.

Varicose veins should improve or disappear after delivery.

—**Sore Breasts:** Your breasts will get larger, heavier, and possibly sore. A good supporting bra, sometimes worn 24 hours a day, may help you feel better.

You also may find liquid coming from your nipples. It may be clear or milk-like, but in either case is perfectly normal.

Your nipples may be sore. Wash them only with water. Applying lanolin may help the soreness.

—**Constipation:** Pregnancy can make your bowel movements hard to pass. To remedy the problem, drink plenty of liquids and eat foods such as bran cereal, raisins, fruits, and raw vegetables. Daily exercise may also help you. Check with your doctor before taking a laxative.

—**Hemorrhoids (HEM-uh-roids):** These are enlarged veins in the rectal area which cause pain and itching. They occur when the growing uterus puts pressure on rectal veins.

Eating fiber-filled foods, drinking liquids, and exercising will help keep bowel movements soft and help prevent this problem.

—**Heartburn:** This is a common complaint during pregnancy. As the baby grows, acid from your stomach is pushed up into your esophagus (ee-SOF-uh-gus) or food tube, causing a burning sensation.

Eating small, frequent meals rather than 3 large meals can help. Don't eat greasy or spicy foods or lie down after eating. Bending over or lying flat can make the problem worse. Ask your doctor about taking antacids.

—**Vaginal Discharge:** You may have thicker and heavier vaginal discharge, which could have an odor. Most of the time this is not a health problem. But you could have a vaginal infection. Check with your doctor if the discharge is accompanied by burning or itching.

—**Frequent Urination:** You will urinate more often as the growing uterus presses on the bladder. You could also pass urine when you cough, sneeze, or move.

—**Urinary Infections:** Infections in the urinary tract are more common during pregnancy. Call right away if you have burning or pain when you urinate. You will be given antibiotic medicine to treat the infection.

—**Moodiness:** Your moods may quickly change from joy to sadness or mild depression. These changes are caused by variations in your body's hormones. Talk to your doctor or someone close to you if you feel very sad or have feelings that could harm you.

—**Skin:** You may have red marks, called stretch marks, on your skin. There is nothing that you can do to keep from getting them. They often fade after pregnancy.

Your skin may feel dry and itchy. Applying lotion will help to remedy this problem.

The skin on your face may darken. You can prevent this by using a sunscreen or staying out of the sun.

You also may notice that the skin around your nipples and below your belly button is darker. After you have your baby, your skin will likely return to normal.

—**Edema (eh-DEEM-uh):** Your fingers, feet, and ankles may swell later in pregnancy. Lying down 2 or 3 times a day and raising your legs above your heart for 10 or 15 minutes will reduce the swelling. Your legs will also feel better.

Lie on your left side while sleeping. In this position the blood flow is better from your legs back to your heart; and this helps prevent swelling.

Cooking without salt can help reduce swelling. Even though you are retaining water, continue to drink plenty of liquids. Do **not** use water pills.

You may want to wear elastic support stockings. They will help your legs feel better.

—**Bleeding Gums:** Brushing and flossing during pregnancy will keep your gums and teeth healthy. You can see your dentist during pregnancy; but be sure to tell him that you are pregnant.

—**Round Ligament (lig-uh-ment) Pain:** On each side of your uterus are bands of tissue called ligaments. These hold the uterus in place. As the uterus grows, these ligaments are pulled and may cause abdominal pain. This is normal and you should not be concerned. Lying on your sore side may help the pain.

—**Toxoplasmosis (tox-o-plas-MO-sis):** This is an infection pregnant women can get from eating raw meat or being around cat litter. It can cause birth defects and other pregnancy problems.

Wash your hands after touching raw meat and make sure it is well-cooked. Let someone else clean your cat's litter box. Do not garden in soil that cats use as a bathroom.

Douching
• Do not douche during pregnancy. Talk to your doctor if you have questions about douching.

Exercise
• Regular exercise during pregnancy is important. It will help you feel better and keep you in good physical shape, making your labor and delivery easier.
• Start exercising slowly if you weren't active before pregnancy. Walking and swimming are great choices. Don't do any exercise that could hurt you or the baby. Check with your doctor if you are not sure whether an exercise is safe.

Hot Tubs
• Do **not** sit in a hot tub or sauna while you are pregnant.

Sex
• You can have sex until shortly before your labor starts unless there are complications. Your doctor may tell you to limit or not have sex if you are bleeding from the vagina or having pain in your abdomen or vagina.

Work
• If you are healthy, you can work until just before labor. Check with your doctor if you work around poisonous or harmful substances. After delivery, your doctor will let you know when you can return to work.

Smoking
• Your baby may weigh less at birth if you smoke during pregnancy. Smoking also increases the chances of your baby being born too early or not growing well. Do not smoke tobacco or marijuana during pregnancy.

Alcohol
• Do **not** drink alcohol while pregnant. Alcohol can cause birth defects and other problems. Your baby will have a better chance of being born healthy if you stop drinking now.

Medicines
• Do **not** take any medicine without first checking with your doctor. This includes drugs that can be bought over-the-counter such as aspirin or acetaminophen.

Street Drugs
• Do **not** use any street drugs such as cocaine, marijuana, or heroin while pregnant. These drugs can harm the baby.

Travel
• The most comfortable time to travel is during the 4th to 6th months. Your morning sickness should be gone and you may have more energy during this time. Ask your doctor for advice before taking a trip. The following tips may be helpful:
  —Wear your seat belt if taking a road trip. Fasten the lap belt under your belly and across your upper leg. Loose-fitting clothes will help you feel better. Stop every hour to get out of the car and walk around.
  —It is safe to fly during pregnancy. An aisle seat will make it easier for you to get to the bathroom or walk around. Check with your doctor before flying during the last month of pregnancy.
  —Travel can upset your stomach. Do **not** take medicines without checking with your doctor. This includes laxatives (medicine to help you have a bowel movement) and motion sickness pills.

Clothing
- Wear loose, comfortable garments. Wearing flat or low-heeled shoes may help you keep your balance.

Call Your Doctor Immediately If . . .
- You have blood or liquid coming from your vagina.
- You have swelling and puffiness of your face, fingers, or feet.
- You have frequent headaches or headaches that will not go away.
- You vomit more than 3 to 4 times daily.
- You have dizziness, fainting, or blurred vision.
- Your baby has not moved for 8 to 10 hours.
- You have chills or a high temperature.
- You have burning when you urinate or are urinating less.
- You are having frequent regular contractions before the 36th week.

Seek Care Immediately If . . .
- You have bright red, painless vaginal bleeding.
- The umbilical (um-BILL-ih-cull) cord is hanging out of your vagina.
- Early in the pregnancy you have dull or sharp lower abdominal pain, spotty or heavy vaginal bleeding, or pain in the back or right shoulder.

Pregnancy, Tubal

See Ectopic Pregnancy

Premenstrual Syndrome

WHAT YOU SHOULD KNOW

Premenstrual syndrome (pree-MEN-strul SIN-drome)—also known as PMS—is a common group of symptoms that can happen about one or two weeks before a woman starts her period. These symptoms can affect the body and the way a woman acts and feels. They go away after the period begins. There is no cure for PMS, but medicines may help reduce some of the symptoms.

Causes
The cause of PMS is unknown. It is thought to be related to changes in chemicals in the body called hormones. About half of all women have PMS at some time. It becomes more common with age. We do not know why some women have more severe cases than others. Stress seems to encourage the problem.

Signs/Symptoms

Many different changes can occur. Most women have only a few.

- **Changes in how you act or feel:** Feeling mad, tense, nervous, or sad; feeling hungry; changes in mood; crying spells; wanting to be left alone; craving foods like chocolate, sugar or salt. Some women have trouble with thinking or concentration. You may feel very tired or have trouble sleeping.
- **Changes in your body:** Weight gain and swollen breasts, belly, ankles, hands, and face are common. Acne (pimples) and headaches can also occur. Some women feel dizzy or may faint. You may have changes in your bowels such as constipation or diarrhea. You may not urinate as often as usual.

Care

There is no cure. Medicines that help the body get rid of water can sometimes reduce the swelling. Taking hormones (birth control pills) and other medicines works for some women. Getting counseling or joining a support group can help you understand the problem and help you and your family to deal with it. You may need to make changes in your life like eating differently, exercising more, and reducing your stress level.

WHAT YOU SHOULD DO

- Write down the date your periods start and end and what your symptoms are each day. Do this for at least two or three menstrual periods. Knowing when you are likely to have PMS symptoms will help you plan your activities to keep the premenstrual time as free from stress as possible. Stress often makes the symptoms worse.
- Avoiding foods that have a lot of salt will help prevent your body from feeling so swollen. Read the "Nutrition Facts" label on every food or drink package to find out how much salt (sodium) is in it. Don't have more than 3000 mg of sodium a day.
- Try to avoid foods and beverages that have caffeine in them, including coffee, colas, tea, and chocolate. Too much caffeine can make you feel more nervous or moody.
- Eat well-balanced meals. Don't smoke or drink alcohol for 1 week before your period, and get plenty of sleep.
- Exercising every day can help relieve PMS symptoms. It can make you feel better and reduce stress. Yoga, relaxation exercises, and biofeedback may also help cut stress. A counselor may be able to help you learn to lessen stress and handle possible conflicts in your life. Ask your doctor for sources of help or look in the telephone book under Mental Health Services.

• Learn as much as you can about PMS. Books on the subject can be found in bookstores and libraries. There are support groups for women with PMS. You also can get information from a national PMS association at the following address: PMS Access, PO Box 9326, Madison, WI 53715; or call toll-free 1-800-222-4767.

Pressure-Equalizing Ear Tubes

WHAT YOU SHOULD KNOW

Doctors sometimes insert a pressure-equalizing (PE) tube into an incision or opening in the eardrum to prevent middle ear infections. These infections, known medically as otitis media, are particularly common in young children. The operation is known as a myringotomy (mir-ing-GOT-oh-mee). The tubes (also called ventilation tubes, tympanoplasty tubes, or transtympanic tubes) resemble very small spools of thread.

The PE tubes remain in the eardrums for between 6 and 18 months. During this time, they gradually work their way out of the eardrums and into the ear canals. A small amount of blood may ooze from the ears when the tubes finally come out. Because the tubes are very tiny, it's unlikely that you will see them when they fall out.

If the tubes remain in the eardrums longer than five years, they should be removed. Otherwise, scar tissue might form around them.

Risks

There is a small chance that the tubes could cause scarring or injury to the eardrum, leading to hearing problems. In addition, pus may drain from the ear.

IF YOU'RE HEADING FOR THE HOSPITAL . . .

Before You Go

• Your doctor will tell you when you or your youngster should stop eating or drinking. Follow these directions exactly.
• Be sure to remove glasses, contact lenses, and false teeth before the surgery. Jewelry should also be taken off.

What to Expect While You're There

You may encounter the following procedures and equipment during your stay:
• **Emotional:** If your child is having the operation, you may stay to give comfort and support. Children feel safer in the hospital with a parent nearby.
• **Taking Vital Signs:** These include temperature, blood pressure,

pulse (counting the heartbeats), and respirations (counting the breaths). A stethoscope is used to listen to the heart and lungs. Blood pressure is taken by wrapping a cuff around the arm. There is no pain when taking vital signs.

- **IV:** A tube placed in a vein for giving medicine or liquids. It will be capped or have tubing connected to it.
- **During the Surgery . . .**
  —Children are usually put to sleep during this operation. Adults may receive numbing medication instead.
  —The doctor will make a tiny hole in the eardrum to drain out fluid that has accumulated inside the ear.
  —The PE tube will then be put into the hole in the eardrum so that the fluid can continue to drain.
  —To fight possible infection, the doctor will put antibiotic medicine in the ear.
  —After the surgery, patients are allowed to wake up in the recovery room before being returned to their room or sent home.

After You Leave

- Medications given during the operation will cause drowsiness. Do not plan on driving immediately afterward.
- After PE tubes are put in, there may be a mild earache for 2 to 3 hours, and clear fluid may drain from the ears for up to 24 hours.
- Your doctor may suggest medicine to ease the pain.

Call Your Doctor If . . .

- Pain persists despite the operation.
- Blood or pus drains from either ear.
- A fever develops.

Proctitis

WHAT YOU SHOULD KNOW

Proctitis (proc-TIE-tus) is swelling in the last part of the bowel—the rectum and the tissues around the anus.

Causes

Proctitis can result from a number of diseases spread by sex, infections from certain kinds of bacteria, and radiation therapy.

Signs/Symptoms

Typical symptoms include rectal pain, a constant urge for a bowel movement, blood or mucus from the rectum, and cramps on the left side of the abdomen.

Care

You may need tests done on your blood and stool, and your doctor may need to examine the anus and rectum through a flexible tube. You also may need to be tested for diseases spread by sex. Treatment will depend on the cause.

WHAT YOU SHOULD DO

- If you have an infection, your doctor may prescribe an antibiotic medicine to kill the germs. Take it exactly as directed and finish the entire prescription, even if you begin to feel better.
- You may take medicine for pain and swelling, including oral pain-killers and products applied to the anus.
- If you have a sexually transmitted infection:
  —Don't have sex, including anal intercourse, until your doctor tells you the infection is cured.
  —Tell your sexual partner that you have this infection so that he or she can be treated.
  —Use a latex condom during sex. This helps protect against catching or spreading proctitis and other infections.
- Keep the anal area clean and dry. After every bowel movement, clean the area with a moistened tissue, cotton ball, or soft washcloth. Then gently pat the area dry.
- To help relieve pain, sit in a tub of comfortably hot water for 10 to 15 minutes. Do this several times a day.
- To prevent constipation, eat a high-fiber diet (vegetables, fruits, whole grains) and drink at least 8 glasses (soda-can size) of water a day.
- Avoid foods and beverages that may irritate the rectum. These include beer, tea, coffee (regular and decaffeinated), milk, cola, tomatoes, citrus fruits, nuts, chocolate, and spicy foods.
- Avoid frequent use of laxatives.

Call Your Doctor If . . .

- You start having really bad stomach pain, chills, joint pain, rash, swelling of the testicles, or a high temperature.
- Your symptoms come back after treatment.

Proctoscopy

See Sigmoidoscopy

Prolapsed Disk

See Slipped Disk

Prostate, Enlarged

See Enlarged Prostate

Prostatitis

WHAT YOU SHOULD KNOW

Prostatitis (PRAH-stuh-TIE-tus) is an inflammation and swelling of the prostate (PRAH-state), the donut-shaped gland that sits at the base of the bladder and surrounds the urinary canal (urethra). Prostatitis occurs most often in older men whose prostates have grown larger than normal.

Causes

The problem is sometimes the result of infection by bacteria, which can travel up the urethra or reach the prostate through the blood. In some cases, no specific cause can be found.

Signs/Symptoms

Typical symptoms include the urge to urinate right away and a burning sensation during urination. Other signs are frequent urination (of only small amounts) and difficulty starting urination, with failure to completely empty the bladder.

You may also have a fever and chills, or notice blood in your urine or semen. You may experience pain between the scrotum and the anus, in your lower back, or in your muscles and joints. Bowel movements may also be painful.

Care

Your doctor may prescribe antibiotics to fight infection. Medications may also be needed to make your stools soft, or lower fever.

WHAT YOU SHOULD DO

• If you are taking antibiotics to fight infection, finish the entire prescription, even if you feel better. Some bacteria may survive and re-infect you if you stop the drug too soon.
• You may take acetaminophen, aspirin, or ibuprofen for pain.
• Rest in bed until fever and pain go away. When you feel better, you may resume regular activities.

• Drink 8 to 10 soda-can size glasses of water a day to encourage urination. Be sure not to let your bladder become too full.
• Do not drink any alcohol or eat spicy foods until the infection is cured; they irritate the urinary tract.
• There is no need to give up sex. In fact, being sexually active may lower your risk of developing the infection again.

Call Your Doctor If . . .
• You find blood in your urine.
• You cannot urinate.
• There is no improvement after a few days.
• You have any problems (redness, swelling, trouble breathing, or a bad upset stomach) that you think may be caused by the medicine you are taking.
• Your symptoms come back after treatment.

Seek Care Immediately If . . .
• You get a high temperature or shaking chills.

Pubic Lice

See Crabs

Pulled Elbow

WHAT YOU SHOULD KNOW

Pulled elbow, a mild dislocation that occurs in children, is often called a "nursemaid's elbow." It happens when a sudden yank on the child's arm pulls the two forearm bones out of line. It occurs most frequently in children 1 to 4 years old. Because the chances of the dislocation recurring are high for 3 to 4 weeks after this injury, it is important to avoid pulling the child's arm during this period.

Causes
The dislocation usually results from pulling the child's arm—even just to swing the youngster around. The problem is more likely in children with a birth defect that causes the elbow to pull out of its socket easily.

Signs/Symptoms
Pain and swelling of the elbow may make the child unwilling to move the injured arm.

Care

An x-ray of the elbow will probably be needed. Your doctor may then have to reset the bones by pulling on the youngster's arm. This will be painful until the elbow has popped back into place. The child may need to wear a sling until the elbow has healed. A cast is rarely necessary. If the problem occurs repeatedly, the child may need surgery to fix the joint.

WHAT YOU SHOULD DO

- Try to put ice on the injury for 15 to 20 minutes each hour for the first 1 to 2 days. Put the ice in a plastic bag and place a towel between the bag of ice and the skin.
- After the first 1 to 2 days, you may put heat on the injury to help ease the pain. Use a heating pad (set on low), a whirlpool bath, or warm, moist towels for 15 to 20 minutes every hour for 48 hours.
- If your child is given a sling, keep it on until the doctor says you can remove it. This will make the youngster more comfortable and will help keep the problem from recurring. It's often difficult to keep a younger child in a sling. If the child objects, don't force the issue.
- For pain relief, you may give the child acetaminophen.
- Do not pull the child by the hand, wrists, or forearms. Use the upper arms or armpits to lift the child.
- If the youngster is given a cast, remember that it should never get wet.
  —When giving the child a bath, cover the cast with a plastic bag and secure the top with tape or a loose rubber band. Remove the plastic bag as soon as the youngster gets out of the water.
  —If the cast gets really wet and soft, call your doctor right away. Sometimes the wet part of a cast can be dried with a hair dryer set on low.

Call Your Doctor If . . .

- The child still refuses to use the arm 6 hours after it is put back into place.
- The child still has pain after 24 hours.
- The child's fingers get numb and tingly.
- The child's elbow comes out of the socket again.

Pulled Muscle

See Muscle Strain

Pulmonary Edema

WHAT YOU SHOULD KNOW

When extra fluid collects in the lungs, the condition is known as pulmonary (PULL-mon-air-ee) edema (eh-DEE-ma).

Causes
Many things can cause this illness. Among them are heart disease, allergies to drugs, lung injuries, strokes, head injury, infection, fever, drug overdose, or excess body fluid.

Signs/Symptoms
Early signs may include coughing and restlessness during sleeping. Later you may experience trouble breathing when awake and at night. Coughing usually brings up white or pink-tinged frothy sputum.

Noisy breathing (wheezing and bubbly sounds), bluish nailbeds and lips, sweating, and a fast heartbeat are other signs. You also may feel very anxious.

Care
You will need a stay in the hospital. It is important to get rid of the extra fluid in your lungs, while making sure they get enough oxygen.

Risks
This is a serious, life-threatening illness, and treatment should not be delayed or avoided. Untreated, this condition can be fatal.

WHAT YOU SHOULD DO

Call Your Doctor If . . .
- You are light-headed or dizzy, sweaty, or nauseated after you take your medicine.
- You have gained 2 to 3 pounds in 1 or 2 days.
- You cough up yellow, green, or pink frothy sputum.
- You are wheezing (a high-pitched noise when breathing in or out).
- You have trouble breathing, have swelling in your feet or ankles, or feel more tired than usual.
- You have a high temperature, muscle aches, headache, and dizziness. These are signs of an infection.

Seek Care Immediately If . . .
- You have these signs of fluid in your lungs or heart failure:
  —You have more trouble breathing than usual, feel weak, cannot

sleep or rest because of trouble breathing, or have a fast or uneven heartbeat.
—You have noisy or bubbly breathing and cough up pink frothy sputum.
—You have increased swelling in your legs, feet, and abdomen. You feel dizzy. Your lips and nailbeds are a white or blue color.
• You have chest pain that spreads to your arms, jaw, or back, and you are sweating, feel sick to your stomach, and have trouble breathing. These are signs of a heart attack.
• **These are emergencies. Call 911 or 0 (operator)** to get to the nearest hospital or clinic. **Do not drive yourself!**

IF YOU'RE HEADING FOR THE HOSPITAL . . .

What to Expect While You're There

You may encounter the following procedures and equipment during your stay.
• **Ventilator:** Also called a respirator. This is a special machine to help with breathing.
• **ET Tube:** A tube, placed in either the mouth or nose, that goes into the lungs. It's usually hooked up to a breathing machine. With this tube in place, you will not be able to talk, but can hear normally.
• **Medicines:** There are many different medicines that can help remove extra fluid from your lungs, help you breathe easier, and ease your pain.
—**Diuretics** (dy-u-RET-iks): Often called "water pills." This medicine helps remove extra water from the body. It may be given by mouth or in your IV.
—**Morphine:** Opens up veins to help remove extra fluid, may help relax breathing, and lower anxiety.
—**Antibiotics:** Used to fight infection if it is causing the illness.
—**Heart Medicines:** May be needed to make the heartbeat stronger.
—**Lung Medicine:** May be needed to open the airways in the lungs so you can breathe easier.
• **Heart Tubes/Wires:** You may be attached to many different tubes and wires. Some may enter your body under your collarbone or in your groin and be threaded into your heart. They are attached to monitors that measure your heart while it's working. These readings help your doctor guide your treatment.
• **Chest X-ray:** This picture of your lungs and heart will help your doctor determine the seriousness of the problem.
• **Taking Vital Signs:** These include your temperature, blood pressure, pulse (counting your heartbeats), and respirations (counting

your breaths). A stethoscope is used to listen to your heart and lungs. Your blood pressure is taken by wrapping a cuff around your arm.

- **Oxygen:** You may need extra oxygen during your stay. It is given either by a mask or nasal prongs. Tell your doctor if the oxygen is drying out your nose or if the nasal prongs bother you.
- **Pulse Oximeter:** While you are getting oxygen, you may be hooked up to a pulse oximeter (ox-IM-uh-ter). It is placed on your ear, finger, or toe and is connected to a machine that measures the oxygen in your blood.
- **ECG:** Also called a heart monitor, an electrocardiograph (e-LEK-tro-CAR-dee-o-graf), or EKG. The patches on your chest are hooked up to a TV-type screen or a small portable box (telemetry unit). This screen shows a tracing of each heartbeat. Your heart will be watched for signs of injury or damage that could be related to your lung congestion.
- **12 Lead ECG:** This test makes tracings from different parts of your heart. It can help your doctor decide whether a heart abnormality is part of the problem.
- **Blood Gases:** Blood is taken from an artery in your wrist, elbow, or groin. It is tested for the amount of oxygen it contains.
- **Blood:** Usually taken from a vein in your hand or from the bend in your elbow. Tests will be done on the blood.
- **IV:** A tube placed in your vein for giving medicine or liquids. It will be capped or have tubing connected to it.

After You Leave

- Rest in bed until you are breathing easier and feel stronger. Then, slowly return to your normal activities.
- Get at least 7 hours of rest each night. Take a nap during the day if you feel tired. As you get stronger, you will need less rest during the day.
- Exercise daily. It helps make the heart stronger, lowers blood pressure, and keeps you healthy. If your exercise plan seems too hard or too easy, talk to your doctor.
- Always take your medicine as directed by your doctor. If you feel it is not helping, call your doctor. Do not quit taking it on your own.
- If you are taking antibiotics, continue to take them until they are gone—even if you feel better.
- If you have other illnesses such as diabetes or high blood pressure, it is important to control them also. Take medicines for these illnesses as directed. Because of your other illnesses, you have a higher chance of getting fluid in your lungs if you don't take care of yourself.

- Quit smoking. It harms the heart and lungs. If you have trouble quitting, ask your doctor for help.
- Weighing too much can make the heart work harder. If you need to lose weight, ask your doctor for the plan that's best for you.
- Weigh yourself every day, before breakfast. Weight gain can be a sign of extra fluid in your lungs or body. Call your doctor if you have gained 2 to 3 pounds in a day.
- To prevent fluid build-up, your doctor will probably put you on a low-salt diet. Reducing fat and cholesterol is also important. Ask your doctor what you should and should not eat.
- Do not drink alcoholic beverages. Alcohol makes the heart and lungs work harder.

Pulmonary Embolism

WHAT YOU SHOULD KNOW

A pulmonary embolism is a blood clot or piece of fat blocking an artery in the lung. Clots can develop in any vein, break loose, and go to the lungs.

Causes

Most pulmonary embolisms are clots that come from deep veins in the legs or pelvis. Fatty embolisms usually come from a break in a bone or, during pregnancy, from amniotic fluid. This type of embolism occurs less frequently.

Chances of a blood clot forming increase if you sit or lie in one spot for a long time. Surgery, heart problems, and taking birth control pills also increase your chances of forming a clot.

Signs/Symptoms

The most common symptoms are trouble breathing and sudden chest pain that worsens with deep breathing. Other signs are faintness or fainting, coughing (sometimes with blood), a fast heartbeat, and a low fever.

Care

While in the hospital, you will have tests to find the blood clot. These may include a chest x-ray, pulmonary angiogram, venogram, or lung scan (also called a VP scan). These are all types of pictures of the chest, arteries, veins, and lungs.

You may be given oxygen, blood thinners, and pain medicine, and surgery may be needed to remove the clot.

Risks

If the pulmonary embolism is not treated it can cause part of the lung to die. Thousands of people a year get a pulmonary embolism and some do die. But if you see your doctor right away, you can be treated safely with fewer problems. Without treatment, your chances of getting another potentially fatal embolism increase.

WHAT YOU SHOULD DO

- To keep blood clots from forming in your legs, do not rest in bed for long periods of time during an illness. If you must stay in bed, change the position of your legs frequently. Start walking as soon as possible, especially after surgery.
- Do not wear tight garters or girdles, and avoid tight pants as well. Do wear tight knee socks, especially when you must stay in bed.
- When traveling, stand and walk every 1 or 2 hours. Don't cross your ankles or legs for long periods of time. Don't smoke, especially if you're taking birth control pills.

Call Your Doctor If . . .

- While taking blood thinning medication for the embolism, you find yourself bruising easily and often, develop bleeding from your gums or nose, or have blood in your urine or stools.
- You have swelling or pain in the calf of your leg. This may be a sign of a leg clot. Inform your doctor immediately.

Seek Care Immediately If . . .

- You have sudden chest pain, have trouble breathing, or begin coughing-up blood. You may have another embolism. **Call 911 or 0 (operator)** to get to the nearest hospital.

IF YOU'RE HEADING FOR THE HOSPITAL . . .

What to Expect While You're There

You may encounter the following procedures and equipment during your stay.

- **Taking Vital Signs:** These include your temperature, blood pressure, pulse (counting your heartbeats), and respirations (counting your breaths). A stethoscope is used to listen to your heart and lungs. Your blood pressure is taken by wrapping a cuff around your arm.
- **Oxygen:** Your body may need extra oxygen at this time. It is given either by a mask or nasal prongs. Tell your doctor if the oxygen is drying out your nose or if the nasal prongs bother you.
- **Pulse Oximeter:** While you are getting oxygen, you may be hooked up to a pulse oximeter (ox-IM-uh-ter). It is placed on your ear,

finger, or toe and is connected to a machine. It measures the oxygen in your blood.

- **Activity:** At first you may need to rest in bed with your head and feet slightly raised.
  - —Be sure to slowly move your legs around often. This keeps the blood from settling in your legs and causing more blood clots.
  - —You may be given tight knee socks or leg wraps. They keep blood from pooling in your legs and forming clots.
  - —Don't cross your legs or ankles.
- **Blood:** Usually taken from a vein in your hand or from the bend in your elbow. Tests will be done on the blood.
- **Blood Gases:** Blood is taken from an artery in your wrist, elbow, or groin and tested for oxygen.
- **IV:** A tube placed in your vein for giving medicine or liquids. It will be capped or have tubing connected to it.
- **Medicines:** You may be given any of the following medications.
  - —**Heparin:** This drug keeps the blood thin so no other clots form. It is given in an IV.
  - —**Other Blood Thinners:** Drugs that can be taken by mouth, such as aspirin or warfarin, will eventually be substituted for heparin. These also keep clots from forming.
  - —**Clot Busters:** These drugs break apart existing clots. They are given in your IV, usually at the same time as heparin. This medicine can make you bleed or bruise easily.
- **ECG:** Also called a heart monitor, an electrocardiograph (e-lec-tro-CAR-dee-o-graf), or EKG. The patches on your chest are hooked up to a TV-type screen or a small portable box (telemetry unit). This screen shows a tracing of each heartbeat. Your heart will be watched for signs of injury or damage.
- **12 Lead ECG:** This test makes tracings from different parts of your heart. It can help your doctor decide whether there is a heart problem.
- **Chest X-ray:** This picture of your lungs and heart will help doctors decide whether there is a clot.
- **Other Tests:** One test is called a Ventilation-Perfusion scan. Another is called pulmonary (PULL-mun-air-ee) arteriography (r-tear-e-OG-ruf-e). Both tests help your doctor see whether your lungs are working normally and whether there is a clot blocking blood flow. The doctor may also get an x-ray of your veins (a venogram) to check for additional clots.

After You Leave

• Be certain to take your medicine exactly as directed by your doctor. If you feel it is not helping, call the doctor. Do not quit taking it on your own.

• If you are taking a blood thinner:

—Wear a medic-alert bracelet to warn people that you are taking a blood thinner.

—Notify your dentist and other caregivers that you are taking a blood thinner.

—Watch for bleeding from your gums or nose, or in your urine or stools.

—Avoid contact sports since you will bruise more easily.

• Every couple of hours take 2 or 3 deep breaths.

• Quit smoking. It harms the lungs. If you're taking birth control pills, it also increases the chances of a clot.

Puncture Wound

WHAT YOU SHOULD KNOW

Puncture wounds are perforations made by sharp, pointed objects. The object may carry dirt and germs deep into the tissues. This kind of wound usually takes from 2 days to 2 weeks to heal, depending on its depth. Most of the time these wounds are not stitched closed because of the danger of infection.

Causes

Nails, needles, teeth, ice picks, bullets—any sharp, pointed object can cause a puncture.

Signs/Symptoms

Puncture wounds are accompanied by pain, bruising, bleeding, and swelling. Bleeding is beneficial because it helps carry dirt out of the wound. However, some puncture wounds may cause very little bleeding.

Care

Because puncture wounds are especially prone to infection, it is extremely important to clean the wound well and to keep it clean by soaking it several times a day. Your doctor may give you a tetanus shot if you have not had one in the past 5 to 10 years. If you think there might still be something in the wound, you will probably need an x-ray.

WHAT YOU SHOULD DO

- Soak the wound in warm water for 10 to 20 minutes 2 to 3 times a day. After soaking, put a fresh bandage over it.
- Keep the bandage clean and dry. If it gets wet and must be changed, unwrap it slowly and carefully. If the bandage sticks or starts to hurt, use warm water to loosen it gently. Pat the area dry with a clean towel before putting on another bandage.
- If possible, keep the wound lifted above the level of your heart for 24 to 48 hours. This will help reduce the pain and swelling and promote healing.
- Do not go swimming and, if the wound is on your hand, do not wash dishes until the puncture has healed (usually 3–5 days).
- If you are given a tetanus shot, your arm may get swollen, red, and warm to the touch at the site of the shot. This is a normal reaction to the medicine.

Call Your Doctor If . . .
- You have a high temperature.
- Blood soaks through the bandage.
- The pain in the wound gets worse.
- You feel numbness or see swelling of the skin below the wound.
- You have redness, swelling, pus, a bad smell, or red streaks coming from the wound. These are signs of infection.

Rape

See Sexual Assault

Raynaud's Syndrome

WHAT YOU SHOULD KNOW

Raynaud's (Ray-KNOWS) Syndrome is a circulation problem affecting the fingers and, sometimes, the toes. It is more common among women, especially those between the ages of 20 and 40.

Causes
When the small arteries that bring blood to the fingers and toes are exposed to cold, they spasm and contract, reducing the blood supply. The arteries may be extra-sensitive to the cold because of problems in your immune system. People with Raynaud's Syndrome frequently have other diseases such as lupus (LEW-pus) and arthritis.

Signs/Symptoms

Fingers turn pale with cold or stress, then turn bluish, and, finally, red. Pain, numbness, and tingling accompany these color changes. Warming your hands or feet usually helps relieve these symptoms.

Care

You may have tests done on your blood and x-rays of your hands and feet. You also may have a cold challenge test in which your hands are plunged in cold water. You may be given medicine that expands your blood vessels so that blood flows more easily to your fingers and toes. You also may be given medicine to help you relax. Surgery may be needed, but this is rare.

Do's and Don'ts

To keep from getting Raynaud's Syndrome, stop smoking and stay away from cigarette smoke. Also, try not to get stressed-out. Make sure you follow your doctor's care plan for diseases, such as Lupus and arthritis, that are known to lead to Raynaud's.

WHAT YOU SHOULD DO

- Always take your medicine as directed by your doctor. If you feel it is not helping, call your doctor. Do not quit taking it on your own.
- Don't let your hands or feet get cold. Keep your whole body warm and dry. Wear mittens or gloves when handling ice or frozen food and when outdoors. Use holders for glasses or cans containing cold drinks. If possible, stay indoors during very cold weather.
- Limit your use of caffeine. Switch to decaffeinated coffee, tea, and soda pop. Avoid chocolate.
- Don't smoke. This makes your symptoms worse. Avoid staying around people who smoke.
- Wear loose fitting socks and comfortable, roomy shoes.
- Avoid using tools and machinery that vibrate.
- Whenever possible, avoid stressful situations and emotional upset. Exercise, meditation, and yoga may help you cope with stress.
- Many people with Raynaud's syndrome often find biofeedback training helpful. It teaches them a way to control attacks.

Call Your Doctor If . . .

- Your pain becomes worse, despite treatment.
- You get sores on your fingers and toes that do not heal.

Rectal Bleeding

WHAT YOU SHOULD KNOW

The rectum is the last part of the bowel; just inside the anus. Bleeding in the rectum can range from mild to life-threatening.

Causes
Bleeding can be caused by rips in the lining of the rectum; infection; hemorrhoids (HEM-uh-roids), which are swollen veins of the rectum; polyps (POL-ips), which are lumps of tissue that bulge out from the lining; or tumors.

Signs/Symptoms
Typically, you will notice bright red blood coming out of the rectum or appearing on the stool. Blood may be found in a test of the stool. Other possible symptoms are dizziness, light-headedness, or fainting from loss of blood.

Care
Depends on the cause of bleeding. You may need surgery or other treatment to stop the bleeding. You may be given antibiotic medicine to treat an infection. If there is a lot of bleeding, you may need a blood transfusion.

Risks
Without treatment, you may continue to bleed and may even die.

WHAT YOU SHOULD DO

- Be sure to see your doctor. It's important to find the cause of the rectal bleeding and start treatment.
- Take any medicine the doctor prescribes exactly as directed. If you feel it is not helping, call your doctor. Do not quit taking it on your own.
- You may eat your regular diet. Drink 8 glasses (soda-can size) of liquids each day.

Call Your Doctor If . . .
- You have a high temperature.
- You start having stomach pain or swelling, nausea, or vomiting.
- You see a small amount of bright red blood on your stool or in the toilet water.

Seek Care Immediately If . . .

- You see more than a streak of blood on the toilet paper after wiping your bottom.
- You have black stool.
- You feel dizzy, weak, or faint.

IF YOU'RE HEADING FOR THE HOSPITAL . . .

What to Expect While You're There

You may encounter the following procedures and equipment during your stay.

- **Colonoscopy** (co-lin-OS-ko-pee): To locate the source of the bleeding, the doctor may order this test, which gives a view of the inside of the colon (large intestine). A soft tube with a light and camera lens on the end of it is inserted through the rectum and pushed into the colon.
- **Sigmoidoscopy** (sig-moid-OS-ko-pee): This test gives the doctor a view of only the lower end of the colon, called the sigmoid, and the rectum. A short, flexible tube with a light and camera lens is used for the test.
- **Taking Vital Signs:** These include your temperature, blood pressure, pulse (counting your heartbeats), and respirations (counting your breaths). A stethoscope is used to listen to your heart and lungs. Your blood pressure is taken by wrapping a cuff around your arm.
- **Pulse Oximeter:** While you are getting oxygen, you may be hooked up to a pulse·oximeter (ox-IM-uh-ter). It is placed on your ear, finger, or toe and is connected to a machine that measures the oxygen in your blood.
- **Blood:** Usually taken from a vein in your hand or from the bend in your elbow. Tests will be done on the blood.
- **IV:** A tube placed in your vein for giving medicine or liquids. It will be capped or have tubing connected to it.
- **Blood Transfusion:** If you are losing too much blood, you may receive a transfusion.
- **Oxygen:** Your body may need extra oxygen at this time. It is given either by a mask or nasal prongs. Tell your doctor if the oxygen is drying out your nose or if the nasal prongs bother you.
- **ECG:** Also called a heart monitor, an electrocardiograph (e-lec-tro-CAR-dee-o-graf), or EKG. The patches on your chest are hooked up to a TV-type screen or a small portable box (telemetry unit). This screen shows a tracing of each heartbeat. Your heart will be watched for signs of injury or damage that could be related to your illness.
- **NG Tube:** Also called a nasogastric (naz-o-GAS-trik) tube. It is

passed through your nose or mouth and down into your stomach. The tube is attached to suction which will keep the stomach empty.

- **Strict Intake and Output:** Caregivers will carefully watch how much liquid you are getting and how much you are urinating.
- **Activity:** You may need to rest in bed. Once you are feeling better, you will be allowed to get up.

Rectal Thermometer Use

WHAT YOU SHOULD KNOW

Measuring a small child's temperature with a thermometer inserted into the rectum is the most exact way of determining whether the child has a fever. Special thermometers with short stubby tips are made for this purpose. They are recommended for use in children under 5 years old.

Rectal temperatures generally run higher because the rectum is a warm area. The normal rectal temperature of a child is 99.6 degrees F (37.5 degrees C).

WHAT YOU SHOULD DO

- You must start by shaking the thermometer down below the 97 degrees F mark (36.1 degrees C). Hold the thermometer by the end opposite the tip and sharply snap your wrist and hand. Keep the thermometer over a couch or bed so that, if it slips from your hand, it won't break.
- Cover the tip of the thermometer with lubricating or petroleum jelly.
- Place the child on his or her stomach to limit struggling.
- Spread the buttocks and gently insert the thermometer about an inch into the rectum. Never force it. Hold the buttocks together to keep the thermometer from falling out.
- Leave the thermometer in place for 3 minutes. DO NOT leave the child unattended during this period.
- To read the temperature, slowly turn the thermometer until you can see the line of mercury. Each long line represents 1 full degree. Short lines are read as 0.2 degrees.
- Wash the thermometer carefully in soap and warm water after each use. Store in a safe place.

Seek Care Immediately If . . .
- The child has a high temperature.

Reflux Esophagitis

See Heartburn

Removing Stitches

WHAT YOU SHOULD KNOW

The stitches (sutures) often used to close a cut or wound must be taken out by your doctor. Once the stitches are out, be careful not to bump or hurt the wound. It still needs several days to heal completely, and any injury may cause it to open up again.

WHAT YOU SHOULD DO

- If the doctor puts small strips of tape across the wound, leave them on as long as instructed. You don't need to replace them if they fall off after a few days.
- Take care to avoid bumping the wound
- If you have a scalp wound, you may wash your hair gently.
- You may wash your wound as you would normally wash your skin. You may want to be careful for the first few days.

Call Your Doctor If . . .
- You have a high temperature.
- The wound begins to bleed, or the edges begin to come apart.
- You have constant and increased pain in the injured area.
- You have signs of infection (redness, swelling, pus, a bad smell, or red streaks leading away from the wound).

Renal Calculi

See Kidney Stones

Renal Failure, Acute

See Kidney Failure, Acute

Renal Failure, Chronic

See Kidney Failure, Chronic

Respiratory Infection, Upper

See Common Colds

Rib Fracture

WHAT YOU SHOULD KNOW

Broken ribs are more common in older adults than younger people. The ribs may be fractured in more than one place. They generally take from 3 to 8 weeks to heal.

Causes
Causes range from a fall or a blow to the chest to hard coughing or sneezing.

Signs/Symptoms
You'll suffer pain, especially when taking a breath. Other symptoms are tenderness and shallow breathing. You may feel as though you have to hold your chest to relieve the pain. There may be bruising at the place of injury.

Care
The break will need to heal naturally. To speed healing, follow the guidelines listed below.

WHAT YOU SHOULD DO

- Avoid strenuous activity. Be careful not to bump the injured rib.
- Eat a normal, well-balanced diet. Drink plenty of fluids to avoid constipation.
- Take deep breaths several times a day to keep the lungs free of infection.
- Do not wear a rib belt or binder.
- You may apply heat to the injury to help relieve pain. Use a warm heating pad, whirlpool bath, or warm, moist towels.
- You may use over-the-counter pain-killers such as aspirin, acetaminophen, or ibuprofen.

Call Your Doctor If . . .
- You develop a high temperature.
- You develop a cough.
- You cough up thick or bloody sputum.

Seek Care Immediately If . . .
- You have trouble breathing.
- You develop nausea, vomiting, or abdominal pain.
- Your pain gets worse.

Ringworm of the Body

WHAT YOU SHOULD KNOW

Ringworm of the body, known medically as tinea corporis (TIN-ee-uh kor-POR-us), is a fungal infection of the skin. Even with treatment, it may take weeks or sometimes months to go away; and you can contract the disease repeatedly.

Causes

The fungus that causes ringworm is easily spread from person to person. You can get it by sharing towels or shoes, and from using public shower stalls. Pets who are infected can spread the disease to people.

Signs/Symptoms

Ringworm can appear just about anywhere. On the body, it produces red, round, flat sores, sometimes accompanied by scaly skin. Sores may cause an itchy, scaly rash under the beard.

Care

The problem is treated with medicines applied to the infected skin or taken by mouth.

WHAT YOU SHOULD DO

- Your doctor will probably prescribe a therapeutic cream or ointment. If you are using an ointment, wash and dry infected skin completely before applying it.
- Do not scratch the sores.
- If your pet has the same skin infection, have it treated by your veterinarian.

Call Your Doctor If . . .

- The ringworm patch continues to spread after 7 days of treatment.
- The rash is not gone in 4 weeks.
- The area beyond the patch becomes red, warm, tender, and swollen.
- You develop a high temperature.

Ringworm of the Scalp

WHAT YOU SHOULD KNOW

Ringworm of the scalp, known medically as tinea (TIN-ee-uh) capitis (cap-IH-tis), is a fungal infection particularly common among

school-age children. Even with treatment, it may take weeks or sometimes months to go away; and it can be contracted repeatedly.

Causes
The fungus that causes ringworm is easily spread from person to
person. You can also catch it from infected towels, hair brushes,
combs, barrettes, or hats. Infected pets are another source of the
problem.

Signs/Symptoms
You'll notice patchy hair loss and scaling of the scalp, sometimes
with itching.

Care
The problem is usually treated with medications taken by mouth.

WHAT YOU SHOULD DO

- Take prescribed medication exactly as directed. Be sure to finish the
  prescription, even if the scalp seems to improve. If you fail to finish
  the treatment, some of the fungus may survive and cause a new
  infection.
- Do not share brushes, combs, barrettes, or hats. Do not share towels
  used on the infected area. Use a clean towel to dry washed hair, and
  be sure to dry the hair completely.
- Do not scratch your scalp.

Call Your Doctor If . . .
- The ringworm patch continues to spread after 7 days of treatment.
- The patch is not gone in 4 weeks.
- The area beyond the patch becomes red, warm, tender, and swollen.
- You or your child develops a high temperature.

Rotator Cuff Injury

WHAT YOU SHOULD KNOW

The rotator cuff is a group of muscles that hold the top of the arm in
its socket in the shoulder. Either the entire rotator cuff or a small por-
tion can be torn. Healing time depends on the severity of the tear or
injury. Most torn rotator cuffs occur in the arm used the most frequently, and most victims are men over the age of 40.

Causes
In many cases, the rotator cuff is torn during an attempt to break a fall
with an outstretched hand. Other common causes include throwing,

heavy lifting, or falling on your arm. Rotator cuff injuries happen frequently to skiers, and baseball, tennis, and football players.

Signs/Symptoms
Symptoms typically include pain, weakness, numbness, and tingling in the shoulder, and weakness in the arm. You will also have difficulty moving your arm, especially out from your body.

Care
Your doctor will probably order an x-ray of your shoulder. You will probably need to wear a sling or immobilizer so the shoulder can heal. A severe injury may require surgery to repair the tear.

WHAT YOU SHOULD DO

- Apply ice to the injury for 15 to 20 minutes each hour for the first 1 to 2 days. Put the ice in a plastic bag and place a towel between the bag of ice and your skin.
- After the first 1 to 2 days, you may put heat on the injury to help ease the pain. Use a heating pad (set on low), a whirlpool bath, or warm, moist towels for 15 to 20 minutes every hour for 48 hours.
- If you are wearing a sling, keep it on all the time until your doctor says you can remove it. If you take it off to dress or bathe, be sure to avoid moving or lifting your arm.
- If you have a shoulder immobilizer (sling and straps), do not remove it until your doctor says you can take it off, or until your follow-up examination. If you must take it off, move your arm as little as possible.
- You may want to sleep on 2 or 3 pillows at night to reduce the swelling.
- If pain medicine prescribed by the doctor makes you drowsy, don't drive. You also may use over-the-counter medicines for pain. Take all medications exactly as directed.

Call Your Doctor If . . .
- The pain in your shoulder gets worse, or new pain starts in your arm, hand, or fingers.
- The hand or fingers on the side with the injury are colder than on the other side.
- The arm, hand, or fingers on the side with the injury feel numb or tingly, become swollen, or turn white or blue.

Round Ligament Pain

WHAT YOU SHOULD KNOW

Round ligaments on each side of the uterus attach it to the abdomen and hold it in place. During pregnancy, the uterus gets bigger to make room for the growing baby. This puts strain on the round ligaments and may cause pain. The problem is not serious. It is a normal part of pregnancy.

Causes
Stretching of the round ligaments during pregnancy.

Signs/Symptoms
Pain on one or both sides of your abdomen, usually in the lower part.

Care
Lie on the sore side to help relieve the pain.

WHAT YOU SHOULD DO

• Don't worry. Nothing is wrong. This is a normal part of pregnancy. It will not hurt your baby.

Call Your Doctor If . . .
• The pain in your abdomen changes.

Seek Care Immediately If . . .
• The pain in your abdomen gets worse.
• You have any discharge from your vagina such as blood or a watery liquid.

Rubella

See German Measles

Rubeola

See Measles

Ruptured Disk

See Slipped Disk

Ruptured Eardrum

See Perforated Eardrum

Ruptured Tendon Repair

WHAT YOU SHOULD KNOW

If you tear a tendon, your doctor may need to sew it back together. This may or may not require an overnight stay in the hospital, depending on which tendon you need repaired and how badly it was injured. For 2 weeks after surgery, you may need a splint or cast to protect the tendon and help it heal. When the splint is removed, you'll need to begin special exercises to build strength in the area of the injury.

Risks
Without treatment, you are more likely to have a lasting injury, and you may have difficulty using the injured area.

IF YOU'RE HEADING FOR THE HOSPITAL . . .

Before You Go
- Prior to the operation, you will need to stop eating or drinking anything (even water). Your doctor will tell you exactly when this will become necessary.
- If you take pills, swallow them with only a sip of water on the day of surgery.
- A few days before the operation, your doctor will probably tell you to stop taking over-the-counter pain killers such as aspirin or ibuprofen.
- If you have a splint or cast, take care of it exactly as the doctor tells you to.
- If you are going to be put to sleep during surgery, an anesthesiologist (AN-is-THEE-se-OL-o-gist) may give you a call the night before surgery.
- If you are going home after the surgery, have someone come with you or pick you up afterwards. Do not plan on driving yourself home.

What to Expect While You're There
You may encounter the following procedures and equipment during your stay.
- **Taking Your Vital Signs:** These include your temperature, blood pressure, pulse (counting your heartbeats), and respirations (counting your breaths). A stethoscope is used to listen to your heart and lungs. Your blood pressure is taken by wrapping a cuff around your arm.

- **Oxygen:** May be given to you during your surgery. You may need it as you wake up from your surgery, as well.
- **Pulse Oximeter:** While you are getting oxygen, you may be hooked up to a pulse oximeter (ox-IM-uh-ter). It is placed on your ear, finger, or toe and is connected to a machine to determine the amount of oxygen in your blood.
- **Blood:** Usually taken from a vein in your hand or from the bend in your elbow and sent to a laboratory for testing.
- **IV:** A tube placed in your vein for giving medicine or liquids. It will be capped or have tubing connected to it.
- **ECG:** Also called a heart monitor, an electrocardiograph (e-LEK-tro-CAR-dee-o-graf), or EKG. The patches on your chest are hooked up to a TV-type screen or a small portable box (telemetry unit). This screen shows a tracing of each heartbeat. Your heart will be watched to make sure your body is handling the surgery well. It will also be watched for signs of injury or damage during surgery.
- **Chest X-ray:** This picture of your lungs and heart is used to check their condition before surgery.
- **ET Tube:** During surgery, a tube may be inserted through your mouth or nose and into your windpipe. This tube will protect the windpipe during surgery and allow your doctor to give you the oxygen you need. The ET tube may leave you with a sore throat after the operation.
- **Medicines:**
  —**Prior to surgery** you may be given medicine to make you sleepy just before being taken to the operating room. Your splint or cast may be taken off and the area cleaned with special liquid.
  —**Antibiotics** may be given by IV, in a shot, or by mouth to prevent an infection from the surgery.
  —**Pain medicine** may be given in your IV, as a shot, or by mouth. If the pain does not go away or comes back, tell a doctor right away.
- **Splint/Cast:** After the operation, your doctor may put a cast or splint on the injury to protect it and keep it from moving while it heals.
- **Crutches:** If you have a leg injury, you may need to walk with the aid of crutches for a while. Make sure you learn how to use them the right way. If you lean on your armpits, you may damage some of the nerves in the area.
- **Urinating:** Before you leave, your doctor may want to make sure you can urinate on your own. This is especially important if you were put to sleep during surgery.

After You Leave

- Do not use the injured tendon until the doctor says it is all right to do so.
- The doctor will tell you how long to rest the tendon. Do not use it for lifting heavy things or walking. Do not drive until your doctor gives the go-ahead.
- To reduce swelling and pain, keep the injury lifted above the level of your heart as much as possible for the first 1 to 2 days.
- Leave the splint or bandage in place until you return to your doctor for a wound check.
- If you have a bandage, be sure to keep it clean and dry.
- If you have a cast:
  —Do not get it wet. If you need to take a bath, cover the cast with plastic. Do not put the cast into the water.
  —If you have a fiberglass cast and it gets wet, you may dry it with a hair dryer.
  —Do not push or lean on the cast; it may break.
- If you have a splint that is held in place with an ace bandage, make sure the bandage is not too tight. If you feel numb or tingly below the injury, loosen the bandage by gently unwrapping and rewrapping it. Be sure the splint stays in exactly the same place.
- Always take your medicine exactly as directed by your doctor. If you feel it is not helping, call your doctor, but do not stop taking it on your own.
- If you are taking antibiotics, finish all your medication even if you feel well. If you stop the drug too soon, some germs may survive and cause additional problems.
- If you are taking medicine that makes you drowsy, do not drive or use heavy equipment.

Call Your Doctor If . . .

- You notice yellow, smelly drainage coming from the injury.
- The pain and swelling get worse.
- You develop a high temperature.
- Your bandage gets wet or dirty and needs to be changed before your next visit.
- Your cast or splint breaks or gets very wet and soft.

Seek Care Immediately If . . .

- The area below the injury becomes numb or tingly.

Safe Sex

WHAT YOU SHOULD KNOW

Safe sex is way of lowering your chances of catching a sexually transmitted disease. This class of diseases, called STDs for short, includes any infection spread during sex. STDs include gonorrhea, syphilis, HIV (the AIDS virus), chlamydia, trichomoniasis, herpes, pubic lice, and genital warts.

Many sexually transmitted diseases can be cured with a week or two of treatment. If not treated, however, some of these diseases can cause infertility. Others eventually can be fatal. You can't tell by looking whether someone has an STD, and many people don't know they are infected.

Practicing safe sex keeps you and your partner from sharing body fluids, such as vaginal fluids and semen. These fluids typically carry STDs. Safe sex does not guarantee that you'll avoid infection. The only 100-percent certain way to protect yourself is to never have sex or to sleep with only one person who is completely faithful to you. However, if you do have sex with more than one person, having safe sex EVERY TIME will improve your odds of remaining infection-free.

WHAT YOU SHOULD DO

- Limit your activity to things that do not involve exchange of body fluids. For example, safe sex includes:
  - —Hugging and body-to-body rubbing
  - —Masturbation alone or with someone else
  - —Massage
  - —Dry kissing
  - —Sex with the use of a condom
- Avoid activities that will result in an exchange of body fluids. The following things are NOT safe:
  - —Mouth-to-mouth kissing (French kissing)
  - —Sharing sex toys
  - —Using saliva as a lubricant
  - —Sex without the use of a condom
- Latex condoms help to prevent the spread of the AIDS virus. They do not make vaginal, oral, or anal sex completely safe because they can break. For greatest safety, here are some important steps to follow:
  - —Use only condoms made from latex rubber. Never use a condom made from animal membranes because germs can get through

them. Birth control pills, diaphragms (DIE-uh-frams), sponges or foams may stop pregnancy, but they do not stop diseases.

—Use a sperm-killing gel (spermicide) along with the condom. The spermicide should contain at least 5 percent nonoxynol-9, which can kill the AIDS virus. Some condoms come with it already on them. Check the package. Never use a spermicide alone; you cannot rely on it to kill all the germs.

—If you use a lubricant, choose a water-based brand such as K-Y Jelly, Foreplay, or Wet. Don't use Vaseline, Crisco, baby oil, or cooking oil; they could make the condom break.

• If you have oral sex, it is best to use a dry condom. If you have oral sex without a condom, don't brush or floss your teeth first. Small cuts in the gums make it easier for germs to get into the body. You should not let the person getting oral sex finish in your mouth. To be completely safe, do not have oral sex at all.

• Do not have sex with anyone who is at high risk of getting AIDS or who has had a positive AIDS test. People at high risk include those who have lots of sex partners and those who use IV drugs.

• If you are infected with the AIDS virus, you owe it to your partners to let them know about it. You should avoid oral, anal, and vaginal intercourse. If you do have sex, you must always use a latex condom lubricated with a spermicide containing at least 5 percent nonoxynol-9.

Safety Seats

WHAT YOU SHOULD KNOW

All states have laws that require children to be in an approved car safety seat when in a moving car. A car safety seat is a padded chair that holds the child's body at each shoulder and hip and between the legs. Any child who weighs less than 60 pounds should be put in a safety seat **every** time the child is in the car. You may be able to rent a car seat from your hospital or an outlet in your community.

WHAT YOU SHOULD DO

• Use only safety seats labeled: "This child restraint system conforms to all applicable Federal motor vehicle safety standards." The label should have a stamp stating that the seat was manufactured after January 1, 1981.

• Whenever possible, put the safety seat in the back seat of the car. Fasten the harnesses on the car seat over the child's shoulders with less than one inch of space. Do **not** put small infants in seats with rigid shields.

- The following age and weight guidelines will help you choose the right car seat. Consult the manufacturer's instructions for exact figures.

  —BIRTH TO 9 TO 12 MONTHS (OR 20 POUNDS): Use an infant or convertible seat facing backward.

  —9 TO 12 MONTHS (OR 20 POUNDS) TO 4 YEARS (OR 40 POUNDS): Use a convertible or toddler seat in the forward-facing position.

  —4 YEARS (OR 40 POUNDS) TO 8 YEARS (OR 70 POUNDS): Keep your child in a convertible or toddler seat as long as he or she will fit. When your child has outgrown the seat, use one of the following:

  If the car has a lap/shoulder belt in the rear seat, use a booster seat that positions the lap/shoulder belt correctly. Secure the lap belt across the child's hips. The shoulder belt should not cross the face or front of the neck.

  Use the rear lap/shoulder belt alone **if** it fits properly. It should not cross the face or neck or ride up across the stomach. The belt should fit across the child's hips.

  If no rear lap/shoulder belt is available, use a shield-type booster seat restrained by the lap belt in the car.

  If no other type of restraint is available, use the lap belt. Position it low on the hips and adjust snugly.

  —8 YEARS AND OLDER (OR 70 POUNDS AND MORE): You can use the car's protection system without a booster seat.

- Check the seat's temperature before you place your child in it. Hot straps and belts may cause burns. Cover the car seat with a towel or sheet in hot weather and whenever you park in direct sunlight.

- Praise your child often for appropriate behavior in the car. Never let a fussy child out of the car seat or safety belt while the car is moving. If your child tries to get out of the seat or unbuckles the seat belt, pull over and stop the car. Firmly, but calmly, explain that the car won't go until the child is buckled in the car seat or seat belt.

Salmonella Food Poisoning

WHAT YOU SHOULD KNOW

Salmonella (sal-muh-NEL-uh) is a type of bacteria often found in tainted food. The germs usually settle in your stomach and intestines and cause diarrhea.

Causes
Salmonella infection usually stems from undercooked meat and poultry, raw eggs, or water containing live salmonella bacteria. Pet turtles and other animals can carry the bacteria. Infection can also spread from person-to-person.

Signs/Symptoms
Typical symptoms include watery or bloody diarrhea, stomach cramps, throwing-up, fever, headache, chills, sweats, fatigue, and lack of appetite.

Care
You will probably need medicine to treat your diarrhea. If the infection is severe, you may be given an antibiotic to fight it.

Risks
The greatest danger lies in loss of body fluids and salts (dehydration) from prolonged diarrhea. This can lead to shock and can be deadly, especially in infants and people over 60. If the bacteria get into the bloodstream, other parts of the body may become infected.

WHAT YOU SHOULD DO

- If you are taking antibiotics, continue to take them until they are all gone—even if you feel well. Always take medicine as directed. If you feel it is not helping, call your doctor. Do not quit taking it on your own.
- Rest in bed at least 3 days after your symptoms go away. You may get up to go to the bathroom. While in bed, move your legs a lot. This helps to prevent blood clots from forming.
- Use a heating pad or hot water bottle to help relieve stomach cramps.
- Drink plenty of liquids that have a lot of minerals and vitamins in them until the diarrhea stops. Then eat healthy, soft, bland foods such as bananas, rice, applesauce, and toast.
- To keep from getting another infection, cook all meat and poultry thoroughly. Do not eat dishes containing raw eggs.
- Follow directions on food labels on how to properly store and refrigerate foods known to be carriers of the salmonella bacteria.
- Wash your hands after handling uncooked foods and before handling cooked foods.

Call Your Doctor If . . .

• You have diarrhea, stomach cramps, fever, or a headache that last longer than a few days.
• You have a dry mouth; dry, wrinkled skin; dark urine, less urine than usual; dry eyes without tears; or if you feel sleepier than usual. These are signs of the dehydration that can develop from prolonged diarrhea.
• You develop a rash, itching, or swelling of your abdomen (belly) or legs. This condition may be caused by your medicine.

Seek Care Immediately If . . .

• You can't drink fluids or keep food down.
• You have high temperature, yellow color to the skin or eyes, cough up blood, or worsening diarrhea.

IF YOU'RE HEADING FOR THE HOSPITAL . . .

What to Expect While You're There

You may encounter the following procedures and equipment during your stay.

• **Taking Vital Signs:** These include your temperature, blood pressure, pulse (counting your heartbeats), and respirations (counting your breaths). A stethoscope is used to listen to your heart and lungs. Your blood pressure is taken by wrapping a cuff around your arm.
• **Pulse Oximeter:** While you are getting oxygen, you may be hooked up to a pulse oximeter (ox-IM-uh-ter). It is placed on your ear, finger, or toe and is connected to a machine that measures the oxygen in your blood.
• **IV:** A tube placed in your vein for giving medicine or liquids. It will be capped or have tubing connected to it.
• **Blood:** Usually taken from a vein in your hand or from the bend in your elbow. Tests will be done on the blood.
• **Antibiotic Medicines:** You may need antibiotics to fight your infection. They may be given through the IV, in a shot, or by mouth.
• **Stool Sample:** You may be asked to save a sample of your diarrhea in a cup. Your doctor will send it to the lab. This sample will help the doctor determine the exact cause of the illness. It will also help the doctor choose the medicine you need.
• **Activity:** Stay in bed at least 3 days after diarrhea, fever and other symptoms go away. Don't get out of bed if you are feeling dizzy or light-headed.

Salpingitis

See Pelvic Inflammatory Disease

Scabies

Scabies (SKAY-bees) is a skin infection with a tiny insect called a mite. The problem spreads from person to person through shared clothing and bed linen. It affects the hands, wrists, armpits, breasts, elbows, genital area, and buttocks.

Causes
The scabies mite burrows under the skin and lays eggs. Scratching spreads both the insect and its eggs.

Signs/Symptoms
You'll begin to notice itchy, pin-point sized, red, water-filled blisters. (If infected, the blisters may fill with pus.) The itching may continue for several days.

Care
If you apply medication, the problem will disappear in 1 to 2 weeks.

- Use the scabies medicine exactly as directed. To reduce swelling and itching, you may use over-the-counter medicines such as diphenhydramine syrup. Do not drink or drive while taking this medication.
- Wash your body thoroughly. While infected, do not share towels or clothing or sleep in the same bed with others.
- Machine wash bedding, towels, pajamas, and underwear in hot water and either dry them on the hot cycle of a dryer or iron them until they are dry. Wash toys. Store blankets and hard-to-clean items for 4 days. You do not need to clean coats, jackets, furniture, or floors.
- You may return to school or work after one treatment with scabies medicine.

Call Your Doctor If . . .
- The rash or itching lasts for more than 1 week after treatment.
- You develop new or unexplained symptoms.

- Other family members, close contacts, or sexual partners develop symptoms.
- You have any problems that may be related to the medicine you are taking.

Scapular Fracture

See Broken Shoulder Blade

Scoliosis

WHAT YOU SHOULD KNOW

Scoliosis (SKO-lee-O-sis) is a sideways curvature of the spine most commonly found among teenage girls. The condition is painless, but may cause twisting of the shoulders, hips, chest, back, and rib cage.

Causes

Scoliosis may result from a birth defect, poor posture, uneven leg length, or polio. It tends to run in families. In most cases, no specific cause can be found.

Signs/Symptoms

There are usually no early warning signs. Later, back pain and curving of the upper body may appear, and the back may become S-shaped. Other signs include a sunken chest, uneven hips and shoulders, and rounded shoulders.

Care

You may need physical therapy to strengthen your back muscles; and your doctor may suggest you wear a back brace or a shoe lift. In severe cases, surgery may be necessary to correct the condition.

WHAT YOU SHOULD DO

- It may not be advisable to participate in sports activities. Check with your doctor beforehand.
- Scoliosis can be corrected if treated early. You'll need to follow your doctor's program very carefully, however, and make it to all follow-up appointments.

Call Your Doctor If . . .

- You develop back pain that is not relieved by aspirin or other nonprescription pain relievers.

Scrapes

WHAT YOU SHOULD KNOW

A scrape or abrasion is a wound that occurs when the skin is rubbed off.

Causes
Abrasions are usually caused by a fall, a car accident, or a sports injury.

Signs/Symptoms
You'll have pain, redness, rash, swelling, and bleeding where the skin is rubbed off. Dirt or gravel may get into the wound.

Care
It's important to keep the wound clean and protected. Check with your doctor if the wound seems serious or develops signs of infection.

WHAT YOU SHOULD DO

- Clean the wound gently with a cotton swab dipped into a small amount of water mixed with an equal amount of hydrogen peroxide. Then apply a bandage. Be sure to keep the bandage clean and dry.
- Clean the wound and change the bandage several times a day. Take the bandage off slowly and carefully. If it sticks or starts to hurt, use warm water to gently loosen it. Pat the area dry with a clean towel before putting on another bandage.
- Keep the wounded area raised above the heart as much as possible. This will relieve the pain and swelling and help the wound heal.
- Let the wound dry for several hours.
- You may take over-the-counter medications for the pain.
- Continue using a bandage until a scab forms.

Call Your Doctor If . . .
- You develop a high temperature.
- Blood soaks through the bandage.
- Pain in the injured area becomes worse.
- You have numbness or swelling at a point below the wound.
- You have redness, swelling, pus, a bad smell, or red streaks coming away from the wound. These are signs of an infection that needs immediate treatment.

Seatworm

See Pinworms

Seizures

WHAT YOU SHOULD KNOW

A seizure, also called a convulsion or a fit, is a sudden attack of brain activity that causes a loss of control over movement. The attacks last anywhere from a few seconds to several minutes. People of any age can be affected.

Causes

The most common type of seizure is idiopathic (ID-ee-o-PATH-ik) epilepsy, a form of epilepsy whose cause is not known. This brain disease causes recurrent attacks. Seizures can also be caused by head injury, withdrawal from alcohol or other drugs, a high fever, a brain tumor, or an infection. Sometimes, no cause can be found.

Signs/Symptoms

People with epilepsy often know when they are about to have a seizure. When the seizure starts, the victim may lose consciousness. The face, arms, and legs may begin to jerk. Victims may lose control of their bladder and bowels or vomit without knowing it. After the episode, the victim may feel irritable, confused, or sleepy.

Care

The doctor can prescribe medicine to prevent further convulsions.

WHAT YOU SHOULD DO

• Instructions for the seizure patient:
  —If your doctor prescribes medicine to prevent seizures, take it exactly as directed. Do not stop taking the medicine without talking to your doctor first.
  —Avoid activities in which a seizure would cause danger to yourself or to others. Do not operate dangerous machinery, swim alone, use ladders, or climb in high or dangerous places such as roofs or girders. Do not drive until your doctor says it's okay.
  —Wear an emergency medical identification bracelet with information about your condition. If you have a seizure, people around you will be able to tell what's wrong and get appropriate help.
  —If you have any warning that you may have a seizure, lie down in a safe place where you can't hurt yourself.

—Teach your family and close friends what to do if you have a seizure.
• Instructions for others if a seizure occurs:
—Stay calm. To keep the person from falling onto hard or sharp objects, move these potential hazards out of the way.
—Don't force anything into the person's mouth or try to open clenched jaws. Turn the person on his or her side when the violent movement stops or the victim begins vomiting.
—When the seizure is over, the person may be confused or drowsy and may need reassurance that everything is all right. Help him or her to rest and relax.

Call The Doctor If . . .
• You have any problems that may be related to the medicine you are taking.
• You are caring for someone who has had a seizure and he or she:
—Does not wake shortly after the seizure.
—Has new problems (such as difficulty seeing, speaking, or moving).

Seek Care Immediately If . . .
• You are caring for someone who has had a seizure and he or she:
—Is injured during the seizure.
—Develops a high temperature.
—Vomits and breathes the vomit into the windpipe.

Separated Shoulder

WHAT YOU SHOULD KNOW

This problem occurs when an accident forces the shoulder and collar bones out of position. The connecting tissue that normally holds the bones in place is stretched or torn, causing these bones to separate. The injury is known medically as acromioclavicular (a-kro-MY-oh-kla-VIC-ku-lar) separation.

Causes
Separation is usually the result of falling on your shoulder or receiving a strong blow to your upper body.

Signs/Symptoms
You can expect to feel pain, swelling, stiffness, or numbness. You may have problems moving the arm on the side that is injured.

Care

You will need to keep the affected arm in a sling for several weeks. Ice packs, heat, and medications can be used to relieve the pain.

WHAT YOU SHOULD DO

- Apply ice to the injury for 15 to 20 minutes each hour for the first 1 to 2 days. Put the ice in a plastic bag and place a towel between the bag of ice and your skin.
- After the first 1 to 2 days, you may apply heat to the injury to help relieve pain. You may use a heating pad set on "low," a whirlpool bath, or warm, moist towels. Apply the heat for 15 to 20 minutes every hour for 48 hours.
- Wear your sling constantly for several weeks (your doctor will tell you how long). If you remove the sling to dress or bathe, be sure to keep your arm in the same position as it is when the sling is on. Do not lift your arm.
- You may use over-the-counter medicines such as acetaminophen or ibuprofen. Take all medications exactly as directed by your doctor.

Call Your Doctor If . . .

- You have more pain or swelling from the injury.

Seek Care Immediately If . . .

- Your arm becomes numb, pale, or cold.

Sepsis

WHAT YOU SHOULD KNOW

Sepsis is a bacterial infection that has spread throughout the body. The infection damages the tissues and causes them to become swollen. If you develop sepsis, the sooner you are given antibiotic medicine, the better your chance of getting well without other problems.

Causes

Sepsis develops when bacteria from a small, localized infection enter the bloodstream and spread throughout the body, causing a widespread infection. The infection can begin anywhere, including the teeth, gallbladder, or even a cut.

Signs/Symptoms

You may have a fever, dizziness, fast breathing, and a fast heart rate. Tests may show that you have bacteria in your blood.

Care
You will need to be treated in the hospital with antibiotic medicine, IV fluids, and possibly blood pressure medicine. The doctor will watch closely for signs of other problems that can be caused by the infection.

Risks
Without treatment you could die. Your body may go into shock, and organs such as the lungs, heart, and kidneys may stop working.

WHAT YOU SHOULD DO

• It is important to take proper care of small infections so they do not spread in the body and cause sepsis. Symptoms of a small infection in one part of the body are redness, swelling, and tenderness.

Seek Care Immediately If . . .
• You or a family member develops the symptoms of sepsis: fever, fast breathing, dizziness, and a fast heart rate.
• You feel confused or have trouble breathing.

IF YOU'RE HEADING FOR THE HOSPITAL . . .

What to Expect While You're There
You may encounter the following procedures and equipment during your stay.

• **Taking Vital Signs:** These include your temperature, blood pressure, pulse (counting your heartbeats), and respirations (counting your breaths). A stethoscope is used to listen to your heart and lungs. Your blood pressure is taken by wrapping a cuff around your arm.

• **Oxygen:** The body may need extra oxygen at this time. It is given either by a mask or nasal prongs. Tell the doctor if the oxygen is drying out your nose or if the nasal prongs are bothersome.

• **Pulse Oximeter:** If you are getting oxygen, a pulse oximeter (ox-IM-uh-ter) may be placed on your ear, finger, or toe and connected to a machine that measures the oxygen in your blood.

• **Blood:** Usually taken from a vein in your hand or from the bend in your elbow. Tests will be done on the blood.

• **Blood Gases:** Blood is taken from an artery in your wrist, elbow, or groin. It is tested for the amount of oxygen it contains.

• **Chest X-ray:** This picture of your lungs and heart shows the doctor how they are handling the illness.

• **Sputum Sample:** If you are coughing up sputum, the doctor may need to send a sample to the lab. This sample may show what is causing the illness and will also help the doctor choose what medicine you need.

- **IV:** A tube placed in your vein for giving medicine or liquids. It will be capped or have tubing connected to it.
- **ECG:** Also called a heart monitor, an electrocardiograph (e-LEK-tro-CAR-dee-o-graf), or EKG. Patches on your chest are hooked up to a TV-type screen or a small portable box (telemetry unit). This screen shows a tracing of each heartbeat. The heart will be watched for signs of injury or damage sustained from the infection.
- **Foley Catheter:** This tube may be threaded into your bladder to drain urine until you can urinate on your own.
- **Medicine:**
  —**Antibiotics** may be given by IV, in a shot, or by mouth to fight the infection.
  —**Fever medicines** such as acetaminophen or ibuprofen will be given by mouth or in the rectum.

After You Leave
- Get lots of rest while you are ill. Slowly restart your usual activities as you feel better.
- Always take your medicine as directed by your doctor. If you feel it is not helping, call your doctor. Do not quit taking it on your own.
- If you are taking antibiotics, continue to take them until they are all gone, even if you feel well. If you stop too soon, some germs may remain and re-infect you.
- To keep from getting sick again, stay away from people who have illnesses that can spread. Also, get shots against pneumonia and the flu.
- Get lots of rest and eat healthy foods to help keep up your resistance to infection.
- Wash your hands after going to the bathroom and before eating. This will keep you from spreading the infection or becoming infected by germs that live in body wastes.

Call Your Doctor If . . .
- You have a high temperature.
- You have fever, swelling, pain, or redness while you are being treated. These are signs of continuing infection.
- You plan to have surgery or work done on your teeth after you have had sepsis. You may need to be started on antibiotics first.
- You have a rash, swelling, hives, or trouble breathing. These may be caused by the medicine you are taking.

Seek Care Immediately If . . .
• You feel confused or have trouble breathing.
• You or a family member develops the symptoms of sepsis: fever, fast breathing, dizziness, and a fast heart rate.

Septic Shock

WHAT YOU SHOULD KNOW

Septic shock is a life-threatening reaction to a severe infection. During septic shock, the body tissues and organs do not get enough blood and oxygen.

Causes
The problem may start with a small infection that overwhelms the body's defenses and spreads. In some severe infections, the germs make harmful toxins that can cause fluid to leak from blood vessels out into the tissues. The toxins may also prevent the heart from beating strongly enough. Together, these reactions lower blood pressure.

If blood pressure gets too low, the body and its organs become deprived of oxygen. The body tries to help itself, but without enough oxygen, it makes too much of certain waste products. These extra wastes can do additional harm.

Signs/Symptoms
If you develop a small infection in one part of the body, the symptoms may include redness, swelling, and tenderness. Signs that the infection has spread throughout the body are fever, fast breathing, dizziness, and fast heart rate.

Care
Septic shock is an emergency that requires treatment in the hospital. While there, you will get medicine to treat your infection, plus IV fluids, oxygen, and possibly medicine to raise the blood pressure.

Risks
Without treatment, septic shock is usually a killer. The sooner you receive treatment, the better your chances of recovery.

IF YOU'RE HEADING FOR THE HOSPITAL . . .

What to Expect While You're There
You may encounter the following procedures and equipment during your stay.

- **Taking Vital Signs:** These include your temperature, blood pressure, pulse (counting your heartbeats), and respirations (counting your breaths). A stethoscope is used to listen to your heart and lungs. Your blood pressure is taken by wrapping a cuff around your arm.

- **Oxygen:** Your body may need extra oxygen at this time. It is given either by a mask or nasal prongs. Tell the doctor if the oxygen is drying out your nose or if the nasal prongs are bothersome.

- **Pulse Oximeter:** While getting oxygen, you may be hooked up to a pulse oximeter (ox-IM-uh-ter). It is placed on an ear, finger, or toe and is connected to a machine that measures the oxygen in the blood.

- **IV:** A tube placed in the vein for giving medicine or liquids. It will be capped or have tubing connected to it.

- **Blood:** Usually taken from a vein in a hand or from the bend in an elbow. Tests will be done on the blood.

- **Blood Gases:** For this test blood is taken from an artery in a wrist, elbow, or groin. It is tested for oxygen.

- **ET Tube:** This tube is passed through either the mouth or nose and down into the windpipe. It is often hooked up to a breathing machine. With the tube in place, you will not be able to talk.

- **Ventilator** (VENT-ih-lay-ter): A special machine used to help with breathing. This will help you save energy that your body needs to get better.

- **Chest X-ray:** This picture of the lungs and heart shows how they are handling the illness.

- **ECG:** Also called a heart monitor, an electrocardiograph (e-LEK-tro-CAR-dee-o-graf), or EKG. The patches on your chest are hooked up to a TV-type screen or a small portable box (telemetry unit). This screen shows a tracing of each heartbeat. The heart will be watched for signs of injury or damage that could be related to the illness.

- **Foley Catheter:** This tube drains urine from the bladder until you can urinate on your own.

- **Coughing and Deep Breathing:** It is important to do this often because it helps keep the lungs from getting infected.
  - —To ease the pain during coughing and deep breathing, a 6-inch elastic bandage can be loosely wrapped around the rib cage.
  - —Holding a pillow tightly against the chest when coughing can help ease any pain.

- **Medicines:**
  - —**Antibiotics** will be used to fight the infection. They may be given by IV, in a shot, or by mouth.
  - —**Blood pressure medicine** may be given through your IV in order

to bring your blood pressure up to normal. Once the infection is under control and the body can take care of itself, this medicine can be stopped.

- **Heart Tubes/Wires:** You may be attached to many different tubes and wires. Some may enter your body under the collarbone or in the groin and be threaded into the heart. They are attached to monitors that measure the heart while it's working. These readings help the doctor guide your treatment.

Sexual Assault

WHAT YOU SHOULD KNOW

Sexual assault is another word for rape. It means somebody was made to have sex or perform sexual acts when she or he did not want to. It could have been done by someone that they knew, such as a date or a relative, or by a stranger. It usually happens to women, but can also happen to men and to children.

Causes
Rape is not the fault of the person it happens to. It is not provoked by the victim and could not have been kept from happening by the victim.

Signs/Symptoms
Physical injuries such as cuts and bruises, tears of the vagina and rectum. You may get more symptoms such as bruises and muscle pain in the next 2 or 3 days.

People may react to rape in many different ways. These include fear, anger, crying, shaking, talking a lot, not talking at all, and smiling or laughing. Some people show no signs at all when it happens. Later on, many people feel guilty, sad, or angry; have sleep problems; are anxious, afraid of being alone, or want to be alone all the time; or do not want to have sex anymore.

Care
Your doctor will want to examine you to see if you have been hurt. Samples of your blood, the fluid inside your vagina or rectum, and urine may be taken. If you reported the sexual assault to the police, findings from your examination will be used as evidence. You may be given antibiotic medicines to keep you from getting an infection from the person who attacked you. Women may also be given a medicine to keep them from getting pregnant.

Do's and Don'ts

Do tell your doctor everything that happened to you. It might be embarrassing, but a doctor needs to know what happened in order to give you the best care. Don't feel guilty. You did nothing to cause the sexual assault. Don't be afraid to talk to someone and get counseling.

WHAT YOU SHOULD DO

- You may be given antibiotic medicines to keep you from getting an infection from the person that attacked you. You may also be given a medicine to keep you from getting pregnant. Always take your medicine as directed by your doctor. If you feel it is not helping, call your doctor. Do not quit taking it.
- If you are taking antibiotics, take them until they are all gone even if you feel well. If you have an infection, you may not know it.
- Don't wash any clothes that you wore during or right after the assault. The police may use them to get evidence.
- Your doctor will tell you when to call to get the results of tests that were done during your examination.
- It is important that you work through your emotions. Talk to family or friends. People at a rape assistance center can provide support and counseling to help you. Many community agencies have a 24-hour crisis line available for counseling.

Sexually Transmitted Diseases

WHAT YOU SHOULD KNOW

This class of diseases, called STDs for short, includes any infection spread by having sex. STDs include gonorrhea, syphilis, HIV (the AIDS virus), chlamydia, trichomoniasis, herpes, pubic lice, and genital warts.

Many sexually transmitted diseases can be cured with a week or two of treatment. If not treated, however, some of these diseases can cause infertility. Others eventually can be fatal. You can't tell by looking whether someone has an STD, and many people don't know they are infected.

Causes

Most of these diseases are caused by bacteria or viruses and are spread by having oral, vaginal, or anal (rectal) sex.

Signs/Symptoms

Symptoms vary, but often include a discharge from the penis, vagina, or rectum and pain when urinating or having sex. You may get blisters, sores, a rash, or swelling in the genital or anal area or in the mouth. You may also have flu-like symptoms (fever, headache, body aches, or swollen glands) that don't go away.

Care

Your doctor can perform tests to see what kind of infection you have. You may need antibiotic medicine to fight the infection.

WHAT YOU SHOULD DO

- Always take your medicine as directed. If you feel it is not helping, call your doctor. Do not quit taking it on your own. If you are taking antibiotics, continue to take them until they are all gone, even if you feel well. If you stop treatment too soon, some germs may survive to reinfect you.
- Don't have sex (including oral sex) while you and your partner are being treated for a STD.
- Tell all your sex partners that you are being treated for a STD. They may be infected also and need treatment.
- Wash your hands often, especially after you urinate or have a bowel movement. To avoid spreading an STD to your eyes, do not touch them with your hands.
- If you are pregnant, tell your doctor that you have a sexually transmitted disease. Your STD could spread to your unborn child.
- Women should wear cotton underwear or pantyhose with a cotton crotch so that wetness will not be trapped in the vaginal area.
- Ask your doctor for the instructions on practicing safe sex and using condoms.
- If you have had a test, be sure to call your doctor for the results.
- To keep from getting an STD, you should practice safe sex or avoid all sexual contact. The only completely safe sex occurs between two faithful partners who do not have STDs.
- You can improve your chances of avoiding an STD by using condoms. Although condoms do not provide foolproof protection, they reduce your risk of being infected. Other kinds of birth control (pills and diaphragms, for instance) can help prevent pregnancy, but they do not stop infections.
- The more people you have sex with, the greater your chance of developing a sexually transmitted disease. The fewer your sexual partners the better.

Call Your Doctor If . . .

- You have a rash, itching, or swelling after taking your medicine.
- The symptoms or problems for which you were seen get worse or come back after treatment.

Shingles

WHAT YOU SHOULD KNOW

Shingles, also known as herpes (HER-peas) zoster (ZOS-ter), is a nerve infection that usually affects people over 50 years of age. The pain and discomfort usually disappear when the rash is gone—anywhere from a few days to a few weeks. However, some people with shingles continue to suffer pain, itching, or burning of the skin for months or even years.

Causes

The disease is caused by varicella (VARE-ih-SELL-uh), the same virus that causes chickenpox. Someone with shingles can give chickenpox to an individual who has not had the disease before.

Signs/Symptoms

You'll notice small fluid-filled blisters on a red base. The blisters usually appear in a wide band of reddened skin on one side of the body. Other potential symptoms are chills, fever, nausea, stomach pain, diarrhea, chest and face pain, and burning pain in the skin.

Care

Although there is no cure, certain prescription medications can help relieve symptoms if you begin taking the drugs as soon as you notice the rash. Over-the-counter medicines also can be used for fever and pain.

WHAT YOU SHOULD DO

- If your doctor prescribes medication, take it exactly as directed. To relieve pain, you may use over-the-counter medicines, such as acetaminophen or ibuprofen, and put heat on the sore areas. Use a heating pad set on low or apply warm, moist towels for 10 to 20 minutes every hour for 48 hours. Applying calamine lotion may also provide relief.
- Do not bandage the sores.
- Get plenty of rest and drink a lot of liquids.
- When bathing, wash blisters gently. Try not to open the blisters; this could lead to infection.
- Until the rash is healed, avoid persons who have never had chickenpox or who are ill.
- Keep your hands away from your eyes.

Call Your Doctor If . . .
• You have difficulty seeing.
• You develop blisters on your eyelids.
• Your pain does not get better, even with treatment.
• You develop new or unexplained symptoms.

Seek Care Immediately If . . .
• You develop neck stiffness or confusion, or have trouble walking or moving.

Shock

See Septic Shock

Shoulder Blade Fracture

See Broken Shoulder Blade

Shoulder Dislocation

See Dislocated Shoulder

Shoulder Separation

See Separated Shoulder

Sickle Cell Crisis

WHAT YOU SHOULD KNOW

Sickle cell anemia, a blood disease that affects black people, usually begins at about the age of 6 months. The red blood cells become sickle-shaped, rather than round, and may block off small blood vessels, causing pain. An attack of pain is called "sickle cell crisis." Although there is no cure for sickle cell anemia, the symptoms can be treated.

Causes
Sickle cell anemia is an inherited disease.

Signs/Symptoms
Typical symptoms include pain and swelling in joints, hands or feet. Other possible symptoms are chest, stomach, or back pain; shortness of breath; paleness; fatigue; weakness; and difficulty walking.

Sickle Cell Crisis

To treat sickle cell crisis, your doctor may prescribe medicine, give you oxygen, and have you drink a lot of liquids. You may need to be hospitalized for tests and care. It is extremely important to follow your doctor's treatment plan.

WHAT YOU SHOULD DO

- Always wear a medic-alert bracelet or necklace stating you have sickle cell anemia.
- Drink at least 8 glasses of water a day—more if you have a fever. This helps keep the cells from blocking blood vessels.
- During a pain crisis:
  —Stay warm.
  —Apply warm compresses to painful parts of your body.
  —Rest in bed.
- To prevent a crisis:
  —Avoid high altitudes. (Don't drive in the mountains or use air travel.) If you have to fly, take oxygen while you are in the air.
  —Avoid activities that may cause injury.
  —See your doctor immediately if injury or infection occurs.
  —If you become pregnant, see your doctor regularly.
  —Avoid difficult exercise.
  —Avoid cold temperatures.
  —Make sure you or your child gets all the necessary shots, especially the shot protecting you against pneumonia.

Call Your Doctor If . . .

- You have signs or symptoms of pain crisis.
- You have a sore that won't get better.

Seek Care Immediately If . . .

- You have severe chest pain, with or without a cough.
- You have severe stomach pain, abdominal pain, or constant vomiting.
- You have severe pain in a bone or joint.
- You have blood in your urine or urine that appears cloudy.
- You have fainting spells.

Sigmoidoscopy

WHAT YOU SHOULD KNOW

Sigmoidoscopy (sig-moid-OS-co-pee)—also known as a proctoscopy —gives a view of the inside of your bowel. During the procedure, the doctor will be able to inspect the anus, rectum, and sigmoid (the lowest end of the bowel).

Risks
It is possible that your bowel could be injured during the test. To avoid problems, follow your doctor's instructions carefully.

IF YOU'RE HEADING FOR THE HOSPITAL . . .

Before You Go
• You will need to clean out your bowel to get ready for this test. To do this, you will be given medicine and allowed to drink only liquids before the test.
• To help clear the bowel, you may be given a laxative to take the night before the test.
• You also may need to have an enema the night before and the day of your test.
• You can eat a small breakfast (mostly liquids) on the morning of the test.

What to Expect While You're There
• **Taking Vital Signs:** Before the test, a nurse will take your temperature, blood pressure, pulse (counting your heartbeat), and respirations (counting your breaths). A stethoscope is used to listen to your heart and lungs. Your blood pressure is taken by wrapping a cuff around your arm.
• **During the Sigmoidoscopy . . .**
  —You will be asked to lie on your side. You may need to raise one or both knees toward your chest. Your lower body will be covered with a sheet.
  —A soft tube with a light and camera lenses on its tip will gently be put into your rectum. Pictures from the inside of the bowel will show up on a TV-like screen. To improve the view, air may be pumped into the bowel.
  —A sample of the tissue inside the bowel may be taken. The doctor may also take a stool sample.
  —Your test will take about 15 to 30 minutes.

After You Leave
• You may resume normal activities and begin drinking or eating as soon as you feel up to it.

Call Your Doctor If . . .
• You have a generally ill feeling, headache, chills, and muscle aches.
• You have a high temperature.

Seek Care Immediately If . . .
• You have bright red bleeding from your rectum.
• You feel dizzy or short of breath, or you faint.
• You have nausea, vomiting, and severe pain in your stomach.

Sinusitis

WHAT YOU SHOULD KNOW

Sinusitis (SINE-uh-SI-tis) is swelling and irritation in the sinuses (the air spaces behind and above the nose), especially the sinuses located behind the forehead and cheekbones. Treatment should relieve the problem within a few days.

Causes

The problem usually starts during or just after a cold, when bacteria grow in your sinuses, causing an infection. It may also be caused by smoking, allergies (hay fever), swimming in dirty water, staying outside in cold damp weather, or spending a lot of time in dry indoor heat.

Signs/Symptoms

Typically, you'll have pain, pressure, or swelling around the forehead, cheeks, or eyes that sometimes gets worse when you bend over. You may have a headache, fever, chills, or other cold symptoms, a dry cough or tooth pain. The discharge from your nose may be thick and yellow or green in color.

Care

If an infection is the cause, your doctor is likely to prescribe an antibiotic. Without treatment, the infection will continue, and could cause long-term problems. Decongestants and pain-killers may also be advised.

WHAT YOU SHOULD DO

• Use a cool-mist vaporizer or humidifier to add moisture to the air. This will help thin the nasal discharge, allowing it to drain more easily.
• To help ease the pain, put heat on your face and nose with a warm wash cloth or an electric heating pad (set on low).
• Blow your nose gently. In very young children, use a bulb syringe to empty the nose. Place your thumb on top of the bulb and squeeze it down. Insert the tip of the syringe into the nose while you hold the bulb with your thumb. Slowly take your thumb off the bulb. Repeat

this 2 or 3 times in each nostril. Do not hold the child's nose closed over the syringe.
- You may need decongestant medicine to unplug your nose and ease the pain. Over-the-counter pain-killers, such as acetaminophen and ibuprofen, will also help. Always take these medicines exactly as directed.
- If your doctor has prescribed antibiotics, finish all the medication even if you feel better. If you stop treatment too soon, some bacteria may survive and cause a second infection.
- If you do not have to limit the amount of liquids you drink, drink 8 to 10 (soda-can size) glasses of water each day.
- To prevent future attacks, wash your hands after touching a person who has a cold. Don't smoke or swim in dirty water.

Call Your Doctor If . . .
- You develop a high temperature.
- Your nose bleeds.
- You have a really bad headache that is not eased by over-the-counter medication.
- You have swelling over the forehead, eyes, side of the nose, or cheek.
- Your vision becomes blurred.

Seek Care Immediately If . . .
- You have trouble breathing and develop a rash, itching, or swelling after taking your medicine.

Skier's Thumb

WHAT YOU SHOULD KNOW

Skier's thumb is a tear in one of the ligaments connecting the bones of the thumb. It's particularly common among skiers. The injury can happen suddenly or over a long period of time and may take 6 to 8 weeks to heal. If the tear is bad, surgery may be necessary to repair it.

Causes
The injury occurs when you force the joint in your thumb closest to the hand to move in a certain way over and over again. This causes a tear in the ulnar (UL-ner) collateral (ko-LAT-er-ul) ligament.

Signs/Symptoms
You may have difficulty holding things between your thumb and finger. Moving your thumb will be painful.

Care

You may need an x-ray to make sure there is no break in the bones near the injury. The doctor may apply a splint or cast to keep the thumb from moving and protect it so the ligaments can heal.

WHAT YOU SHOULD DO

- Apply ice to the injury for 15 to 20 minutes each hour for the first 1 to 2 days. Put the ice in a plastic bag and place a towel between the bag of ice and your skin.
- After the first 1 to 2 days, you may put heat on the injury to help ease the pain. You may use a heating pad (set on low), a whirlpool bath, or warm, moist towels for 15 to 20 minutes every hour for 48 hours.
- If your thumb is not in a splint or cast, do not use it until your doctor gives the okay.
- If you're given a plaster or fiberglass cast:
  —Do not try to scratch the skin under the cast using a sharp or pointed object.
  —Check the skin around the cast every day. You may put lotion on any red or sore areas.
  —Keep the cast dry. Wrap it in a plastic bag to protect it during bathing.
  —If your fiberglass cast gets a little wet, you can dry it off with a hair dryer.
- If you're given a plaster splint:
  —Do not get the splint wet. Use a plastic bag for protection while bathing.
  —If your fingers start to get numb or tingly, loosen the elastic bandage (ace wrap) around the splint.
  —Wear the splint until your doctor says you may take it off or until your follow-up examination.
- You may use over-the-counter medications for pain.

Call Your Doctor If . . .

- Your thumb or fingers change color or the pain increases. Your cast or splint may be too tight.
- You have continued numbness or tingling in your thumb or fingers.

Skin Biopsy

WHAT YOU SHOULD KNOW

A biopsy (BYE-op-see) is removal of a small piece of tissue for study in a laboratory.

Risks
There will be a small amount of bleeding and a slight possibility of infection.

IF YOU'RE HEADING FOR THE HOSPITAL . . .

Before You Go
• Tell your doctor if you are taking aspirin or a medicine to thin your blood.
• Tell your doctor if you have had surgery on your heart.
• Eat a light meal shortly before your biopsy.

What to Expect While You're There
You may encounter the following procedures and equipment during your stay:
• **Taking Your Vital Signs:** These include your temperature, blood pressure, pulse (counting your heartbeats), and respirations (counting your breaths). A stethoscope is used to listen to your heart and lungs. Your blood pressure is taken by wrapping a cuff around your arm.
• **During the Biopsy . . .**
  —You will need to lie still and move as little as possible. Your doctor will give you numbing medicine, so you will feel little pain. The area where the tissue (skin) is to be removed will be washed with soap and water.
  —Your doctor will carefully remove the tissue and send it to the lab for tests. Sutures (stitches) may be used to close the wound. A bandage will be put on the wound.
  —The skin biopsy may take about 15 to 30 minutes.

After You Leave
• Keep the area clean and dry for 24 hours. Do not shower without covering the wound.
• Cover the incision site with a sterile bandage or gauze dressing for 1 to 2 days.
• Your doctor will tell you when to return to have your stitches taken out.
• You may resume normal activities and begin eating and drinking as soon as you feel up to it.

Call Your Doctor If . . .
• The area of the biopsy is red and tender.
• There is any more bleeding than a spot on the bandage.

- You have severe pain in the area of the biopsy for more than 24 hours.
- You develop a high temperature.

Skin Cryosurgery

WHAT YOU SHOULD KNOW

Cryosurgery (CRY-o-SIR-jer-ee) gets rid of abnormal or diseased tissue by freezing it, usually with liquid nitrogen. Growths on the skin such as warts, moles, and some kinds of skin cancer are often removed with cryosurgery. In most cases, liquid nitrogen is put on the growth with a large cotton-tipped swab until freezing destroys it. Sometimes liquid nitrogen is sprayed on the area.

Shortly after the procedure, the treated area becomes red and swollen, and within 2 or 3 days, a blister forms over it. The blister, which may contain a small amount of blood, will break by itself in about 2 weeks, and may leave a scab. After the area is totally healed, you should have little or no scarring.

WHAT YOU SHOULD DO

- Keep the treated area dry and covered with a bandage for 2 or 3 days. If the bandage gets wet, change it right away.
- After the blister forms, do not pick at it or try to break it open. This could cause an infection or leave a scar.
- Do not put any medicine, creams, or lotions on the area.

Call Your Doctor If . . .
- Pain, swelling, redness, drainage, or bleeding in the treated area gets worse.
- The blister on the treated area becomes large and painful.

Slipped Disk

WHAT YOU SHOULD KNOW

A slipped disk—also known as a herniated or prolapsed disk—occurs when the ligaments that support and surround the flat, platelike cushions between the vertebrae in the spine begin to weaken. A back strain may cause one of these ligaments to break, allowing the disk material to squeeze out from between the vertebra and press on nearby nerves. Slipped disks become increasingly common with age.

Causes

The ligaments may give way under the stress of regular lifting, or tear open during a sudden injury. The odds of this happening increase when you are overweight.

Signs/Symptoms

A slipped disk in the lower back can put pressure on the sciatic (sigh-AT-ik) nerve, causing sciatica—sharp, shooting pain from the buttock down the back of the leg to the foot. You may notice weakness, numbness, or loss of muscle strength in the affected leg.

If a disk slips in the neck, the pain will get worse when you move your neck. It may also extend across the shoulder or down one arm. Your arm may feel weak or numb, or may lose muscle strength.

Care

Your doctor may prescribe pain medications or muscle-relaxing drugs. Physical therapy will help to strengthen your muscles and prevent future strains. Surgery may be necessary if a disk has ruptured.

WHAT YOU SHOULD DO

- If your doctor prescribes medication to control pain or to relax the muscles in your back, take it exactly as directed.
- It is important that you rest your back and give the irritated nerves and muscles a chance to recover. Your doctor may suggest you rest in bed to take the weight off your back. You may read or watch TV, but you should get up only to go to the bathroom and eat meals.
- Use a firm mattress or put a piece of plywood between the mattress and box spring. Don't use a water bed; it will not support your back correctly. When resting or sleeping, lie on your side with your knees slightly bent.
- For the first day or two, apply ice to your back to help relieve pain. Put the ice in a plastic bag and place the bag on your back. You can also have someone rub the ice directly over your back 4 times a day for 30 minutes.
- After 2 days, applying heat to your back may help relieve pain. For 30 minutes every 3 or 4 hours, use an electric heating pad set on low, or a hot water bottle wrapped in a towel.
- After your period of bed rest, limit your activities until your symptoms improve; then gradually resume your normal activities. Avoid motions and activities that cause back strain, including heavy exercise and lifting, or sitting in a slumped position.
- After you feel better, do exercises, such as walking and swimming, that will strengthen your back muscles. Avoid exercises, such as

rowing and jogging, that will put stress on your back. Check with your doctor before starting any exercises or sporting activities.

Call Your Doctor If . . .
• The pain in your back, legs, or arms gets worse or fails to improve with treatment.

Seek Care Immediately If . . .
• You develop weakness or numbness in your legs or arms.
• You lose control of your bladder or bowels.

Smoke Inhalation

WHAT YOU SHOULD KNOW

Short of sustaining burns, smoke inhalation is the greatest danger posed by a fire. Smoke from a fire may contain poison gases or may be hot enough to burn your throat and airways, resulting in serious breathing problems.

Signs/Symptoms
After inhaling too much smoke, you may develop such symptoms as coughing, breathing difficulties, upset stomach, vomiting, sleepiness, and confusion.

Care
If you have inhaled a lot of smoke or it has burned your airways, you may need to be hospitalized so you can be given oxygen. You may also need medication.

WHAT YOU SHOULD DO

• Get out of a smoky area as quickly as possible.
• Once you've reached fresh air, rest while taking deep breaths.
• Do not return to a burning building until the fire has been put out and all smoke is gone.
• Buy smoke detectors for your home.
• Make an escape plan in case there is a fire in your home. Practice it with your family.

Call Your Doctor If . . .
• You develop a high temperature.

Seek Care Immediately If . . .
- You have wheezing, trouble breathing, a continuous cough, an upset stomach, or vomiting.
- You become confused, irritable, or unusually sleepy. Have someone drive you to the hospital or **call 911 or 0 (for the operator). DO NOT drive yourself!**

Snake Bite

WHAT YOU SHOULD KNOW

A snake may bite when it is surprised or feels trapped. Bites from nonpoisonous snakes are more common than those from the poisonous variety. Fortunately, even poisonous snakes do not always leave their venom when they bite. Most snake bites are sustained on the arms and legs; the most harmful ones are on the head or chest.

Signs/Symptoms
You'll have pain and swelling around the bite. If you've been poisoned, you may also develop red skin with blisters, dark areas under the skin, and nausea and vomiting. In addition, you may suffer fever, headache, chills, sweating, and blurred vision. Your hands, feet, and the area around the mouth may tingle or have no feeling. The most dangerous symptoms include trouble breathing, fainting, and seizures.

Care
See a doctor at once if you show any signs of poisoning. You may need an antidote. You also may need medication for pain.

WHAT YOU SHOULD DO

- Stay calm and lie down.
- Wash the bite area with soap and water.
- Do not apply ice or drink alcohol.
- Never cover the bite so tightly that the area becomes numb.
- Keep the bite area clean and dry. Wash it daily with soap and water and apply an adhesive or gauze bandage.
- You will be given a tetanus shot that may make your arm swollen, red, and warm to the touch at the site of the injection. This is a normal response to the medicine in the shot.

Seek Care Immediately If . . .
- You develop any symptoms of poisoning (increased pain, redness and swelling, blood blisters or purple spots in the bite area, nausea,

vomiting, numbness or tingling, excessive sweating, breathing difficulty, or blurred vision).
• You have any signs of infection such as redness, swelling, pain, tenderness, pus, or red streaks running from the wound.
• You develop a high temperature

Soft Tissue Foreign Body

See Splinters

Soft Tissue Infection

See Cellulitis

Sore Throat

WHAT YOU SHOULD KNOW

Sore throats are painful, but usually clear up in a few days unless there is a more serious problem.

Causes

Infection with viruses, bacteria, or a fungus can cause a sore throat, as can allergies or irritation from smoking, alcohol use, or chemical fumes.

Signs/Symptoms

Typical symptoms include pain, swelling, redness, and a tickle or lump in the throat, a cough, and swollen glands in the neck. You may have a fever or headache. People with a really bad sore throat may drool or have trouble swallowing and talking.

Care

If the doctor suspects a bacterial infection, you may receive antibiotics. To relieve symptoms, follow the instructions below.

WHAT YOU SHOULD DO

• Gargle with mouthwash or warm salt water (1 teaspoon salt in 1 cup water) several times a day. DO NOT SWALLOW the mouthwash or salt water.
• Sucking on throat lozenges or hard candy may ease the pain. You also can take over-the-counter medications, such as acetaminophen and ibuprofen, and use a nonprescription antiseptic throat spray. Take all medicines exactly as directed.

- If your doctor has prescribed antibiotics, finish all the medication even if you feel well. If you don't, the infection may return.
- Use a cool-mist humidifier (vaporizer) to increase air moisture and help relieve the tight, dry feeling in your throat. Do not use hot steam.
- Do not smoke or drink alcoholic beverages while your throat is sore.
- You may be more comfortable only eating soft foods or just drinking liquids.
- Do not share food, drinks, or eating utensils while your throat is sore.

Call Your Doctor If . . .
- Your throat pain gets worse or is not better in a few days.
- You develop a high fever.
- You get a rash anywhere on your skin or the inside of your mouth.
- You have swollen, tender lumps in your neck.
- You have a thick discharge from your nose.
- You have a really bad headache.
- You cough up green, yellow, brown, or bloody sputum.

Seek Care Immediately If . . .
- You have trouble breathing or swallowing.
- You have really bad throat pain or start to drool.

Spastic Colon

See Irritable Bowel Syndrome

Spinal Tap

WHAT YOU SHOULD KNOW

In a spinal tap—also known as a lumbar (LUM-bar) puncture—the doctor removes a small amount of the fluid from the spine for testing in a laboratory.

Risks
There is a possibility of headache, backache, or infection following a spinal tap. Other risks include bleeding, an injury to a disk in your spine, or leakage of the spinal fluid. There is a very small chance of problems that could hurt the brain and spinal cord.

IF YOU'RE HEADING FOR THE HOSPITAL . . .

Before You Go
- You may follow your normal diet before this procedure.

What to Expect While You're There

You may encounter the following procedures and equipment during your stay:

- **Taking Your Vital Signs:** These include your temperature, blood pressure, pulse (counting your heartbeats), and respirations (counting your breaths). A stethoscope is used to listen to your heart and lungs. Your blood pressure is taken by wrapping a cuff around your arm.

- **Urinating:** You will be asked to empty your bladder before the test begins.

- **During the Lumbar Puncture:**
  —Typically, you will be asked to lie on your side with your knees pulled up to your chest. You may have a pillow under your head and will be covered with a sheet. Alternatively, the doctor may want you to sit in a chair with your head bent toward your knees.
  —You will be asked not to move. Your lower back will be washed with a cleaning agent. To lessen your pain, you will be given a shot of numbing medicine.
  —Your doctor will carefully put a needle into a space between the vertebrae (VER-tuh-bray) in your lower back. You may feel some pressure as the needle enters your back. Tell the doctor if you feel pain.
  —The doctor will test the pressure in your spinal canal. Before the procedure continues, you can stretch your legs out.
  —A sample of your cerebrospinal (SER-ee-broh-SPINE-ul) fluid will be taken and sent to the laboratory for testing. (This fluid is also called "CSF" or spinal fluid.)
  —The lumbar puncture will take about 15 to 20 minutes. A small dressing will be put on your back after the test.
  —To avoid a headache, you must lie flat for several hours after the test. You may eat and drink.

After You Leave

- You may resume normal activities as soon as you feel better.
- Keep the area clean and dry for 24 hours. When you shower, place a piece of waterproof material, such as plastic, over the bandage. Keep the area covered with a bandage or gauze dressing for 1 to 2 days.
- Drink 6 to 8 glasses of water a day for 1 to 2 days.

Call Your Doctor If . . .

- You feel severe pain in your back.
- You have any bleeding other than a small spot on your bandage.

- You develop a high temperature.
- You have a headache for longer than 24 hours.

Seek Care Immediately If . . .
- You have a severe headache that is not relieved by lying down.
- You have any numbness or tingling in your legs.

Spitting Up in Infants

WHAT YOU SHOULD KNOW

When babies spit up, the problem is known medically as gastro-esophageal (gas-trow-e-sof-uh-GEE-ul) reflux.

In this condition, food in your child's stomach backs up into the esophagus (ee-SOF-uh-gus), the tube that leads down to the stomach. The problem typically starts in the first weeks of life, is rarely seen in children more than 1 year old, and often disappears between the ages of 6 and 12 months.

Causes
The opening between the esophagus and stomach fails to close completely.

Signs/Symptoms
Soon after eating, your child may spit up 1 to 2 mouthfuls of food. This can occur with or without force. If the condition becomes serious enough, it can cause the child to choke or vomit blood. Because of the vomiting, the baby may not gain enough weight.

WHAT YOU SHOULD DO

- Do not overfeed your child; it makes the problem worse. At each feeding, give at least 1 ounce less than you have been giving. Wait at least 2-1/2 hours between feedings.
- Burp the baby several times during each feeding. This will get rid of air in the stomach and help prevent the spitting up.
- Keep your child in an upright position for a while after each feeding. You may hold the baby or use a frontpack, backpack, or swing. Avoid using an infant seat.
- For sleeping, place the baby on the stomach or side—not flat on the back. If possible, raise the head end of the crib a bit. DO NOT put the child on a pillow.
- Don't hug or play hard with the baby right after meals. When you change diapers, be careful not to push the child's legs up against the stomach. Don't close the diapers too tight.

Call Your Doctor If . . .
• Your child continues to spit up.
• Your child isn't gaining weight normally.

Seek Care Immediately If . . .
• The spitting up causes coughing or choking.
• Your child spits up blood.
• Your child vomits forcefully.

Splinters

WHAT YOU SHOULD KNOW

A splinter stuck under the skin can be painful and may become infected, whether it's stuck just under the skin or deep beneath the surface. The problem is known medically as a soft tissue foreign body.

Causes
The trouble can be caused by a wood splinter, a sliver of metal or
glass, a thorn, or any other small object that lodges beneath the skin.

Signs/Symptoms
There will be an opening in the skin where the object entered. The
splinter itself may or may not be visible. The area may bleed, bruise,
swell, or cause pain. It may remain sore for 2 to 3 days after the object is removed.

Care
The most important part of your care is to get the object out. If it is not
visible, your doctor may order an x-ray to locate it. For a foreign body
very deep under your skin, numbing medicine may have to be applied
to the area before the object is removed. A deep cut may be required
to reach the object; and you will need to care for this wound as outlined below.

Your doctor may give you a tetanus shot if you have not had one
in the past 5 to 10 years. You may also need to take antibiotic medicine to prevent infection in the wound.

WHAT YOU SHOULD DO

• Keep the wound dry for 24 hours.
• Keep the bandage covering the wound clean and dry. If the bandage
  gets wet and must be changed, unwrap it slowly and carefully. If it
  sticks or starts to hurt, use warm water to loosen it gently. Pat the
  area dry with a clean towel before putting on another bandage.

- If possible, keep the injury raised during the first 1 to 2 days to reduce pain and swelling and promote healing.
- Clean the wound gently 3 to 4 times a day:
  —Use soap and water or a cotton-tipped swab dipped in a mixture of half water and half hydrogen peroxide.
  —You may also keep the wound clean by soaking it 3 to 4 times a day in clean, warm water.
- If your doctor puts small strips of tape across the wound, you'll be told when to remove them. It's all right if they fall off by themselves after a few days.
- If you are given a tetanus shot, your arm may get swollen, red, and warm to the touch at the site of the shot. This is a normal response to the medicine.
- If your doctor has prescribed antibiotics, keep taking them until they are all gone. If you stop taking them too soon, an infection could still develop.

Call Your Doctor If . . .

- You have a high temperature.
- More and more blood is coming from the wound.
- You have any signs of infection (redness, swelling, pus, a bad smell, or red streaks leading from the wound).
- You develop a rash, itching, or swelling after taking your antibiotic.
- You have pain or numbness in the injured area that gets worse and won't go away.

Seek Care Immediately If . . .

- You develop swelling, have trouble breathing, or feel as if your throat is closing after taking your medicine.

Sponge Bathing Your Baby

WHAT YOU SHOULD KNOW

It's best to sponge bathe your baby for the first few weeks until the cord heals and falls off. When the cord comes off, you may tub bathe the baby.

How often you bathe the baby depends on his or her skin, the baby's activities, and the weather. Babies with dry skin and those who sleep most of the day may need a bath only 1 or 2 times a week. If the baby has normal skin, is active, and the weather is hot, a daily bath may be needed.

WHAT YOU SHOULD DO

Follow these steps when bathing your baby:
- **Never** leave your baby unattended during a bath.
- Put the baby on a towel.
- Use water that is warm to your skin, **not** hot.
- Wash the face first and the bottom area last.
- Use a wet washcloth with no soap to clean the baby's face. Rinse off the eyelids with fresh water. Wash the ears with a cloth. Do not put cotton swabs in the baby's ears. This will push the wax back into the ear. A mild shampoo may be used on the head.
- For boys, wash the bottom with a mild antibacterial soap or with plain water. Be sure to lift the scrotum and wash underneath it.
- For girls, wash the bottom with plain water. Wipe from front to back to keep from spreading germs from the rectum to other parts of the bottom.
- When you are finished bathing, make sure all the soap is rinsed off the baby's skin. Soap left on it can be irritating.
- You may apply lotion after the bath once the baby is 3 to 4 weeks old. Use only lotion suggested by your doctor. Lotion can be warmed by putting the container in warm water before the bath.
- Do not use baby powder because it contains talc and may irritate your baby's lungs. You may use cornstarch.

Spontaneous Abortion

See Miscarriage

Sporotrichosis

WHAT YOU SHOULD KNOW

Sporotrichosis (SPOR-o-trick-O-sis) is a type of skin infection. It usually strikes people who work around plants and soil. With treatment, the infection is usually cured within 1 to 2 months. Full recovery may take 6 to 7 months.

Causes

Sporotrichosis is caused by a fungus that lives in soil, weeds, and rotting garden material. It will not spread from person to person.

Signs/Symptoms

The infection starts as a small, movable bump under the skin of the finger. The bump grows slowly and may change to a pink color. An open sore may form. In a few days or weeks, a darker bump may show up on your arm.

Care

Medicine may be needed to treat this infection. You may need hospitalization for more tests and treatment.

WHAT YOU SHOULD DO

- If your doctor prescribes medication, use it exactly as directed.
- Protect the sore with a loose-fitting bandage.
- To speed healing, place a warm, wet cloth or warm heating pad (set on low) on the sore for 20 to 30 minutes 2 to 4 times a day.
- To avoid another infection, wear gloves, a long-sleeved shirt, long pants, and shoes when working with plants and soil.

Call Your Doctor If . . .

- You develop any new symptoms during treatment, including cough, unexplained weight loss, joint pain, or swelling.
- You develop a high temperature.
- You have pain, swelling, pus, or red streaks in the affected area.
- The sore is not better within 2 weeks after treatment begins.
- You have problems that may be related to the medicine you are taking.

Sprained Ankle

WHAT YOU SHOULD KNOW

A sprain occurs when the ligaments that hold together the bones in the ankle are suddenly stretched or torn. With care, the sprain should heal in 4 to 6 weeks.

Causes

Most sprained ankles result from a sudden wrench. Some common causes are tripping or bending your ankle the wrong way.

Signs/Symptoms

Typically, you'll have pain, tenderness, swelling, or bruising of the injured ankle. You also may have trouble moving the ankle.

Care

The doctor may x-ray the ankle. You'll need to wear a splint or an elastic bandage on the ankle until it heals.

WHAT YOU SHOULD DO

- Put ice on the injury for 15 to 20 minutes each hour for the first 1 or 2 days. Put the ice in a plastic bag and place a towel between the bag of ice and your skin.
- After the first 1 or 2 days, you may put heat on the injury for the next 48 hours to help relieve the pain. Apply the heat for 15 to 20 minutes every hour. You may use a heating pad (set on low), a whirlpool bath, or warm, moist towels.
- For 48 hours, keep your foot lifted above the level of your heart whenever possible. This will reduce pain and swelling.
- Activity:
  —Stay off your feet for 24 hours. You can then begin to slowly walk more on the injured ankle as the pain allows.
  —You may walk on your ankle until it begins to hurt too much to continue.
- Use crutches or a cane until you can stand on your ankle without having pain.
- If you have a plaster splint:
  —Wear it until your doctor says you may take it off or until your follow-up visit.
  —Do not push or lean on it or it may break.
  —Do not get it wet. You may take it off to take a shower.
- If you have an air splint:
  —You may blow more air in it or take some out to make it more comfortable.
  —You may take it off at night and when bathing.
- You may have been given an elastic bandage (ace wrap) to use either alone or with a plaster splint. If your foot or ankle feels numb or tingly, the bandage is too tight. You can rewrap it to make it comfortable.
- You may take over-the-counter medications such as acetaminophen or ibuprofen to help ease the pain.

Call Your Doctor If . . .
- Your bruising, swelling, or pain is getting worse.
- Your toes below the injury are cold when you touch them, feel numb, or turn blue or grey.

Sprained Knee

See Knee Injury

Sprained Ligament

WHAT YOU SHOULD KNOW

Sprains occur when ligaments (the tissues that hold bones together) are suddenly stretched or torn. Most sprains happen around joints such as the ankles, knees, or fingers. With rest, a sprain usually takes 6 to 8 weeks to heal; really bad sprains may take longer.

Causes

Sprained ligaments usually result from falling or twisting the joint. You may also get a sprain if you are in an car accident. The ankle is the most common site of this kind of injury.

Signs/Symptoms

Symptoms typically include pain, tenderness, and swelling in the injured area. Movement may be difficult.

Care

Your doctor may order an x-ray of the injury to make sure you have not broken a bone. If you have a severe sprain, you may need a splint to keep the injured area immobile so it will heal. If you scratched or tore some skin, you may also need a tetanus shot.

Do's and Don'ts

To prevent sprains and strains, warm up your muscles and ligaments before you exercise. Gently stretching your muscles is one good warm-up; your doctor can show you others. Before heavy exercise, wrap weak joints with support bandages.

WHAT YOU SHOULD DO

- Your doctor will tell you how long to rest the injured area. Then slowly start using the joint as the pain allows.
- Keep the joint above the level of your heart if possible. This will reduce swelling.
- Apply ice to the injury for 15 to 20 minutes each hour for the first 1 to 2 days. Put the ice in a plastic bag and place a towel between the bag of ice and your skin.
- After the first 1 to 2 days, you may put heat on the injury to help ease the pain. Use a heating pad (set on low), whirlpool bath, or warm, moist towels for 15 to 20 minutes every hour for 48 hours.
- If you are given a splint, keep wearing it until the doctor says you can remove it.
- If you are given an elastic bandage (ace wrap), your doctor will tell

you how long you must wear it. You can rewrap it if it becomes uncomfortable. Take it off at least once a day. If you have numbness or tingling below the injury, the bandage is too tight. Take it off and rewrap it more loosely.
• You can take off the splint or bandage when bathing.
• You may use over-the-counter medicines to relieve the pain. Take all medications exactly as directed.
• If you are given a tetanus shot, your arm may get swollen, red, and warm to the touch at the site of the shot. This is a normal reaction to the medicine.

Call Your Doctor If . . .
• Bruising, swelling, or pain gets worse.
• You have cold, numb or blue toes or fingers (depending on the location of the injury).

Sprained Neck

See Whiplash

Sprained Wrist

See Wrist Injury

STD

See Sexually Transmitted Diseases

Stings, Insect

See Insect Stings

Stings, Marine Life

See Marine-Life Stings and Bites

Stitch Removal

See Removing Stitches

Stomach Flu in Children

WHAT YOU SHOULD KNOW

The disease we call stomach flu is known medically as gastroenteritis. It's an irritation of the stomach and intestines. The throwing up and diarrhea it causes usually go away in 2 to 5 days.

Causes

The problem is often caused by viruses, bacteria, or parasites from infected food or water. Other causes include poisonings (food or heavy metal), use of strong laxatives to relieve constipation, or toxins in some plants or seafood.

Signs/Symptoms

The chief symptoms are an upset stomach, stomach cramps, vomiting and diarrhea. The child may have a fever, feel weak, and not feel like eating. Most other symptoms are caused by water loss from the body.

Care

The child may need tests done on blood and stool. If the cause is an infection, the doctor may prescribe antibiotics. Make sure the child gets plenty of fluids. If a child loses too much body water, he or she may need to be put in the hospital and given IV fluids.

Risks

The greatest danger is loss of too much water and salt from the body. This dehydration can make the illness worse—and even become life-threatening.

WHAT YOU SHOULD DO

- Do NOT give your child any medicines for diarrhea and vomiting without first checking with your doctor.
- Give the child an oral rehydration solution that you can buy at a drug, grocery, or discount store without a prescription. It has the right amounts of water, salts, and sugar to replace the lost water. Some solutions come in fruit and bubble gum flavors.
    —Use the solution as it comes. Don't add water or sugar.
    —Give small, frequent feedings. Use a teaspoon, especially if the child is vomiting.
    —Give the child 1/2 to 1 cup of fluid for each diarrheal stool. Start with 1 teaspoon of fluid every 2 or 3 minutes. Then gradually give more.
    —Keep giving the child the rehydration solution until the diarrhea stops. Do NOT give this solution for longer than 24 hours.
- Do NOT give the child other clear liquids, such as apple juice, soft drinks, tea, chicken broth, or sports drinks, instead of the rehydration solution. They have the wrong amounts of water, salts, and sugar. Some even may make the diarrhea worse. DO NOT GIVE PLAIN WATER.

- If the child can't keep anything down, have him or her suck on ice chips to supply water to the body.
- If you are either breast- or bottle-feeding your child, continue to do so while giving the rehydration solution. Wait 2 to 3 days before giving milk to an older child.
- Continue to feed the child his or her usual diet along with the rehydration solution.
  —Good foods to give are cooked cereal, rice, noodles, potatoes, cooked meats, crackers, soup, yogurt, fruits, and vegetables.
  —Don't give your child sugary foods such as soft drinks, undiluted apple juice, presweetened cereals, and flavored gelatin. Also avoid fried and spicy foods.
- Continue bed rest until the child feels better or until 24 hours after the vomiting and diarrhea have stopped.
- Check the child's temperature in the morning, at night, and every 4 hours during the day.
- Wash your hands after changing diapers and before fixing food. Have your child wash hands after using the toilet and before eating.
- Keep a supply of oral rehydration solution at home at all times. You should start giving the solution as soon as diarrhea begins.

Call Your Doctor If . . .
- Your child has a high temperature.
- Diarrhea or vomiting lasts more than 24 hours.
- You have any questions about feeding the child.

Seek Care Immediately If . . .
- The child's diarrhea or vomiting gets worse, there is blood in the diarrhea, or the vomit is bloody or green.
- The child is not drinking enough fluids and has signs of water loss: sunken eyes, less urination, no tears when crying, dry mouth, unusual sleepiness or fussiness, extreme thirst.
- The child has not urinated in quite a few hours.
- A high temperature continues to climb.

IF YOU'RE HEADING FOR THE HOSPITAL . . .

What to Expect While You're There
You may encounter the following procedures and equipment during your stay.

- **Taking Vital Signs:** These include the child's temperature, blood pressure, pulse (counting heartbeats), and respirations (counting breaths). A stethoscope is used to listen to the heart and lungs. Blood pressure is taken by wrapping a cuff around the arm.

- **Pulse Oximeter:** Your child may be hooked up to a pulse oximeter (ox-IM-uh-ter). It is placed on the child's ear, finger, or toe and is connected to a machine that measures the oxygen in the blood.
- **IV:** A tube placed in your child's veins for giving medicine or liquids. It will be capped or have tubing connected to it.
- **Blood:** Usually taken from a vein in the hand or from the bend in the elbow. Tests will be done on the blood.
- **Daily Weight:** Your child will be weighed every day to check for weight loss.
- **Strict Intake/Output:** Your child's nurses will carefully watch how much liquid the child is getting and how much urine is passing.
- **Activity:** At first, bed rest may be necessary. Once the child is feeling better, he or she can get up.
- **Medicines:**
  —**Antibiotics** may be given by IV, in a shot, or by mouth to fight infection.
  —**Anti-nausea medicine** may be given to get rid of an upset stomach and keep the child from throwing up. This will prevent dangerous loss of body fluids.

Stomach Ulcers

See Ulcers

Strained Cervical Spine

See Whiplash

Strained Knee

See Knee Injury

Strained Muscle

See Muscle Strain

Strained Wrist

See Wrist Injury

Strep Throat

WHAT YOU SHOULD KNOW

When streptococcal (STREP-toe-COCK-ul) bacteria attack the throat, the infection is known as streptococcal pharyngitis (FAIR-in-JIE-tis), or strep throat. With care, you will begin to feel better in 2 or 3 days. Although the sore throat may go away without treatment, you may develop other problems, such as ear, sinus, or kidney problems or rheumatic (ru-MA-tick) fever.

Causes

Streptococcal bacteria can easily spread from person to person in the home, at school or day care, or at work. Smoking, fatigue, and exposure to cold, wet weather can increase your chances of developing a strep infection.

Signs/Symptoms

Typically, you'll have pain, swelling, redness and, perhaps, a tickle or lump in the throat; plus swollen glands in the neck. You may also have a fever and a headache. People with a severe strep throat may drool or have trouble swallowing and talking. Children with the infection may be fussy and cry, have trouble swallowing, and refuse to eat, drink, or sleep.

Care

See your doctor for a throat culture. If strep is found, the doctor will prescribe antibiotics.

WHAT YOU SHOULD DO

• To ease the pain in your throat, suck on hard candy or cough drops. Adults and children over 8 years of age should gargle with 1 teaspoon salt in 8 ounces of warm water or strong tea (warm or cold). Younger children can be given a teaspoon of honey or corn syrup several times a day. (Do not give honey to children under 1 year of age.)

• Using a cool-mist humidifier in the sickroom may also help.

• For swollen and tender lumps in the neck, apply a moist, warm towel to the area several times a day for 30 to 60 minutes. To prevent burns, keep the compresses warm but not hot.

• Drink 8 to 10 (soda-can size) glasses of water each day. If your throat is too sore to eat solid food, drink milk, milk shakes, and soups. Resume a normal diet as soon as you feel better.

- To relieve fever and pain, you may use over-the-counter medicines such as acetaminophen and ibuprofen. Always follow directions.
- If your doctor has prescribed antibiotics, be sure to finish all the medication. If you stop treatment too soon, some bacteria may survive and cause additional problems.
- Do not smoke or drink alcohol. Try not to cough, clear your throat, sing, or talk a lot.
- Try to get as much rest and sleep as possible.
- Don't share food or drinks with anyone until your treatment is finished. Get a new toothbrush.
- Family members with a sore throat or fever should see their doctor or have a throat culture.
- You may return to work or school 24 hours after starting antibiotics.

Call Your Doctor If . . .
- You develop a high temperature, or your fever lasts more than 48 hours.
- You have large and tender lumps in your neck.
- You get a rash, cough, or pain in your ears.
- You cough up green, yellow-brown, or bloody sputum.

Seek Care Immediately If . . .
- You have any new symptoms such as throwing up, really bad headache, stiff neck, chest pain, shortness of breath, or trouble breathing or swallowing.
- You develop really bad throat pain, drooling, or changes in your voice.
- A child with strep becomes increasingly sleepy, is unable to wake up completely, or grows irritable.

Stress

WHAT YOU SHOULD KNOW

Although most people feel tense at one time or another, what seems stressful to one person may not bother another person at all. Stress tolerance also varies. If you are overstressed, you may feel depressed and have less resistance to illness. Learning to prevent or reduce stress can improve the quality of your life.

Causes
Any major change in your life will be stressful. Sickness or death of a friend or family member causes great stress. So do conflicts with your spouse or partner; moving; having a baby; dealing with money

problems; and trying to do more than you have time for. Getting fired puts you under major stress, and so does starting a new job. Injury and illness are very stressful. Even lack of rest is a source of stress.

Signs/Symptoms

People under stress are typically anxious, tense, and moody. You may also have skin rashes, stomach pain, diarrhea, wheezing, changes in your period, headaches, back pain, or trouble having sex.

Care

There is no instant cure for excessive stress. Your doctor may suggest meditation or muscle relaxation exercises to relieve the problem. You may need some counseling in stress-management techniques.

WHAT YOU SHOULD DO

- Talk things over with your family and friends; it often helps to share your concerns and worries. If you feel your problem is really bad, you may want to get help from a counselor.
- Don't blame yourself if things don't always go right.
- Learn what things make you feel tense and either avoid them or learn how to deal with them better.
- Deal with your problems one at a time instead of lumping them all together. Trying to take care of everything at once may seem impossible. List all the things you need to do and then start with the most important one.
- Do not use alcohol or drugs to relieve stress. Although you may feel better for a short time, they do not solve the underlying problems— and can be habit forming.
- Clean your house or your work space. Get rid of things you don't need.
- Exercise at least 3 times a week. Exercise helps to reduce tension.
- Take a short time-out period when you feel stressed out during the day. Close your eyes and take some deep breaths.
- Try using muscle relaxation. Start with the muscles in your face: Tense them, hold them this way for a few seconds, and then relax. Repeat this with the muscles in your neck, shoulders, hands, belly, back, and legs.
- Take good care of yourself. Eat a balanced diet and get plenty of sleep.
- Make time for fun. Take a break from your daily chores to relax.

Call Your Doctor If . . .

• You feel your problems are getting the best of you and you can no longer deal with them on your own.

Seek Care Immediately If . . .

• You feel an urge to hurt yourself or someone else.

Stroke

WHAT YOU SHOULD KNOW

A stroke is known medically as a cerebrovascular (SER-ee-broh-VAS-q-lar) accident, or CVA for short.

A stroke occurs when the supply of blood to the brain is suddenly interrupted. This can be caused by the buildup of fat or by a clot (air or blood) that gets stuck in a blood vessel. A broken blood vessel can also cause a stroke.

When the flow of blood stops, oxygen no longer reaches a part of the brain. This can cause brain damage.

Causes

High blood pressure, diabetes, high amounts of fat in the blood (high cholesterol), excess weight, and smoking.

Signs/Symptoms

Trouble feeling or moving on one side of the body; trouble speaking or swallowing; blurred, double, or lost vision; a headache; or becoming dizzy, confused, or unconscious.

Symptoms may appear in the first few minutes after a stroke, or may take hours to appear. They continue past the first 24 hours.

Only one side is affected because each side of the brain controls the other side of the body. That is why, when the right side of the brain is damaged, the left side of the body has symptoms.

Care

Hospital care is usually needed so the doctor can find out if a stroke has occurred and why. During the stay, you will be watched carefully to make sure that any brain damage doesn't get worse.

When you are better, you may need therapy. This may include physical, occupational, and speech therapy.

Risks

About 20 percent of patients who have a stroke die. Others have some kind of permanent problems (like trouble moving arms or legs). The sooner care starts, the better your chance of getting back to normal.

WHAT YOU SHOULD DO

If you are going to a special hospital or "skilled nursing facility" before going home

• The caregivers there will help you re-learn to dress and feed yourself, and use the toilet.

If you are going home

• You may need to put in special ramps and side rails in your home. This will help you get around the house safely.

• You may need to have physical, occupational, and speech therapy when you get home. Arrange your therapy sessions during the time of day when you are least tired.

• Work closely with the therapists. It is important to do the exercises they teach you.

• Always take your medicine as directed by your doctor. If you feel it is not helping, call your doctor. Do not quit taking it on your own.

• If you take aspirin regularly, continue taking it. Aspirin helps thin the blood so blood clots do not form. Do not take acetaminophen or ibuprofen instead.

• Have your blood pressure checked. You may want to buy a blood pressure cuff. Ask your doctor to show you or a family member how to use it.

• You may not be able to feel hot and cold things as well as you did before your stroke. To keep from burning yourself, test the water before bathing or washing your body.

• If you have other illnesses such as diabetes, high blood pressure, or heart disease, you need to keep them under control. Take medicines as directed. If you don't, you have a greater chance of having another stroke.

• Exercise daily. It helps make the heart stronger, lowers blood pressure, and keeps you healthy. If the exercise is too hard or too easy, call your doctor.

• Quit smoking. It harms the heart and lungs. If you are having trouble quitting, ask your doctor for help.

• Weighing too much can make the heart work harder. If you need to lose weight, ask your doctor about the best way of doing it.

• A diet low in fat, salt, and cholesterol is very important. It helps keep your heart healthy and strong. Ask your doctor what you should and should not eat.

• It may take time getting used to a new diet. Special cookbooks may help the cook in your family find new recipes.

• For more information about strokes, call the **National Stroke Association** at **1-800-STROKES**.

Call Your Doctor If . . .
• During exercise, you have chest pain that doesn't go away with rest.
• You are having trouble with any of your therapy or exercises.
• You are getting pressure sores on your skin.
• You have a high temperature.
• Your blood pressure is high.

Seek Care Immediately If . . .
• You cannot speak, move part of your body, or see; if you have blurred vision; or if you become dizzy, confused, or unconscious. These are signs of a stroke. **THIS IS AN EMERGENCY. Call 911 or 0 (operator)** to get to the nearest hospital or clinic. **Do not drive yourself!**

IF YOU'RE HEADING FOR THE HOSPITAL . . .

What to Expect While You're There
You may encounter the following procedures and equipment during your stay.
• **Taking Vital Signs:** These include your temperature, blood pressure, pulse (counting your heartbeats), and respirations (counting your breaths). A stethoscope is used to listen to your heart and lungs. Your blood pressure is taken by wrapping a cuff around your arm.
• **Pulse Oximeter:** While you are getting oxygen, you may be hooked up to a pulse oximeter (ox-IM-uh-ter). This device is placed on your ear, finger, or toe and is connected to a machine that measures the oxygen in your blood.
• **ECG:** Also called a heart monitor, an electrocardiograph (e-LEK-tro-CAR-dee-o-graf), or EKG. The patches on your chest are hooked up to a TV-type screen or a small portable box (telemetry unit). This screen shows a tracing of each heartbeat. Your heart will be watched for signs of injury or damage that could be related to your illness.
• **12 Lead ECG:** This test makes tracings from different parts of your heart. It can help your doctor decide whether there is a heart problem.
• **Oxygen:** Your body may need extra oxygen. It is given either by a mask or nasal prongs. Tell the doctor if the oxygen is drying out your nose or if the nasal prongs are bothersome.
• **IV:** A tube placed in your vein for giving medicine or liquids. It will be capped or have tubing connected to it.

- **Ventilator (VENT-ih-lay-tor):** A special machine used to help with breathing.
- **ET Tube:** This tube is placed in either the mouth or nose and passed into the windpipe. It is often hooked up to a breathing machine. You will not be able to talk.
- **Breathing Treatments:** A machine may be used to help you breathe in medicine. A doctor will help with these treatments. They are given to help open your airways so you can breathe more easily. At first you may need them frequently. As you get better, you may only need them when you are having trouble breathing.
- **Medicine:**
  —**Heparin:** Keeps the blood thin so no other clots can form. It is given in an IV.
  —**Other Blood Thinners:** These include aspirin and warfarin. They are given by mouth as a replacement for heparin. Like heparin, they keep the blood from forming clots.
  —**Blood Pressure Medicine:** Given for constant high blood pressure. At first it may be given in an IV, and later in a pill.
- **Blood:** Usually taken from a vein in your hand or from the bend in your elbow. Tests will be done on the blood.
- **CT Scan:** Also called a "CAT" scan, this is an x-ray using a computer. It is used to make pictures of your internal organs.
- **Lumbar Puncture:** Also called a spinal tap. Fluid is taken from your spine and sent for tests.
- **EEG:** Also called an electroencephalogram (e-LEK-tro-EN-sef-uh-lo-gram). This is a brain wave study.
- **Chest X-ray:** This is a picture of your lungs and heart. The caregivers use it to see how your heart and lungs are handling the illness.
- **Feedings:** If you can't swallow well, you will be fed either by an IV or by a nasogastric (NG) tube placed into the stomach. When you are able to swallow, food will be given as liquids, then as soft food (mashed).
- **Skin Care:** If you can't move by yourself, you will be turned often by the caregivers. A special mattress (egg crate or air mattress) will be put on your bed. This keeps you from getting bed sores.
- **Foley Catheter:** A tube put into the bladder. The bladder is the organ where urine is kept until you urinate. The catheter will be taken out when you can get up and use the bathroom on your own.
- **Pressure Stockings:** May be put on your legs. This keeps the blood from sitting in the legs for a long time and causing clots.
- **Therapy:** A Physical Therapist and an Occupational Therapist will exercise the arms, legs, and hands. They will also teach dressing and

feeding skills, and how to use the toilet. A Speech Therapist may help you re-learn to speak.

- **Wrist Restraints:** May be used to keep your wrists close to the bed, so you don't pull out the ET tube.

Sty

WHAT YOU SHOULD KNOW

A sty is an infection in a hair follicle gland in the eyelid. A few days after the sty forms, a white or yellow head of pus appears on the swollen area. Within 2 or 3 days, the sty usually bursts and the pus drains.

Causes

Sties are caused by bacterial infections.

Signs/Symptoms

A sty will cause redness, warmth, pain, and swelling of the top or bottom eyelid. You may have a gritty feeling in your eye and may have more tears than usual.

Care

Your doctor can prescribe medication to put on the sty. In some cases, surgery may be needed to drain it.

WHAT YOU SHOULD DO

- To avoid spreading the infection to other parts of the eye, don't touch your eyelid and wash your hands often, drying them with a clean towel.
- To ease pain and speed healing, apply a warm, clean washcloth to your eyelid for 10 to 20 minutes several times a day.
- When the head of pus appears in the swollen area, gently pull out the eyelash. Do not squeeze the sty. Wash the eyelid carefully to remove the pus.

Call Your Doctor If . . .

- Your eye becomes painful.
- Your vision changes.
- The sty does not drain by itself within 7 days.
- The sty comes back within a short period of time even with treatment.
- You notice redness *around* the eye.
- You develop a high temperature.

Subconjunctival Hemorrhage

WHAT YOU SHOULD KNOW

A subconjunctival (SUB-con-JUNK-tie-vul) hemorrhage (HEM-or-ij) occurs when a blood vessel under the conjunctiva (the transparent coating that covers the inner eyelid and the white of the eye) breaks and turns the white of the eye red. The condition is not dangerous, and you will have no permanent damage. In fact, your eye should clear up in 2 to 3 weeks without treatment.

Causes

A broken blood vessel can be caused by an eye injury, coughing, sneezing, or vomiting. Sometimes no cause can be found.

Signs/Symptoms

You'll see a patch of bright red blood over the white of your eye. With time, the color changes to brown or green, then goes away.

Care

No special care is needed.

WHAT YOU SHOULD DO

• Do not worry about the appearance of your eye. You may continue your usual activities.

Call Your Doctor If . . .

• Your eye becomes painful.
• Your vision changes.
• The red patch does not disappear within 3 weeks.

Subtalar Fracture

See Broken Foot

Subungual Hematoma

WHAT YOU SHOULD KNOW

A subungual (sub-UN-gul) hematoma (HE-muh-TOE-muh) is a pocket of blood under a fingernail or toenail.

Causes

Subungual hematomas are usually the result of an injury, such as smashing a finger in a door, or an infection from an object stuck under the nail.

Signs/Symptoms

Symptoms typically include pain, bruising, or bleeding. The blood trapped under the nail usually causes pain. Eventually the nail may fall off.

Care

Your finger may have to be x-rayed to see whether a bone was broken when you injured the nail. If there is an object under the nail, it will have to be taken out. Your doctor may need to put a small hole in the nail to let out the trapped blood and help ease the pain. You may also have to get a tetanus shot.

WHAT YOU SHOULD DO

- Apply ice to the injury for 15 to 20 minutes each hour for the first 1 to 2 days. Put the ice in a plastic bag and place a towel between the bag of ice and your skin.
- After 1 or 2 days, you may use heat to ease the pain. Soak the finger or toe in warm water for about 15 to 20 minutes 3 to 4 times a day.
- For 48 hours, keep your hand or foot above the level of your heart whenever possible to reduce pain and swelling.
- Keep the area clean. You may also need to cover the nail with a bandage. Keep the bandage on until your doctor says you may take it off.
- The nail may fall off. You may want to trim it gently as this occurs to keep it from catching on something and causing the nailbed to bleed or rip.
- You may use over-the-counter medications to relieve the pain.
- If you are given a tetanus shot, your arm may get swollen, red, and warm to the touch at the site of the shot. This is a normal reaction to the medicine.

Call Your Doctor If . . .

- Pain or swelling gets worse.
- You have any signs of infection (redness, swelling, pus, a bad smell, or red streaks leading from the wound).

Sunburn

WHAT YOU SHOULD KNOW

Whether it's from the sun itself or just a sunlamp, a sunburn can be painful and even debilitating. The lighter or fairer your skin, the more likely it is to burn; though even people with darker skin are vulnerable. Clouds offer little protection. You can get a bad sunburn on a cloudy day. Even sunlight reflected from snow, water, sand, or bright clothing can give you a burn.

Sunburns usually take from 3 days to 3 weeks to heal, depending on their severity. Repeated sunburn can eventually cause wrinkles, brown spots on the skin, and skin cancer.

Signs/Symptoms

A typical sunburn includes redness, swelling, pain, blisters and peeling on the burned area. A severe sunburn may lead to fever, headache, upset stomach, vomiting, and dizziness.

WHAT YOU SHOULD DO

- To ease the pain, take cool baths (showers usually are too painful) or put cool wet towels on the skin 3 to 4 times a day. You may add 2 or 3 tablespoons of baking soda to your bath water. An oatmeal bath may also help relieve the pain.
- You may use over-the-counter medicines such as aspirin or ibuprofen to relieve the pain, swelling, or fever caused by the burn. For severe sunburn, one-half percent hydrocortisone cream or spray may be necessary. Later, it also will help reduce peeling and itching. Apply 3 times a day for pain or 1 or 2 times a day for itching.
- Don't put first aid creams or sprays, ointments, or butter on the burn. You may gently rub in cold cream or baby lotion.
- If the skin is badly burned, apply petroleum jelly to the burn so that nothing will stick to the blisters. Do not break the blisters. If they break anyway, wash the area 2 times a day with soap and water, then cover it with sterile gauze to prevent infection.
- Drink at least 6 to 8 glasses of water (soda-can size) a day. Sunburn increases your chances of becoming dehydrated.
- Peeling will begin in about a week. Put a moisturizing cream or baby lotion on the burn 1 or 2 times a day.
- To keep from getting sunburned:
  —Try to stay out of the sun between noon and 3 p.m.
  —Stay in the sun for only short periods of time until you build up a tan. Start with 15 or 20 minutes a day and increase your exposure by 5 minutes a day.
  —If it is not too hot and you burn easily, wear shirts with long sleeves, pants, a hat, and shoes; or if you are going to be outside for a long time, bring this type of clothing with you. Wear sunglasses with ultraviolet (UV) protection. Try not to wear bright-colored clothing on sunny days; it reflects light onto your face.
  —30 to 60 minutes before going outside, apply sunscreen with a sun-protection factor (SPF) of 15 or more. Reapply it every 3 to 4

hours and after swimming or sweating. Many suntan lotions and oils don't protect against sunburn.

—Don't use tanning machines. Over time, they may increase your risk of skin cancer. If you do use them, cover your eyes. Closing your eyes or wearing regular sunglasses or cotton eye patches will not keep the sunlamps from injuring your eyes.

—Some medicines can make your skin more sensitive to sunlight. Ask your doctor about the effects of any medications you are taking regularly.

—If your children have short hair, put sunscreen on the tips of their ears and the back of their necks. And don't forget the tip of the nose; it can get sunburned easily.

Call Your Doctor If . . .

• You develop a high temperature.
• Your pain lasts more than 48 hours.
• You start vomiting or have diarrhea.

Seek Care Immediately If . . .

• You have eye pain or light bothers your eyes.
• You feel confused or dizzy.

Supraglottitis

See Epiglottitis

Supraventricular Tachycardia

WHAT YOU SHOULD KNOW

The heart has 4 chambers. The 2 upper chambers are called atria (A-tree-uh), the 2 lower chambers are known as ventricles (VEN-trick-uls). When the heart "beats," the atria push blood into the ventricles and the ventricles push blood out of the heart. Valves control the flow of blood from the atria to the ventricles.

Supraventricular tachycardia (sup-ruh-ven-TRICK-u-ler tack-uh-CARD-e-uh) is also called atrial tachycardia or SVT. It is a very fast heart rate of 140 to 250 beats per minute (normal is about 70 to 80 beats per minute). It usually starts suddenly.

Your doctor will try to find out the cause of the fast heart rate. Whether the cause is found or not, you may still need to take medicine to control the problem. However, you will still be able to live a normal life.

Causes

Among the possible causes are valve disease, hardening of the arteries, thyroid disease, or heart failure. Other causes include drinking too much alcohol, smoking too many cigarettes, or using too much caffeine.

Signs/Symptoms

You will probably have a fluttery feeling in your chest and may feel light-headed or faint.

Care

- If the fast heart rate does not stop by itself, you will be given oxygen and attached to an ECG (TV-type) monitor. Usually your doctor will try to slow your heartbeat without using medicine. He or she may place your face in ice water, rub an artery in your neck (carotid artery), ask you to strain or "bear-down," or just allow you to sleep.
- If the techniques above don't work, you will need to go to the hospital. There you will be given medicine through an IV tube and later by mouth. If the medicine does not slow your heart rate, you may need to have cardioversion (car-dee-o-VER-shun). This is an electrical shock to your heart.

Risks

If you are not treated, you may have more attacks. If an attack lasts more than a few minutes, you may faint (because your blood pressure is too low) or your heart may fail (which is rare). The sooner you are treated the fewer problems you will have.

WHAT YOU SHOULD DO

- Check with your doctor before taking any over-the-counter cough, cold, or pain medicines. Some of these have medicine in them that will increase your heart rate.
- Always take your medicine as directed by your doctor. If you feel it is not helping, call your doctor. Do not quit taking it on your own.
- If you take aspirin regularly, continue to take it. Aspirin helps thin the blood so blood clots don't form. Do not take acetaminophen or ibuprofen instead.
- If your heart starts beating fast:
  —Try to slow it down by coughing, holding your breath, or bearing down as though you are having a bowel movement.
  —If the above does not work, lie down and relax. Sometimes your heart rate will slow down.

    —If neither of these techniques works, have someone drive you to your doctor's office or the nearest health care clinic or hospital.
- Ask your doctor to teach you how to count your pulse and make sure it is regular and strong.
- A diet low in fat, salt, and cholesterol is very important. It keeps your heart healthy and strong. Try to avoid foods with caffeine in them. Ask your doctor about the right foods to eat.
- It may take time getting used to a new diet. Special cookbooks may help the cook in your family find new recipes.
- Quit smoking. It reduces the amount of oxygen reaching your heart, making your heart work harder. If you are having trouble stopping, ask your doctor for help.
- Exercise daily. It helps make the heart stronger, lowers blood pressure, and keeps you healthy. If your exercise plan seems too hard or too easy, check with your doctor.
- Weighing too much can make the heart work harder. If you need to lose weight, your doctor can recommend a plan for you.
- Since it is hard to avoid stress, learn to control it. Learn new ways to relax (deep breathing, relaxing muscles, meditation, or biofeedback). Try to talk to someone about things that upset you.
- If you have other illnesses such as diabetes or high blood pressure, you need to control them. Take medicines as directed. Because of these illnesses, you have a higher chance of getting a heart attack.
- For more information about the heart, call the **American Heart Association at 1-800-AHA-USA1 (1-800-242-8721)** or call your local **Red Cross**.

Call Your Doctor If . . .
- You have chest pain during exercise that doesn't go away with rest.
- You are dizzy or nauseated after taking your medicine, or you have other problems that you think may be caused by your medicine. Make sure you are taking it as directed.
- Your pulse is slower or faster than usual when counted for 1 minute, and does not return to normal.
- You have trouble breathing while resting, have swelling in your feet or ankles, or feel more tired than usual.

Seek Care Immediately If . . .
- Your pulse is faster than usual when counted for 1 minute, and you feel dizzy or faint, have chest pain, or have trouble breathing. **Call 911 or 0 (operator)** to get to the nearest hospital or clinic. **Do not drive yourself!**

What to Expect While You're There

You may encounter the following procedures and equipment during your stay.

- **Taking Vital Signs:** These include your temperature, blood pressure, pulse (counting your heartbeats), and respirations (counting your breaths). A stethoscope is used to listen to your heart and lungs. Your blood pressure is taken by wrapping a cuff around your arm.

- **Oxygen:** Your body may need extra oxygen at this time. It is given either by a mask or nasal prongs. Tell your doctor if the oxygen is drying out your nose or if the nasal prongs bother you.

- **Pulse Oximeter:** While you are getting oxygen, you may be hooked up to a pulse oximeter (ox-IM-uh-ter). It is placed on your ear, finger, or toe and is connected to a machine that measures the oxygen in your blood.

- **Blood:** Usually taken from a vein in your hand or from the bend in your elbow. Tests will be done on the blood.

- **IV:** A tube placed in your vein for giving medicine or liquids. It will be capped or have tubing connected to it.

- **ECG:** Also called a heart monitor, an electrocardiograph (e-LEK-tro-CAR-dee-o-graf), or EKG. The patches on your chest are hooked up to a TV-type screen or a small portable box (telemetry unit). This screen shows a tracing of each heartbeat. Your heart will be watched carefully until your condition has returned to normal.

- **12 Lead ECG:** This test makes tracings from different parts of your heart. It can help your doctor gauge the seriousness of the problem.

- **Chest X-ray:** This picture of your lungs and heart shows how they are handling the illness.

- **Special Treatments:** These may be needed to slow your heart rate before giving medicine. Do not try them by yourself unless told to do so. They include some of the same techniques you may have been asked to try earlier.
    - —"Pushing or bearing down" as though you are having a bowel movement.
    - —Holding your mouth and nose shut while trying to blow air out (like popping your ears).
    - —Putting your face into cold water or swallowing ice water.
    - —Allowing your doctor to rub an artery (carotid artery) in your neck (called carotid massage).

- **Heart Medicine:**
    - —Drugs will be given in your IV to slow your heart rate. If you get

dizzy, have pain, or feel other side effects after getting your medicine, call your doctor right away.

—After your heart rate is back to normal, you will probably continue to need medicine to keep it under control. Or you may need medicine to control the disease that is causing the rapid beats.

• **Cardioversion:** This may be needed if medicine does not slow your heart rate. The procedure delivers an electric shock to the heart to return it to its normal rate. Before cardioversion, you will be given medicine to make you sleepy. After the procedure, you may need medicine to control your heart rate in the future.

Suture Care

WHAT YOU SHOULD KNOW

Sutures (SOO-churs)—also called stitches—are pieces of thread used to sew the sides of a wound together to help it heal. To avoid infection and minimize scarring, your doctor will remove the stitches when the skin of the wound is strong enough to stay together—usually from 5 to 15 days. If you have stitches in your mouth, they may break apart or dissolve by themselves. Total healing of the skin and tissue in the wound takes months.

Care

Your doctor will tell you how long to keep the wound covered with a bandage, and when to come back to have the stitches removed. Depending on what caused your wound, you may need a tetanus shot unless you have had one within 5 or 10 years.

WHAT YOU SHOULD DO

• Try not to hit the wound on anything, this could cause it to break open.
• Keep the stitches dry for the first 24 hours. After that, you can shower; but be sure to dry the stitches off right away.
• Clean the wound and stitches 3 to 4 times a day:
  —Use soap and water or a cotton tipped swab dipped in a mixture of half water and half hydrogen peroxide.
  —For mouth and lip wounds, rinse your mouth after meals and at bedtime. Ask your doctor what mixture to use. Do NOT swallow the mixture.
• If you have a scalp wound, you may wash your hair gently after you get home. Keep your hair dry until the day you are to have your stitches taken out and then wash it gently.
• Keep your bandage clean and dry. If the bandage gets wet and you

need to change it, unwrap it slowly and carefully. If it sticks or starts to hurt, use water to loosen it gently. Pat the area dry with a clean towel before putting on another bandage.

- If possible, keep the wounded area lifted above the level of your heart to lessen the pain and swelling and help healing.
- Do not soak the wound. Do not go swimming.
- If you have been given a tetanus shot, your arm may get swollen, and red and warm to the touch at the shot site. This is a normal reaction to the medicine in the shot.

Call Your Doctor If . . .
- Bleeding from the wound gets worse.
- You develop a high temperature.
- You have signs of infection (redness, swelling, pus, a bad smell, or red streaks coming away from the wound).
- You have numbness or swelling at a point below the wound.
- You cannot move the joint below the wound.

SVT

See Supraventricular Tachycardia

Swallowed Objects

WHAT YOU SHOULD KNOW

Between the ages of 6 months and 4 years, children tend to put things in their mouths, and sometimes they swallow them. Usually this poses no danger. Some children can cough up the swallowed object. In any case, most objects pass easily through a child's body without causing problems.

Signs/Symptoms
The child could have neck or throat pain or problems swallowing. Vomiting, choking, coughing, noisy breathing, and belly pain are other signs.

Care
Treatment depends on the size and location of the swallowed object. An object that gets stuck in the esophagus (food tube) must be removed as soon as possible.

If the object reaches the stomach, it probably will pass through the body by itself without causing problems. This usually takes several days, but may take as long as 2 or 3 weeks.

X-rays of the chest and abdomen may be done to try to find the object.

Risks
Children rarely die from swallowing a foreign object. The risks of serious illness or death are very small if you follow your doctor's suggestions.

WHAT YOU SHOULD DO

- Your doctor may ask you to look for the object in your child's bowel movements. Putting them in a strainer and running water over them may make the job easier.
- Do **NOT** give your child any medicine such as a laxative to make the object pass sooner.
- There is no need to change your child's diet while waiting for the object to pass.
- To keep this from happening again:
  —Make your home a safe place. Children normally want to climb, touch, taste, and handle everything they can see.
  —Go through each room in your house and look for anything that could be harmful. Keep items such as safety pins, buttons, coins, and toothpicks well out of reach.

Call Your Doctor If . . .
- You do not see the swallowed object in your child's stool within a few days.

Seek Care Immediately If . . .
- Your child has vomiting, gagging, choking, drooling, neck or throat pain, or can't swallow.
- Your child is coughing, wheezing, or breathing noisily.
- Your child has belly pain, blood in the stool, or is bleeding from the rectum.
- Your child has a high temperature.

IF YOU'RE HEADING FOR THE HOSPITAL . . .

What to Expect While You're There
You may encounter the following procedures and equipment during your child's stay.
- **Taking Vital Signs:** These include temperature, blood pressure, pulse (counting heartbeats), and respirations (counting breaths). A stethoscope is used to listen to the heart and lungs. Blood pressure is taken by wrapping a cuff around your child's arm.

- **Blood:** Usually taken from a vein in your child's hand or from the bend in his or her elbow. Tests will be done on the blood.
- **Chest X-ray:** This picture of the upper body may help to locate the object.
- **IV:** A tube put in your child's veins for giving medicine or liquids. It will be capped or have tubing connected to it.
- **Oxygen:** May be given using nasal prongs or a face mask. Your child may be placed in a plastic tent to get moist cool air.
- **Pulse Oximeter:** Your child may be hooked up to a pulse oximeter (ox-IM-uh-ter). It is placed on the ear, finger, or toe and is connected to a machine that measures the oxygen in your child's blood.
- **ECG:** Also called a heart monitor, an electrocardiograph (e-lec-tro-CAR-dee-o-graf), or EKG. The patches on your child's chest are hooked up to a TV-type screen. This screen shows a tracing of each heartbeat. Your child's heart will be watched for signs of injury or damage stemming from the problem.
- **Bronchoscopy:** The doctor may do a test called a bronchoscopy (bron-KOS-ko-pee) if your child is having breathing problems. Before this test is done, the doctor will prescribe medicine to make the child sleepy.
  —It may be possible to remove the object during this test.
  —The child will stay in the hospital until awake and breathing easily.
  —The test may cause a sore throat.
- **Visiting:** You may stay with your child to give comfort and support. The child will feel safer with you nearby.

Swallowed Objects in Adults

WHAT YOU SHOULD KNOW

Once swallowed, a foreign body can get stuck anywhere in the gastrointestinal (GI) tract, from the throat to the stomach and intestines. Pointed objects are more dangerous than round ones. Once the object has reached the stomach, it usually passes through the body by itself without causing problems. This usually takes several days, but may take as long as 2 or 3 weeks. If the object is stuck and must be removed, the doctor may be able to take it out by going down your throat with a tube. Otherwise, you may need surgery.

Causes
In adults, meat and bones are the objects that most commonly get stuck in the GI tract.

Signs/Symptoms

Symptoms range from belly pain or chest pain to anxiety, throwing up, and not being able to swallow.

Care

Depends on what you swallowed and where it is. If you have a piece of meat stuck below your throat, you may be given medicine in an IV to relax your muscles. This may make it easier to swallow the meat or throw it up.

The doctor may order x-rays to find the object. If nothing shows up on the x-ray, your throat and food pipe may be examined through a tube with a scope. Metal detectors can be skimmed over your body to locate metal objects. Once the object is found, your doctor may try to remove it, or you may simply be watched closely in the hospital or at home.

Risks

The degree of danger depends on what you swallowed. Without treatment, sharp objects can damage parts of the gastrointestinal tract and cause major bleeding. Other objects can block part of the GI tract.

WHAT YOU SHOULD DO

- If the swallowed object has not been removed, you should check your stools to make sure it passes. Putting the stool in a strainer and running water over it may make the job easier.
- Eat a high-fiber diet until you pass the object. Good choices are whole grain bread, oatmeal and bran cereals, and fresh fruits and vegetables.
- You may use milk of magnesia to help move the object through your intestines. Do NOT take any other laxatives.
- If the object doesn't pass, you may need more x-rays and other tests.

Call Your Doctor If . . .

- You do not see the swallowed object in your stool within a few days.

Seek Care Immediately If . . .

- You start throwing up, gagging, choking, drooling, have neck or throat pain, or cannot swallow.
- You start coughing, wheezing, or breathing noisily.
- You have a high temperature.
- You start having pain in your stomach, or see bleeding from your rectum or blood in your stool.

IF YOU'RE HEADING FOR THE HOSPITAL . . .

What to Expect While You're There

You may encounter the following procedures and equipment during your stay.

- **Upper GI:** This is an x-ray of your stomach and intestines. You will need to drink a chalky liquid before the test. It blocks x-rays so that an outline of the GI tract will appear on the film.

- **Endoscopy** (end-OS-ko-pee): To locate the object, the doctor may need to pass a soft tube through your mouth and into your GI tract. A light and camera lens at the end of the tube allow the doctor to view the surroundings.

- **CT Scan** (also called a **CAT Scan**): In this test, a computer composes pictures of your GI tract.

- **Chest X-ray:** This picture of your lungs and heart will show whether they have been affected in any way.

- **NG Tube:** Also called a nasogastric (naz-o-GAS-trik) tube, this device is passed through your nose or mouth and down into your stomach. The tube is attached to suction to keep the stomach empty.

- **Taking Vital Signs:** These include your temperature, blood pressure, pulse (counting your heartbeats), and respirations (counting your breaths). A stethoscope is used to listen to your heart and lungs. Your blood pressure is taken by wrapping a cuff around your arm.

- **Pulse Oximeter:** You may be hooked up to a pulse oximeter (ox-IM-uh-ter). It is placed on your ear, finger, or toe and is connected to a machine. It measures the oxygen in your blood.

- **Blood:** Usually taken from a vein in your hand or from the bend in your elbow. Tests will be done on the blood.

- **IV:** A tube placed in your vein for giving medicine or liquids. It will be capped or have tubing connected to it.

- **ECG:** Also called a heart monitor, an electrocardiograph (e-lec-tro-CAR-dee-o-graf), or EKG. The patches on your chest are hooked up to a TV-type screen or a small portable box (telemetry unit). This screen shows a tracing of each heart beat. Your heart is being watched for signs of injury or damage that could be related to the object.

Swimmer's Ear

See Otitis Externa

Swollen Lymph Nodes

WHAT YOU SHOULD KNOW

You're most likely to encounter Lymphadenopathy (limf-AD-en-OP-o-thee), or swollen lymph nodes, in your neck, armpits, or groin. Children are more likely to have swollen nodes than are adults. In children, the problem is usually a sign of infection. When older people develop the condition, there may be a more serious underlying cause.

Causes

Lymphadenopathy is usually caused by a viral or bacterial infection. Other causes include allergic reactions, arthritis, cancer, metabolic diseases, and an overactive thyroid (hyperthyroidism).

Signs/Symptoms

When you're fighting an infection, nearby lymph nodes get bigger and become tender. Normally, lymph nodes are less than 1/2 inch across (about the size of your fingernail). But, with an infection, they can swell to 2 or 3 times their usual size. They will slowly return to normal in 2 to 4 weeks, when the infection is gone. The lymph nodes may also feel hard or firm, and may seem misshapen. The skin near a swollen lymph node may feel warm.

Care

Your doctor will treat the cause of the swelling. If you have an infection, you may need to take an antibiotic or an antiviral medication. If your doctor is not sure what is causing the problem, you may need to have the swollen node biopsied. To perform this procedure, your doctor will insert a needle in the lymph node, remove a sample of tissue or fluid, and send the sample to a laboratory.

WHAT YOU SHOULD DO

- Do not poke or squeeze the swollen lymph nodes. This could keep them from returning to normal.
- You may take acetaminophen for pain and fever, but do NOT take aspirin or give it to children who have an infection.
- Always take your medicine as directed. If you feel it is not helping, call your doctor, but do not stop taking it on your own.
- If you are taking antibiotics, finish the entire prescription even if you feel well. Failure to complete the treatment may leave enough bacteria alive to cause another infection.

- Putting heat on the swollen nodes may help reduce pain. Use an electric heating pad (set on low) or warm, wet towels.
- If you have a sore throat, gargling with warm salt water (1 teaspoon of salt in 1 cup of water) or with double-strength tea may provide some relief.
- If you have a fever, rest until your temperature returns to normal (98.6 degrees F or 37 degrees C). You may resume normal activity slowly after your fever is gone. Be sure to rest whenever you feel tired.
- You may not have much appetite while you are ill, but try to eat as much healthy food as possible. Drink at least 8 soda-can size glasses of liquids each day, especially while you have a fever.

Call Your Doctor If . . .
- You develop a high temperature.
- A swollen node grows to more than 1 to 2 inches across.
- A swollen node remains larger than 1/2 inch for more than 1 month.
- Your lymph nodes continue to feel tender or get worse.
- A swollen node grows more tender to the touch, red streaks develop near it, the overlying skin becomes red, or you develop a rash.

Seek Care Immediately If . . .
- The node interferes with moving your neck, breathing, or swallowing.

Syncope

See Fainting

Syphilis

WHAT YOU SHOULD KNOW

Syphilis (SIF-uh-lis) is an infection that is spread during vaginal, oral, and anal (rectal) sex and sometimes by heavy kissing. Although it may seem to go away without treatment, unless it is cured with antibiotics it will return later, spread, and attack almost any part of the body including the skin, heart, blood vessels, and brain. Antibiotics usually cure the infection in 2 to 3 weeks.

Causes
Syphilis is caused by a type of bacteria called *Treponema pallidum.*

Signs/Symptoms
Syphilis has three stages, each with different symptoms.

During the first stage (3 to 6 days after infection), a red sore appears on the mouth, penis, rectum, vagina, or, sometimes, on another part of the body. It usually doesn't hurt, and many people don't even notice it. Even though this sore goes away in 1 or 2 months without treatment, the infection will remain. During this stage, the germs can be spread to others during sex.

The second stage occurs about 6 to 12 weeks after infection. A small, red, scaly rash appears on the skin, mouth, and sex organs (penis, vagina). Many people also have swollen glands, headache, fever, upset stomach, a stiff neck, and fatigue. During this stage, the infection can be spread to others.

The third stage, which may take place years later, can include many different symptoms such as skin sores and pain in the bones. If the infection spreads to the brain, a person may lose the ability to think clearly. Other symptoms include loss of balance, lack of feeling in the arms or legs, and even paralysis (difficulty moving). Some people have heart problems. During this stage, the infection cannot be spread to others.

Care

To make certain the infection is syphilis, the doctor may do a blood test or take a sample of fluid from a sore. Antibiotic medicine is usually given to fight the infection.

WHAT YOU SHOULD DO

- It is important to follow your doctor's instructions carefully. Syphilis usually can be cured in the early stages, but only if you take antibiotics exactly as prescribed. If your symptoms disappear, do not assume that the infection is cured and stop treatment. The infection can hide in the body for years and must be thoroughly eradicated.
- A few hours after beginning antibiotics, you may get a fever, chills that make you shake, headache, upset stomach, and muscle aches. The rash may get worse. These symptoms last about 24 hours. Rest in bed. Your doctor may tell you to take over-the-counter medicine such as aspirin, acetaminophen, or ibuprofen to reduce the fever and ease the pain.
- Tell all the people you had sex with during the last 3 months that you have syphilis. They may be infected and need treatment.
- Don't have sex until your doctor tells you the infection is cured. This usually takes at least 2 months. After that, use a condom for protection against syphilis and other infections.
- If you are pregnant, be sure to tell your doctor that you have syphilis.

A pregnant woman can pass syphilis on to her baby before it is born, and the infection can cause birth defects or even death.

- After treatment, you must have a blood test every few months for 1 to 2 years to make sure your infection has really been cured.

Call Your Doctor If . . .
- You have a high temperature, a new rash, sore throat, swelling in a joint, or any new symptoms during or after treatment.

Syrup of Ipecac

WHAT YOU SHOULD KNOW

If your child swallows a poison, your doctor may prescribe syrup of ipecac (IP-uh-kak). It will make the child vomit, emptying the stomach of the dangerous material.

WHAT YOU SHOULD DO

Here's what to do after giving the syrup.
- Do not give the child anything to eat or drink for the next 1 to 2 hours. After this time, you may give the child:
    —First, clear liquids such as apple juice or clear sodas.
    —Then, solid foods, if the child keeps down the liquids.
- Keep the child as quiet as possible for the next 2 hours.
- During naptime, the child should lie on the stomach or side in case vomiting occurs.
- For a while after vomiting, the child may have belly pain or loose bowel movements.
- Poison-proof your home. Lock up or put out of reach medicines and other things that could do harm. Keep syrup of ipecac on hand.
- Have the telephone number of your local Poison Control Center handy and call the Center immediately if you think your child has swallowed something dangerous.

Call Your Doctor If . . .
- The child has more than 3 or 4 episodes of vomiting, or if vomiting lasts more than 1 to 2 hours.
- The child has severe stomach cramps or pain or diarrhea lasting longer than 4 to 6 hours.
- The child develops any other sign or symptom that your doctor warned about.

Seek Care Immediately If . . .

• The child is hard to awaken or has trouble breathing. **Dial 911 or 0 (operator) immediately.** Do not try to drive the child to the hospital yourself.
• The child has a seizure.

Tail Bone Injury

See Coccyx Injury

TB

See Tuberculosis

TB Skin Test

See Tuberculin Skin Test

Teething

WHAT YOU SHOULD KNOW

Teething occurs when new teeth begin to come through the gums. Your child's first tooth should appear between 3 and 12 months. The gums may be sore and tender for two or three days as the tooth pushes through. By age three your child will have about 20 teeth.

Signs/Symptoms

Your child may chew on his/her fingers and other things. Drooling and crankiness are additional signs of teething. The child also may not eat or drink as much while teething.

Teething should not cause diarrhea, diaper rash, or change your child's sleeping habits. However, a mild fever of 99 to 99.5 degrees Fahrenheit is a possibility.

WHAT YOU SHOULD DO

To keep your child comfortable while teething:
• Gently rub the swollen gum with a clean finger for 2 minutes. Do this as often as necessary.
• Give your child a clean washcloth to chew. First wet it with cold water and wring it out. Put it in the freezer for 30 minutes.
• Try giving your child a smooth, hard teething ring. Some children like a cold teething ring. Do not tie the ring around the child's neck. It could catch on something and strangle the child.
• Stop breastfeeding briefly since sucking on a nipple may be painful

for the child. You may temporarily want to use a cup to give your child liquids.

- Give frozen juices, a Popsicle, or a frozen banana that has been cut into pieces. The child may also enjoy teething biscuits. Do not use hard foods, such as carrots, that could cause choking.
- You do not need to use special teething gels or lotions. They have a drug in them to which the child could be allergic.
- Acetaminophen may relieve the pain. Your doctor will tell you how much to use and how often to give it. Try to dribble some of the acetaminophen on the baby's gums as you administer it. This will help the gum pain.

Call Your Doctor If . . .
- Your child has a high temperature.
- Your child has signs of infection such as pus or very swollen, reddened gums in the area where the tooth is coming in.

Temporomandibular Joint Disorder

WHAT YOU SHOULD KNOW

Temporomandibular (TEMP-er-o-man-DIB-u-ler) joint disorder, also called "TMJ," affects the joints in front of the ears that serve as hinges for your jaw. In TMJ, one or both of these joints become swollen and painful. The problem is more common in women than in men.

Causes
TMJ is usually caused by tight jaw muscles and grinding of the teeth. Other causes include injury to the jaw, stress, poorly fitting dentures, and arthritis. The condition is sometimes the result of a "bite" problem in which your upper and lower jaw are not lined up correctly. A family history of the disorder puts you at greater risk of developing it.

Signs/Symptoms
You'll typically note a dull, aching pain below the ear on one side of the jaw. This pain will get worse when you yawn. Pain may move to your ear, head, or shoulder. You may hear a clicking or popping noise when you open your mouth. Your mouth may not open all the way, and your teeth may not line up when you close your mouth.

Care
Your dentist may take x-rays of your mouth and feel the action of the joint while you open and close your mouth. You'll probably be given

a prescription to relieve pain and swelling. If the problem is serious, you may need surgery.

WHAT YOU SHOULD DO

- You may take over-the-counter pain relievers such as aspirin or ibuprofen.
- Applying heat may help relieve pain. Use a heating pad set on low, a warm washcloth, or a hot water bottle filled with warm water. Do this for 15 minutes every 2 hours.
- Eat a well-balanced soft diet until the pain disappears. Choose foods such as gelatin, cooked cereal, baby food, ice cream, applesauce, bananas, eggs, pasta, cottage cheese, soups, and yogurt. Don't eat hard chewy foods, such as bagels.
- Your dentist may suggest a nightguard (a plastic mold that fits over the teeth) to wear while sleeping. This helps to prevent you from grinding your teeth.
- Learn methods to relax your muscles.

Call Your Doctor If . . .
- You have new or unexplained symptoms.
- You still have pain after taking your pain medication.

Tendinitis

WHAT YOU SHOULD KNOW

Tendinitis (ten-din-I-tis) is a swelling and irritation of a tendon, the tissue that connects muscles to bones. It may occur in the shoulder, elbow, heel, or hamstring (leg muscle). With treatment, you should be well in about 6 weeks.

Causes
The problem can be caused by many things, including injury, over-exercising, poor posture, and certain diseases such as rheumatoid arthritis and lupus.

Signs/Symptoms
You'll have pain, tenderness, and swelling around the affected tendon. You may also notice weakness in this location.

Care
Follow the directions listed below.

WHAT YOU SHOULD DO

- Use a sling or splint for a few days until the pain decreases.
- Apply ice to the injury for 10 to 20 minutes each hour for the first 1 to 2 days. Put the ice in a plastic bag and place a towel between the bag of ice and your skin.
- After the first day or two, you may apply heat to the injury to help relieve pain. Use a warm heating pad, whirlpool bath, or warm, moist towels for 10 to 20 minutes every hour for 48 hours.
- You may use nonprescription medications such as ibuprofen or acetaminophen to relieve the pain.

Call Your Doctor If . . .
- The pain and swelling increase.
- You develop new, unexplained symptoms.
- You develop a high temperature.

Tendon Repair

See Ruptured Tendon Repair

Tennis Elbow

WHAT YOU SHOULD KNOW

Tennis elbow is pain and swelling of the muscles near the elbow and the tendons that connect them to the bone. Tennis elbow usually affects adults. While it can be cured, it may take 3 to 6 months before the elbow feels better.

Causes
Tennis elbow occurs when stress on the tissues that attach a tendon in the elbow to the muscles in the forearm causes a small tear in the tendon. Moving your forearm in the same pattern over and over again (as you do when playing tennis) can cause this problem. Mechanics or carpenters also may get tennis elbow.

Signs/Symptoms
Hallmarks of the condition are pain, tenderness, or swelling of the elbow. You may also find it difficult to move your elbow.

Care
You need to keep the elbow immobile for a few days and apply ice packs and heat as directed.

WHAT YOU SHOULD DO

- Put ice on the injury for 15 to 20 minutes each hour for the first 1 to 2 days. Put the ice in a plastic bag and place a towel between the bag of ice and your skin.
- After the first 1 to 2 days, you may put heat on the injury to help relieve the pain. Use a heating pad (set on low); a whirlpool bath; or warm, moist towels for 15 to 20 minutes every hour for 48 hours.
- For the first 48 hours, keep your elbow lifted above the level of your heart whenever you can. This will reduce the pain and swelling. Try propping your elbow on the back of the couch while you are sitting down or raising it on some pillows while you are lying down.
- Wear a splint for a few days to keep your elbow from moving.
- You may take over-the-counter pain killers such as acetaminophen, ibuprofen, or aspirin.
- Do not do the activity that caused the problem until your symptoms are completely gone. Then slowly restart your normal activities.
- Do the exercises suggested by your doctor.

Call Your Doctor If . . .
- Your elbow still hurts you after a few weeks.
- You develop a high temperature.

Tension Headache

WHAT YOU SHOULD KNOW

A simple tension headache usually lasts a few hours and has no other symptoms.

Causes
Among the many culprits are tension, stress, eye or muscle strain, depression, allergic reactions, changes in your sleeping pattern, colds and flu, alcohol, caffeine, certain foods and medicines, and weather changes. Changes in hormone levels during a woman's monthly period can also be at fault. Sometimes the cause is unknown.

Signs/Symptoms
Pain from a tension headache can be constant or throbbing, and can be centered anywhere in your head. In addition, muscles in your neck or head may feel tight. You may wake up with a headache and may not be able to sleep.

Care

Take over-the-counter pain-killers. If the pain does not go away, you may need stronger prescription medication.

WHAT YOU SHOULD DO

- You may use aspirin, acetaminophen, or ibuprofen to relieve pain.
- Try some of the following measures to relieve your headache:
  —Stretch and massage the muscles in your shoulders, neck, jaw, and scalp.
  —Take a hot bath.
  —Rest in a quiet, darkened room. Place a warm or cold wet cloth (whichever feels better) over the aching area.
- Don't skip or delay meals. Drink plenty of liquids.
- Avoid alcoholic beverages and cigarette smoking; they often make a headache worse.
- A good night's sleep often is the best way to relieve a headache.

Call Your Doctor If . . .

- Your headache gets worse or lasts longer than 24 hours.
- You develop a high temperature.
- You need to take medicine frequently to relieve headache pain.

Seek Care Immediately If

- Your headache is different from or significantly worse than any headache you ever had before.
- You feel confused or drowsy.
- Your neck feels stiff.
- Your temperature rises very high.
- You have eye problems such as sensitivity to light or blurred or double vision.
- You start to vomit.

Testicular Infection

See Orchitis

Testicular Self-Examination

WHAT YOU SHOULD KNOW

A self-examination of the testicles can detect lumps and other changes that might signal cancer. Regular self-exams help you learn how your testicles normally feel so that you can recognize any changes.

Why do it?

Testicular cancer is one of the most common forms of cancer in men below the age of 40. Its main sign is a lump in the testicle. The best way to beat the disease is to find it early. Learning how to check your testicles can save your life.

Don't put off testicular self-exams because you are "too busy" or "don't know what you are looking for." It's better to find a lump early than to learn about it after cancer has spread.

WHAT YOU SHOULD DO

- Check your testicles once a month. The examination should take about 3 minutes. The best time is after a warm shower or bath, when the scrotal skin is most relaxed.
- Gently roll each testicle between the thumbs and fingers of both hands, feeling for any lumps or changes in the way the testicle feels to the touch.

Call Your Doctor If . . .

- You have aching in your lower belly or groin or find ANY lumps or changes in your testicles.

Tetanus and Diphtheria Vaccine for Adults

WHAT YOU SHOULD KNOW

Tetanus, also called lockjaw, causes your muscles to tighten. Diphtheria (dip-THEER-ee-uh) is a throat infection. You can get tetanus from an injury or a dirty wound. Tetanus is not contagious. Diphtheria, on the other hand, is easily spread from person to person.

You can get a shot for tetanus alone or a combined tetanus/diphtheria ("DT") shot that will prevent you from developing either of these serious diseases.

After getting your first shot, you will need another in 2 months and a third 8 to 14 months later. After this, you will need a "booster" shot at least every 10 years.

WHAT YOU SHOULD DO

- The shot may cause pain, redness, and swelling at the site of the injection (usually the arm). Other potential side effects include chills, fever, and body aches.
  —You may take acetaminophen or ibuprofen for fever and pain.
  —To reduce tenderness and swelling, apply cold compresses to the injection site.

Call Your Doctor If . . .

• The shot site stays tender, red, or swollen for more than 48 hours.
• You develop a high temperature, or the fever lasts more than 48 hours.

Tetralogy of Fallot

WHAT YOU SHOULD KNOW

About 40,000 babies are born in the United States each year with an abnormal heart. Some 4,000 of these babies have a heart defect called tetralogy (tet-RALL-o-gee) of Fallot (fah-LOW), also called TOF. Babies with TOF are also called "blue babies" because their skin does not get enough oxygen and therefore has a bluish tint. Babies with TOF have four problems·

• There is a hole between the lower right and left parts of the heart. This is called a ventricular (ven-TRICK-u-ler) septal (SEP-tul) defect (a VSD).
• The aorta (a-OR-tuh), a major artery that sends blood to the body, gets very big and is pushed out of place.
• There isn't enough blood flowing to the lungs.
• The lower-right part of the heart is larger than normal.

Causes

It is not known what causes TOF. It may be inherited. It can also be caused by an infection or use of drugs or alcohol early in the pregnancy. The heart forms during the first 14 to 60 days of pregnancy.

Signs/Symptoms

Some children have no symptoms. But most have slow growth; tiredness; trouble breathing; poor weight gain; and blue skin, lips, and nailbeds. Symptoms vary from baby to baby.

Care

Treatment depends on how serious the problems are and the age and health of the child. No care may be needed if the heart problem is small. Children with serious problems may need surgery right away. Your child may be put in the hospital to have more tests.

Risks

Tetralogy of Fallot can be fatal. The risks of serious illness or death are smaller if you follow your doctor's suggestions.

WHAT YOU SHOULD DO

- Ask your doctor when you should return for a checkup and make an appointment. Give the child all medicines exactly as directed.
- Your doctor may suggest you give your child oxygen after you go home. You'll be told how often to use it and how long each session should be. Follow these directions exactly.
- Talk to the doctor about your child's activity at home, in day care, or in school.
- If your child is older, he or she will need to take antibiotics before and after dental work. They are needed to prevent infection from developing inside the heart.

Call Your Doctor If . . .
- Your child has a high temperature.
- Your child is not eating or drinking as usual or is fussy.

Seek Care Immediately If . . .
- The child has trouble breathing, the skin between the ribs is being sucked in with each breath, or the lips or nailbeds are turning blue or white. **Call 911 or 0 (operator)** for help.

IF YOU'RE HEADING FOR THE HOSPITAL . . .

What to Expect While You're There
You may encounter the following procedures and equipment during your stay.
- **Taking Vital Signs:** These include the child's temperature, blood pressure, pulse (counting heartbeats), and respirations (counting breaths). A stethoscope is used to listen to the child's heart and lungs. Blood pressure is taken by wrapping a cuff around the arm.
- **Oxygen:** May be given using nasal prongs or a face mask.
- **Pulse Oximeter:** Your child may be hooked up to a pulse oximeter (ox-IM-uh-ter). It is placed on the ear, finger, or toe and is connected to a machine that measures the oxygen in your child's blood.
- **IV:** A tube placed in your child's vein for giving medicine or liquids. It will be capped or have tubing connected to it.
- **Blood:** Is usually taken from a vein in your child's hand or head, or from the bend in the elbow. Tests will be done on the blood.
- **Blood Gases:** Blood is taken from an artery in your child's wrist, elbow, or groin. It is tested to see how much oxygen it contains.
- **Chest X-ray:** This picture of your child's heart and lungs shows how they are handling the illness.
- **ECG:** Also called a heart monitor, an electrocardiograph (e-LEK-

tro-CAR-dee-o-graf), or EKG. The patches on your child's chest are
hooked up to a TV-type screen. This screen shows a tracing of each
heartbeat. Your child's heart will be watched carefully throughout
hospitalization.

- **12 Lead ECG:** This test makes tracings from different parts of your
  child's heart. It can help your doctor gauge the seriousness of the
  problem.
- **ECHO:** Also called an echocardiogram (ek-oh-CAR-dee-o-gram).
  This uses sound waves to view your child's heart while it is beating.
  It can help care givers decide what is causing the heart failure.
- **Cardiac Catheterization (cath-uh-ter-i-ZAY-shun):** A test used
  to study the arteries sending blood to your child's heart.
- **Surgery:** An operation may be needed if the heart problems are
  serious.
- **Emotional Comfort and Support:**
  —You may stay with your child to give comfort and support. Chil-
    dren feel safer in the hospital if parents are close by.
  —As a parent, you may feel scared, confused, and anxious about
    your child's heart problem. You may blame yourself and think
    you have done something wrong. To work out these feelings, talk
    about them with your doctor or someone close to you.
  —Ask your doctor about support groups for parents who have chil-
    dren with heart problems.

Threadworm

See Pinworms

Threatened Miscarriage

WHAT YOU SHOULD KNOW

Bleeding during the first 20 weeks of pregnancy is called a threatened
miscarriage or threatened abortion. Although there is a chance you
could lose the pregnancy, it is not certain to happen. Most women
who have vaginal bleeding or spotting during early pregnancy have
healthy babies.

Causes

Some pregnant women bleed around the usual time of their monthly
period. Bleeding after having sex could be the result of an irritation on
the cervix (bottom part of uterus). Often, no reason for spotting or
bleeding can be discovered.

Signs/Symptoms

Bleeding is the most common sign of a threatened miscarriage. A low backache or cramps in the belly are other signs.

Care

Your cervix will be checked to see if it is closed, starting to open, or open. Your doctor will do a pelvic exam (also called an "internal") to check the size and shape of your uterus (womb).

You may have an ultrasound. It is a painless test done while lying down. A dab of a jelly-like lotion is placed on your belly. The person doing the test will gently move a small handle through the lotion and across the skin, viewing a TV-like screen attached to the handle.

You will need to rest and avoid sex for several days. This will not prevent a miscarriage, but it may reduce your bleeding and pain. There are no medicines that will stop the bleeding and cramping.

WHAT YOU SHOULD DO

Call Your Doctor If . . .

- Your bleeding and cramping get worse. You should not have to use more than one pad each hour.
- You feel weak or faint.
- You have chills or a high temperature.

Seek Care Immediately If . . .

- You pass large clots or other material that looks like tissue. Save the tissue in a clean container or plastic bag. Bring it with you when you come to be checked.

Thrombophlebitis

WHAT YOU SHOULD KNOW

In thrombophlebitis (throm-bo-fluh-BI-tis), a small blood clot forms on the wall of a vein, causing it to swell. The condition occurs most often in leg veins close to the skin.

Signs/Symptoms

The condition is marked by redness, tenderness, and pain in the area of the blood clot. The area may feel hard when you touch it. You may have a fever.

Causes

Thrombophlebitis may result from infection or injury that prompts excessive clotting in the veins. It can also be caused by sitting for long periods on a plane, resting in bed for a long time, or wearing a cast. This immobility prompts blood to pool and, eventually, clot. Smoking while using birth control pills can also lead to more than the usual amount of clotting. Some cases of thrombophlebitis are a result of injury to the wall of the vein from needles or IV fluids or the spread of blood cancer.

Care
Doctors usually recommend resting and keeping the affected arm or leg propped up. You may be given medicines for pain or swelling. If you have an infection, the doctor may also prescribe an antibiotic. You may need to wear elastic stockings. Wrapping towels, soaked in warm water, around your legs may relieve some of the pain. If you follow your doctor's advice, you should be better in about 2 weeks.

Do's and Don'ts
To keep from getting clots, you should not smoke while using birth control pills. Do not abuse IV drugs. If you must rest in bed for a long time, move your legs around as much as possible to keep the blood moving.

Risks
Without treatment, you could get a more serious—possibly fatal—blood clot. Also, if the thrombophlebitis is due to infection, you could get blood poisoning.

WHAT YOU SHOULD DO

Call Your Doctor If . . .
• You see increased swelling in your leg.

Seek Care Immediately If . . .
• During treatment, you start having:
   —Really bad pain in your leg.
   —Trouble breathing.
   —Chest pain.
   —A high temperature.
   —Cough with bloody sputum.

IF YOU'RE HEADING FOR THE HOSPITAL . . .

What to Expect While You're There
You may encounter the following procedures and equipment during your stay.

- **Taking Vital Signs:** These include your temperature, blood pressure, pulse (counting your heartbeats), and respirations (counting your breaths). A stethoscope is used to listen to your heart and lungs. Your blood pressure is taken by wrapping a cuff around your arm.
- **Pulse Oximeter:** You may be hooked up to a pulse oximeter (ox-IM-uh-ter). It is placed on your ear, finger, or toe and is connected to a machine. It tells how much oxygen is in your blood.
- **Blood:** Usually taken from a vein in your hand or from the bend in your elbow. Tests will be done on the blood.
- **Blood Gases:** Blood is taken from an artery in your wrist, elbow, or groin. It is tested for the amount of oxygen in your blood.
- **IV:** A tube placed in your vein for giving medicine or liquids. It will be capped or have tubing connected to it.
- **Venogram:** This is an x-ray study done to see if there are blood clots in your veins.
- **Doppler Study:** In this painless test, sound waves are used to look at your veins on a TV-like screen. Your doctor will be looking for clots in the veins near the area of pain and redness.
- **Chest X-ray:** This is a picture of your lungs and heart. The doctors use it to see how your heart and lungs are handling the illness.
- **Activity:** You may need to rest in bed. Once you are feeling better, you will be allowed out of bed.
- **Pressure Stockings:** These special stockings keep the blood from sitting in the legs for a long time and developing clots. The tightness of the stockings will be increased gradually from leg to leg.
- **Cold or Heat:** A cool towel or heating pad (set on low) placed on the area that hurts may help ease the pain.
- **Medicines:**
  - **Antibiotics:** May be given to fight infection. They may be given by IV, in a shot, or by mouth.
  - **Blood Thinners:** Drugs such as aspirin or warfarin will be given by mouth. They help prevent the blood from forming clots.

After You Leave

- Rest with your leg raised for 1 or 2 days. Move your foot and ankle often. Return to your normal activities slowly after the leg begins to feel better.
- Warm wet soaks may help relieve discomfort. Wring out a towel in hot water and lay it over the affected area. Resoak the towel often to keep it warm.
- Don't sit or stand for long periods of time. Don't cross your legs when you sit. Rest with your leg raised during the day.

• For comfort—and to help prevent further episodes—wear elastic stockings or support hose.
• Stop smoking, especially if you are taking birth control pills.

Thrombosis

See Deep Vein Thrombophlebitis

Thrush

WHAT YOU SHOULD KNOW

Thrush, a yeast infection of the cheeks, gums, and tongue, is seen most often in infants and older people. It can be painful and is known to return after treatment. However, it is not a serious disease; and, with proper care, you should be better in about 3 days.

Causes

Thrush is caused by Candida (CAN-did-uh), a fungus normally found in the mouth. Taking antibiotics can lead to an outbreak of the fungus, especially in older people who use large doses of antibiotics to cure a stubborn bacterial infection. Newborns may get thrush if the mother had a vaginal yeast infection during delivery. The infection can also occur after an injury to the lining of the mouth.

Signs/Symptoms

You'll notice white patches in the mouth that look like milk curds and do not wipe off easily. Other signs may include a dry mouth or pain while eating or swallowing.

WHAT YOU SHOULD DO

• Take prescribed medicine exactly as directed. If the medicine causes problems or doesn't seem to be working, call your doctor. Don't stop taking the medicine on your own.
• You may use over-the-counter medications such as aspirin, acet-aminophen, and ibuprofen to help relieve pain.
• If possible, wash silverware and drinking glasses in an automatic dishwasher. Otherwise, boil them or use plastic items. For infants, soak bottle nipples in hot water for 15 minutes.
• Older children and adults may rinse their mouths with a salt solu-tion. Mix 1/2 teaspoon of salt in 8 ounces of water. Rinse 3 or more times a day after eating. Do not swallow the salt water. Do NOT give salt water to young children.

- Drink lots of fluids and eat foods that are easy to swallow. Use a straw for drinking if your mouth is painful.
- If sucking is painful for your child, reduce sucking time to no more than 20 minutes per feeding. Let the baby use a pacifier only when really needed for going to sleep. Breastfeeding may be continued.

Call Your Doctor If . . .
- A high temperature develops.
- You notice sores on your skin or vagina, or your baby gets diaper rash.
- Your child fails to gain weight or refuses to eat.
- The thrush gets worse or lasts more than 10 days.
- Problems arise that may be related to the medicine you are using.

Seek Care Immediately If . . .
- Your child is not drinking enough fluids and has signs of dehydration, including listlessness, dizziness, dry mouth, increased thirst, and little or no urine.

TIA

See Transient Ischemic Attack

Tic Douloureux

See Trigeminal Neuralgia

Tick Bite

WHAT YOU SHOULD KNOW

The blood-sucking little bugs we call ticks live in tall grasses and trees. They can drop onto you from foliage or latch onto you or your clothes as you pass by. Although most tick bites cause no harm, these insects carry many germs and can pass on many kinds of infections.

Ticks attach to your head, neck, armpits, or groin; bore into your skin; and suck out the blood they need for nourishment. Soft-bodied ticks, which are relatively harmless, let go of the skin by themselves after a few hours. Hard-bodied ticks cause the most serious problems. They may remain attached to the skin for up to 2 weeks.

Signs/Symptoms
You'll first notice redness, pain, and swelling in the area of the tick bite. You may also develop blisters, a rash, and an itch. The bite may cause fatigue, walking difficulties, headache, fever, chills, muscle

weakness, and loss of appetite—all signs of a serious tick-borne disease.

Care
You may need medicine for an infection, pain, swelling, or itching.

WHAT YOU SHOULD DO

- To prevent a tick-borne infection, you must get the tick off of you as soon as possible. To remove the tick:
  —First, disinfect the tick bite site with rubbing alcohol.
  —Grasp the tick as close to the skin as possible. Pull it straight out and up with tweezers or with fingertips protected by a tissue or cloth.
  —Pull gently until the tick lets go. Do not twist the tick or jerk it suddenly; this may leave the tick's head or mouth parts buried in the skin.
  —Do not crush the tick or touch it with your bare hands.
  —Applying a hot match, petroleum jelly, or fingernail polish to the tick is not helpful and may be dangerous.
  —After the tick is removed, wash the bite and your hands with soap and water.
- To keep from getting tick bites when walking through vegetation:
  —Use an insect repellent and wear pants and long-sleeved shirts. Also wear a hat in areas with trees.
  —Put insect repellent on exposed skin and also at boot tops, bottom of pants legs, and sleeve cuffs.
  —Every 2 to 3 hours check your clothing, hair, and skin for ticks. Pay special attention to your hairline, armpits, and waist.
  —If you take a dog with you, check his coat for ticks.
  —As soon as possible, wash and dry clothing worn outside.

Call Your Doctor If . . .
- You cannot remove a tick.
- The tick's head is left in the skin after you remove the body.

Seek Care Immediately If . . .
- You get a fever, rash, headache, or muscle or joint pains. These may be signs of a more serious disease.
- You are having trouble walking or moving your legs. This may be a sign of tick paralysis.

Tinea Capitis

See Ringworm of the Scalp

Tinea Corporis

See Ringworm of the Body

Tinea Pedis

See Athlete's Foot

TMJ Disorder

See Temporomandibular Joint Disorder

Toe Fracture

See Broken Toe

Toenail Removal

See Nail Removal

Tonsillitis

WHAT YOU SHOULD KNOW

Tonsillitis (TON-sill-EYE-tis) is an infection of the tonsils—lumps of tissue at the back of the throat that fight nose and throat infections and keep them from spreading to the neck, lungs, and bloodstream. Tonsillitis is a common problem in young children.

Causes

The infection can be caused by a variety of viruses and bacteria. It is spread from person to person by coughing, sneezing, and touching.

Signs/Symptoms

There may be fever, sore throat, painful swallowing, headache, and sore muscles. The youngster may vomit, have a stomach ache, or be sleepy. The tonsils may look red and swollen and feel tender.

Care

The first step is a throat culture. If the culture is positive for strep germs, the doctor will prescribe the child an antibiotic.

WHAT YOU SHOULD DO

• Have the child rest as much as possible and get plenty of sleep.
• Children older than 8 years may suck on hard candy or frozen juice

bars or gargle with a warm or cold liquid to help soothe the throat. For gargling, use 1 teaspoon salt mixed in 8 ounces of water or strong tea. A younger child can be given a teaspoon of corn syrup or honey several times a day (do not give honey to children younger than 1 year of age).

- Use a cool-mist humidifier to help decrease throat irritation and cough.
- You may give over-the-counter medicines such as acetaminophen to relieve the pain.
- Encourage your child to drink plenty of fluids. While the throat is very sore, feed the child soft or liquid foods such as milk, milkshakes, ice cream, soups, or instant-breakfast milk drinks.
- If the child has swollen, tender lumps in the neck, you may apply a moist, warm towel or wash cloth several times a day for 30 to 60 minutes. Keep the compresses warm, but be careful not to burn the child.
- Family members who develop a sore throat or fever should have a medical exam or throat culture.
- If the child is on antibiotics, wait 24 hours before returning him or her to school or daycare.

Call Your Doctor If . . .
- The child has a high temperature or a fever that lasts more than 48 hours.
- The child has large, tender lumps in the neck.
- A rash develops.
- The child coughs up green, yellow-brown, or bloody sputum.

Seek Care Immediately If . . .
- The child develops new symptoms such as vomiting, earache, severe headache, stiff neck, chest pain, or trouble breathing or swallowing.
- The child develops more severe throat pain along with drooling or voice changes.

Toothache

WHAT YOU SHOULD KNOW

A toothache is usually the result of a cavity formed by the bacteria that cause tooth decay (known medically as dental caries). Cleaning out and filling the cavity brings a quick end to the pain. Without this treatment, however, the pain is likely to get worse.

Causes
Cavities get their start from plaque that sticks to the surface of a tooth and provides food for bacteria. The bacteria and certain acids break through the enamel surface of the tooth, forming a hole that fills with decayed matter. The decay then spreads to the inside of the tooth.

Other causes of toothache are mouth injury, a cracked tooth, a head cold, or sinus or dental infection. You may also have tooth pain after having dental work.

Signs/Symptoms
The pain can be dull, sharp, aching, burning, or throbbing. It may come and go, and may affect the whole mouth or only one part. Hot or cold foods and biting and chewing may increase the pain. Other possible symptoms include fever and swollen gums.

WHAT YOU SHOULD DO

- Until you can see a dentist, use over-the-counter medications such as acetaminophen and ibuprofen to ease the pain.
- Oil of cloves also may help. Clean all food out of the cavity with a toothpick. Soak a small piece of cotton in the oil and pack it into the cavity. Take care to keep the oil off your tongue, where it will sting.
- You may get relief by putting an ice pack on your jaw, but putting heat on it may make the toothache worse.
- To avoid getting another toothache, see a dentist for check-ups every six months, brush your teeth twice a day, and floss once a day.

Call Your Dentist If . . .
- You develop a high temperature.
- Your pain becomes worse.

Seek Care Immediately If . . .
- You have swelling in your face, jaw, cheek, eye, or neck.

Tooth Eruption

See Teething

Tooth Injury

See Damaged Teeth

Torticollis

WHAT YOU SHOULD KNOW

Torticollis (TOR-tih-COLL-is) is a spasm or shortening of the muscles on one side of the neck. A few people are born with the problem, but this is rare. Most often it develops between the ages of 30 and 60 years. It tends to run in families; and women are more likely to get it than men. Healing time may take as long as 5 years, depending on how bad the condition is and what caused it. The problem is also referred to as "wryneck."

Causes
Torticollis may suddenly develop without any accident or injury. You may never know what triggered the pain: It may simply be there when you wake up one morning. Torticollis occasionally results from sleeping on a new bed or new pillow, or on the sofa. The pain sometimes develops gradually over many days.

Signs/Symptoms
The tight muscles on one side of the neck produce neck pain and cause the head to bend and turn to one side. You may find that it hurts to turn your head.

Care
The doctor may take an x-ray, CT scan, or MRI of the neck to make sure nothing else is causing your pain. The doctor may prescribe medications to relax the muscles, and a neck brace or soft collar to keep your neck from moving. You may need to have surgery on these muscles if the torticollis is severe.

WHAT YOU SHOULD DO

- Reduce your activity until the pain abates; rest in bed if needed (your doctor will tell you how long). When you get the go-ahead from the doctor, you can resume your normal activity.
- After the first 1 or 2 days, you may put heat on the area to help ease the pain. You may use a heating pad (set on low), a whirlpool bath, or warm, moist towels. Apply the heat for 15 to 20 minutes every hour. Continue to do this for 48 hours.
- Your doctor can show you how to massage the neck to ease the pain. The doctor can also suggest muscle stretching exercises. Do them regularly as directed.
- If the doctor prescribes a neck brace, continue wearing it until your neck no longer hurts.

- Do not drink or drive while taking pain killers or muscle relaxants. Take your medicine exactly as directed. If you feel it is not helping, call your doctor.
- To keep the neck pain from getting worse:
  —Avoid sleeping in unusual positions.
  —Avoid stressful situations.

Call Your Doctor If . . .
- Your neck pain lasts longer than 1 week.
- You have pain, numbness, tingling, or weakness in your arms or face.

Seek Care Immediately If . . .
- You have trouble breathing or swallowing, or your voice gets hoarse.

Total Hip Replacement

WHAT YOU SHOULD KNOW

Total hip replacement is also called hip joint replacement. It is surgery in which a badly damaged hip joint is replaced with artificial parts. These man-made parts are called a prosthesis (prahs-THEE-sis). The joint is made of metal or a mixture of metal and plastic. The surgery is done to reduce pain and make movement easier and better. It is usually reserved for people with really bad osteoarthritis or rheumatoid arthritis of the hip. Most hip replacements are totally successful. It takes most patients at least 3 to 5 months to get back their strength and energy.

Risks

Without treatment, the pain and problems you have when moving your hip may continue and get worse. Talk with your doctor about the risks of your surgery. To reduce the chances of problems after surgery, be sure to carefully follow your doctor's advice.

IF YOU'RE HEADING FOR THE HOSPITAL . . .

Before You Go
- Do not eat or drink anything (not even water) after the time your doctor recommends.
- You may take pills with a sip of water the morning of surgery.
- Do not take any aspirin or ibuprofen before surgery.
- You may be given a sleeping pill to take the night before surgery to help you sleep.

- Do not forget to bring any papers, given to you by the doctor about this surgery, with you to the hospital (such as consent forms).
- An anesthesiologist (an-is-THEE-se-OL-o-gist) may give you a call the night before surgery. This is the doctor who gives you medicine to make you sleepy during surgery.

When You Arrive
- **Before Surgery:**
  —You may be taught how to cough and deep breathe to lessen your chance of getting a lung infection after surgery.
  —Before surgery, you may learn special exercises to help make your hip stronger. You will also be taught how you will need to roll from side to side after the surgery.
  —You may need to have your hip cleaned with a special liquid before going to surgery. It may make your skin yellow, but it will come off later.
  —You may be given medicine to make you sleepy before you are taken to the operating room. You will be put to sleep during surgery.

What To Expect While You Are There
You may encounter the following procedures and equipment during your stay.
- **Taking Vital Signs:** These include your temperature, blood pressure, pulse (counting your heartbeats), and respirations (counting your breaths). A stethoscope is used to listen to your heart and lungs. Your blood pressure is taken by wrapping a cuff around your arm.
- **Pulse Oximeter:** You may be hooked up to a pulse oximeter (ox-IM-uh-ter). It is placed on your ear, finger, or toe and is connected to a machine that measures the oxygen in your blood.
- **ECG:** Also called a heart monitor, an electrocardiograph (e-LEK-tro-CAR-dee-o-graf), or EKG. The patches on your chest are hooked up to a TV-type screen or a small portable box (telemetry unit). This screen shows a tracing of each heartbeat. Your heart will be watched to make sure your body is handling the surgery well.
- **Blood:** Usually taken from a vein in your hand or from the bend in your elbow. Tests will be done on the blood. You may need to have these done more than once.
- **IV:** A tube placed in your vein for giving medicine or liquids. It will be capped or have tubing connected to it.
- **Chest X-ray:** This is a picture of your lungs and heart. The care givers use it to see how your heart and lungs are doing before surgery.

- **ET Tube:** During surgery, you may have a tube placed in either your mouth or nose that goes into the windpipe. This will protect your windpipe during surgery and allow your caregiver to give you oxygen when you need it. After the tube is taken out you may have a sore throat.
- **Oxygen:** May be given to you during your surgery. You may also need extra oxygen as you are waking up from your surgery.
- **After Surgery:** You will be taken to a recovery room until you wake up. When you wake up or are close to waking up you will be taken back to your room. You will have a bandage over your skin where the surgeon performed the operation. Do not get out of bed until your doctor gives the go-ahead.
- **Activity:** You will need to rest in bed. Your bed will be kept flat at first. Your nurse will show you how far you can raise the head of the bed. Once you are feeling better, you will be allowed out of bed.
- **Turning:** Will need to be done in a special way after surgery. You will need to use pillows between your legs to keep the affected leg in position.
- **Bathroom Needs:** Will have to be taken care of on a special bed pan. Your nurse will tell you how to get on and off the bed pan so you do not hurt your hip.
- **Physical Therapy:** Will be started sometime after surgery. A physical therapist helps you do special exercises to make your hip stronger and move better.
- **Pressure Stockings:** May be put on your legs. They help keep the blood from sitting in the legs for a long time and causing clots.
- **Medicines:**
  - **Antibiotics:** May be given to keep you from getting an infection from the surgery. They may be given by IV, in a shot, or by mouth.
  - **Blood Thinners:** You may be given blood thinners to keep you from getting blood clots, especially if you will be resting in bed for a long time. Heparin, warfarin, or aspirin may be given.
  - **Pain Medicine:** May be given in your IV, as a shot, or by mouth. If the pain does not go away or comes back, tell a caregiver right away.
  - **Anti-Nausea Medicine:** If pain medicine upsets your stomach, you may need additional medication to relieve the problem.

After You Leave

- Always take your medicine as directed. If you feel it is not helping, call your doctor. Do not quit taking it on your own.
- If you are taking antibiotics, take them until they are all gone—even

if you feel well. Ask your doctor if you need to take antibiotics before seeing your dentist.

- If you are taking medicine that makes you drowsy, do not drive or use heavy equipment.
- You will need to use crutches for walking for the first 6 to 12 weeks. Then you may slowly start walking without crutches or a cane.
- For the next 3 months, you must be careful about how you move or place the affected leg.
- Do not cross your legs when you are sitting, lying, or standing.
- Keep the affected leg facing front at all times, even in bed. Never turn your hip or knee outward or inward.
- Put a pillow between your legs when you lie on your side.
- Do not bend over at the hips to reach into cupboards or drawers or to pick things up from the ground.
- Do not sit on low chairs, low stools, or low toilet seats. Do not sit in reclining chairs. You may need to use a firm cushion to raise chair seats. Consider renting or buying a raised toilet seat.
- Sit only in chairs that have arms. When you get up from a chair, move to the edge and use the chair arms to push yourself up. Place the affected leg in front of the other. Push up with the good leg, keeping the affected leg in front while getting up.
- Swimming, golf, walking, and bicycling are usually permitted. Do not do exercises that repeatedly jar the hip joint, such as tennis and jogging.
- Do not drive after your surgery until your doctor gives the go ahead.
- Until you are walking around more often, you may need to wear support socks to help lessen swelling in your legs.

Call Your Doctor If . . .
- You have fever, swelling, or redness at your surgery site.
- You have increased pain in the affected hip or have trouble moving around.

Seek Care Immediately If . . .
- You fall and injure your hip.
- You have trouble breathing.
- The affected leg (or toes) begins to feel numb and tingly or cool to the touch, or looks blue or pale.

Total Knee Replacement

See Knee Joint Replacement

Tracheobronchitis in Adults

See Acute Bronchitis

Tranquilizer Abuse

See Benzodiazepine Abuse

Transient Ischemic Attack

WHAT YOU SHOULD KNOW

A transient (TRANS-e-ant) ischemic (is-SKI-mik) attack, called a TIA for short, is often a warning signal of an impending stroke. Pieces of fat or blood clots can block an artery leading to the brain. When this happens, a part of the brain does not get enough oxygen and the symptoms of a TIA appear.

With a TIA, the artery is only blocked a short time. With a stroke, the blockage lasts much longer, causing brain damage.

Causes
High blood pressure, diabetes, excess weight, high amounts of fat in the blood (cholesterol), and smoking.

Signs/Symptoms
Appear suddenly, last less than 24 hours, and go away completely. Typical signs include seeing double, loss of vision, fainting or dizziness, a weak or numb feeling on one side of the face or body, or trouble swallowing or speaking.

Hospital Care
May include medicines that thin the blood or lower blood pressure. You may need surgery to remove a blockage from the artery.

Do's and Don'ts
To keep from having more TIAs, you may need to take aspirin every day; quit smoking; eat foods low in fat, cholesterol, and salt; lose weight; and start exercising. If you have other illnesses (diabetes, high blood pressure, or heart disease), it is important to keep them under control.

Risks
If you aren't treated, you will have more attacks and maybe a stroke. Most TIAs are caused by other diseases. If these diseases are not

found and treated, you could have a stroke, heart attack, or other serious problems.

WHAT YOU SHOULD DO

- Always take your medicine as directed by your doctor. If you feel it is not helping, call your doctor, but do not quit taking it on your own.
- If you take aspirin regularly, continue taking it. Aspirin helps thin the blood so blood clots don't form. Do not take acetaminophen or ibuprofen instead.
- Have your blood pressure checked. You may want to buy a blood pressure cuff. Ask your doctor to show you or a family member how to use it.
- If you have other illnesses such as diabetes, high blood pressure, or heart disease, you need to control them. Take medicines as directed. If you don't, you will have a greater chance of having another attack.
- Check with your doctor before starting exercise or having sex.
- Exercise daily. It helps make the heart stronger, lowers blood pressure, and keeps you healthy. If the exercise is too hard or too easy, call your doctor.
- Quit smoking. It harms the heart and lungs. If you are having trouble quitting, ask your doctor for help.
- Weighing too much can make the heart work harder. If you need to lose weight, ask your doctor about the best way of doing it.
- A diet low in fat, salt, and cholesterol is very important. It keeps your heart healthy and strong. Ask your doctor what you should and should not eat.

Call Your Doctor If . . .
- You have chest pain during exercise that doesn't go away with rest.
- Your blood pressure is high.
- You feel worse after taking your medicine.
- You feel your medicine is not working.
- You are on a blood thinner and you are bruising easily or have blood in your urine.

Seek Care Immediately If . . .
- You cannot speak, move part of your body, or see; if you have blurred vision, or if you become dizzy, confused, or unconscious. These are signs of a stroke. **THIS IS AN EMERGENCY. Call 911 or 0 (operator)** to get to the nearest hospital or clinic. **Do not drive yourself!**

• You have the above symptoms but they go away. You may be having a TIA. **Call 911 or 0 (operator)** to get to the nearest hospital or clinic. **Do not drive yourself!**

IF YOU'RE HEADING FOR THE HOSPITAL . . .

What to Expect While You're There

You may encounter the following procedures and equipment during your stay.

• **Taking Vital Signs:** These include your temperature, blood pressure, pulse (counting your heartbeats), and respirations (counting your breaths). A stethoscope is used to listen to your heart and lungs. Your blood pressure is taken by wrapping a cuff around your arm.

• **Pulse Oximeter:** While you are getting oxygen, you may be hooked up to a pulse oximeter (ox-IM-uh-ter). It is placed on your ear, finger, or toe and is connected to a machine that measures the oxygen in your blood.

• **ECG:** Also called a heart monitor, an electrocardiograph (e-LEK-tro-CAR-dee-o-graf), or EKG. The patches on your chest are hooked up to a TV-type screen or a small portable box (telemetry unit). This screen shows a tracing of each heartbeat. Your heart will be watched for signs of injury or damage that could be related to your illness.

• **12 Lead ECG:** This test makes tracings from different parts of your heart. It can help your doctor decide whether there is a problem with your heart.

• **Oxygen:** Your body may need extra oxygen at this time. It is given either by a mask or nasal prongs. Tell your doctor if the oxygen is drying out your nose or if the nasal prongs bother you.

• **IV:** A tube placed in your vein for giving medicine or liquids. It will be capped or have tubing connected to it.

• **Blood:** Usually taken from a vein in your hand or from the bend in your elbow. Tests will be done on the blood.

• **Medicine:**

—**Heparin:** Keeps the blood thin so no other clots can form. It is given in an IV. Later, you may get other blood thinners.

—**Blood Thinners:** These include aspirin and warfarin. They are given by mouth as a replacement for heparin. Like heparin, they keep the blood from forming clots.

—**Blood Pressure Medicine:** Given for constant high blood pressure. At first it may be given in an IV, and later in a pill.

• **CT Scan:** It is also called a "CAT" scan. This is an x-ray using a computer. It is used to make pictures of your internal organs.

- **Lumbar Puncture:** Also called a spinal tap. Fluid is taken from your spine and sent for tests.
- **EEG:** Also called an electroencephalogram (e-LEK-tro-en-SEF-uh-lo-gram). This is a brain wave study.
- **Chest X-ray:** This is a picture of your lungs and heart. The caregivers use it to see how your heart and lungs are handling the illness.
- **Surgery:** This may be needed to take out a large blockage in one of your arteries.

Traveler's Diarrhea

WHAT YOU SHOULD KNOW

The loose, watery stools of traveler's diarrhea usually appear after a visit to a country where food and water is not carefully cleaned and cooked. The problem generally lasts 2 to 7 days.

Causes
Bacteria, viruses, and parasites can thrive in unclean food and water. When you swallow the infected material, the germs often take up residence in the bowel, causing diarrhea.

Signs/Symptoms
Typical symptoms include loose, watery, or unformed stools; abdominal cramping and pain; nausea; and a generally ill feeling.

Care
You may take medicine to stop the diarrhea or fight the infection. Be sure to drink lots of liquids. If you have a severe infection or lose too much fluid, you may need a stay in the hospital.

Risks
The greatest danger posed by severe diarrhea is loss of too much of the body's water and salt. This dehydration, if untreated, can be life-threatening.

WHAT YOU SHOULD DO

- You may use Pepto-Bismol to relieve discomfort. Take it according to the directions on the label.
- Take clear liquids, such as defizzed ginger ale or cola, bottled or boiled water, hot tea, or broth during the first 24 hours or until the diarrhea stops. If you are sick to your stomach, suck on ice chips.
- During the next 24 hours, you may eat bland foods such as cooked

cereals, rice, soup, bread, crackers, baked potatoes, eggs, and apple-sauce. Avoid alcohol and caffeine.
- You can return to your regular diet after 2 to 3 days.
- Drink 2 to 3 quarts of fluid a day. Most complications are caused by loss of water.
- To help keep from getting travelers' diarrhea in the future:
  —Take 2 tablets of Pepto-Bismol 4 times a day (with each meal and at bedtime), beginning the day before you leave and continuing for 2 days after arriving home. Continue for up to 3 weeks.
  —Drink only bottled or boiled water or canned or bottled beverages (soft drinks, beer, wine), without ice. Boil water for at least 4 minutes or use purifying tablets to treat the water.
  —Brush your teeth with mouthwash solution. Do not use tap water for this purpose or to wash off food. Always wash your hands before handling or eating food.
  —Avoid all raw fruits and vegetables except those that can be peeled. Also stay away from milk, ice cream, and other dairy products; raw meat and fish; and cold sauces, salsa, and dressings. Relatively safe foods include steaming-hot dishes, grilled foods right off the fire, and dry foods (breads, crackers).

Call Your Doctor If . . .
- Diarrhea lasts for more than 3 days; you find blood, mucus, or worms in your stool, or you have pain in the abdomen or rectum.
- You have a high temperature.
- You have signs of water loss, including dry mouth, extreme thirst, wrinkled skin, little or no urine, or dizziness or light-headedness.

IF YOU'RE HEADING FOR THE HOSPITAL . . .

What to Expect While You're There
You may encounter the following procedures and equipment during your stay.
- **Taking Vital Signs:** These include your temperature, blood pressure, pulse (counting your heartbeats), and respirations (counting your breaths). A stethoscope is used to listen to your heart and lungs. Your blood pressure is taken by wrapping a cuff around your arm.
- **Pulse Oximeter:** You may be hooked up to a pulse oximeter (ox-IM-uh-ter). It is placed on your ear, finger, or toe and is connected to a machine that measures the oxygen in your blood.
- **IV:** A tube placed in your vein for giving medicine or liquids. It will be capped or have tubing connected to it.
- **Daily Weight:** You will be weighed about the same time every day.
- **Strict Intake/Output:** Care givers will carefully watch how much

liquid you are drinking or getting in your IV, and how much you are urinating.

- **Activity:** You may need to rest in bed. Once you are feeling better, you will be allowed to get up.
- **Medicines:**
  —**Antibiotics** may be prescribed to fight the infection. They may be given by IV, in a shot, or by mouth.
  —**Anti-nausea medicine** may be given to get rid of your upset stomach and control vomiting. These medicines will help prevent excessive loss of fluids.

Trichomoniasis

WHAT YOU SHOULD KNOW

Trichomoniasis (TRIK-uh-moe-NEYE-uh-sis)—also called tricho-monas vaginitis in women—is an infection spread by sexual contact. Both men and women can be infected.

Cause
The tiny trichomonas parasite.

Signs/Symptoms
In women, typical symptoms include bad-smelling vaginal discharge, itching, redness, and pain in the vagina. There also may be pain during urination if urine flows on swollen areas. Infected men may have no symptoms at all.

Care
You and your sexual partner will be given medicine to treat the infection.

WHAT YOU SHOULD DO

- Take the entire prescription for this infection. If you stop taking the drug too soon, some parasites may survive and re-infect you.
- Keep your genital area clean and dry. Do not sit around in wet clothing such as swim suits. Take showers instead of tub baths. Use plain, unscented soap. Avoid too much activity, heat, and sweating.
- Avoid feminine hygiene sprays or powders. Do not douche during treatment unless your doctor recommends it. After the infection is cleared up, do not douche more often than once a week.
- Do not have sex during treatment. After treatment, use a condom to help protect against infection.

• Wear underpants and pantyhose that have a cotton lining in the crotch.

Call Your Doctor If . . .

• Your symptoms become worse or last longer than a few days.
• You have vaginal bleeding, and you are not menstruating.
• Your symptoms come back after treatment.
• You have any problems that may be related to the medicine you are taking.

Trigeminal Neuralgia

WHAT YOU SHOULD KNOW

Trigeminal (try-JEM-uh-nul) neuralgia (noor-AL-guh) is a long-term problem marked by sudden attacks of facial pain. The length of the attacks ranges from a few seconds to several minutes. Attacks may occur many times a day or only a few times a month or year. The problem usually affects men older than 40 years of age. It is also called tic douloureux (doll-uh-RUEZ).

Causes

The pain occurs in the trigeminal nerve, a major nerve in the face. Attacks can be triggered by touching, stroking, or shaving your face, brushing your teeth, chewing, yawning, or being exposed to a cold wind.

Signs/Symptoms

The only symptom is severe, knife-like pain in the jaw or cheek—most often on the right side of the face.

Care

Muscle-relaxing medicine may help prevent the attacks. If medical treatment does not help, you may need surgery.

WHAT YOU SHOULD DO

• Take the prescribed medication exactly as directed.
• To help prevent attacks:
  —Chew on the unaffected side of the mouth.
  —Avoid touching your face.
  —Avoid blasts of hot or cold air.
  —To avoid the need for shaving, men may wish to grow a beard.

Call Your Doctor If . . .
- Pain is unbearable and your medicine isn't helping.
- You develop any new, unexplained symptoms.
- You have problems that may be related to the medicine you are taking.

Tubal Pregnancy

See Ectopic Pregnancy

Tub Bathing Your Baby

WHAT YOU SHOULD KNOW

After the cord has come off, you can begin bathing your baby in a tub. At first, the baby may object. But with time, the baby will come to enjoy having his or her clothes off, getting wet, and being washed. When getting a tub bath, the child's safety and comfort are important.

How often you bathe your baby depends on his or her skin, the baby's activities, and the weather. A bath may be needed only 1 to 2 times a week if the baby has dry skin, or sleeps most of the day. In hot weather, an active baby with normal skin may need a bath each day.

WHAT YOU SHOULD DO

- During the first few months, use a baby bathtub or a clean plastic dishpan. The family bathtub may be used once the baby is 6 months old.
- Fill a basin with 2 to 3 inches of warm, **not hot,** water. Slowly put the baby's body in the water. Use one of your hands to support the head. Keep your other hand free to wash the baby.
- Start at the top and move down. You can wash the baby's head and hair 1 or 2 times a week with a gentle shampoo. Rinse with a washcloth to get rid of all shampoo.
- Rinse off the eyelids with fresh water. Wash the ears with a cloth. Do not put cotton swabs in your baby's ears. This will push the wax back into the ear.
- Use either a washcloth or your hands to soap the baby's body. Carefully wash the areas under the neck, between the legs, and under the arms.
- When bathing a boy, wash his bottom with a mild antibacterial soap or with plain water. Be sure to lift the scrotum and wash underneath it.
- If bathing a girl, wash her bottom area with plain water. Wipe from

front to back keep from spreading germs from the rectum to other parts of the bottom.
• When you are finished bathing, make sure all the soap is rinsed off the baby's skin. Soap left on the skin can be irritating.
• You may apply lotion after the bath once the baby is 3 to 4 weeks old. Use only lotion suggested by your doctor. The lotion can be warmed by placing the container in the tub water before the bath.
• Do not use baby powder because it contains talc and may be irritating to your baby's lungs. You may use cornstarch.
• **Never** leave your baby alone in the bath. If you must leave the room, take the child with you.

Tuberculin Skin Test

WHAT YOU SHOULD KNOW

Tuberculosis, also known as TB, is an infection that usually starts in the lungs. The tuberculin (tuh-BER-cue-lin) skin test is used to see if you have the disease. A very small amount of fluid is injected just under the skin. If you have the infection, within 2 or 3 days you will develop a hard, red area around the point where the needle entered your skin.

Tuberculosis can usually be cured completely with 6 to 9 months of treatment. If not treated, the disease can badly damage the lungs, spread to other parts of the body, and eventually lead to death.

Causes
Tuberculosis is caused by bacteria. It can be spread by coughing and sneezing. The people in greatest danger of getting TB are those who have HIV (the AIDS virus), abuse drugs or alcohol, or live in a prison or nursing home. Tuberculosis is also more common among people who work in hospitals and nursing homes, and among those who are black, Asian, Latin American, or native American. Having certain chronic (long-term) diseases or taking certain medicines increases your chances of developing the disease.

Signs/Symptoms
In the early stages of the disease there are often no signs. Some people may have early symptoms that seem like the flu. Later on, you may have fever, lose weight, feel very tired, and sweat a lot (mostly at night). With really bad TB, you can cough up sputum that looks bloody, yellow, thick, or gray; feel pain in the chest; and have trouble breathing.

Care

If the test shows you are infected, your doctor may take a sample of blood and an x-ray picture of your chest. You may also need one or more antibiotic medicines to fight the infection. Your family members and other people with whom you have close contact may need to be tested and treated too.

WHAT YOU SHOULD DO

- RETURN or CALL in 2 or 3 days so the doctor can examine your reaction to the skin test. The test is positive if there is a red bump about the size of a pencil eraser or bigger on your arm.
- A positive test usually means that you are infected with the TB germ. You will need other tests, such as an x-ray picture of your lungs or a sputum sample, to see if you have active TB.
- If you have active tuberculosis, your doctor will give you medicines to fight the infection. Even if you do not have active TB, you may need to take medicine to keep you from developing the disease later.
- If the test is negative, you are probably not infected. However, it takes 2 to 10 weeks after being around a person with tuberculosis for the skin test to be positive. If you have been exposed to someone with TB, you need to get tested again in 2 weeks to make sure you haven't caught the disease.
- If you are infected with HIV (the virus that causes AIDS), your body may not react to a TB skin test. You may need other tests.

Call Your Doctor If . . .

- You have any questions or concerns about the results of your test.
- You have any of the following symptoms of active TB:
  —You start losing a lot of weight.
  —You feel weak or sick.
  —You have a high temperature.
  —You wake up at night covered with sweat.
  —You have chest pain, coughing, or cough up blood.

Tuberculosis

WHAT YOU SHOULD KNOW

Tuberculosis (too-bur-cu-LO-sis)—also called TB—is an infection that can last for years if not treated. Even after treatment, it may come back years later. TB most often infects the lungs, but may be found in almost any part of the body.

Tuberculosis germs are easily spread from person to person through the air. The disease is most common in elderly people, babies, people with AIDS, and drug or alcohol abusers. Living in crowded or unclean housing increases the risk of getting TB.

Causes

Tuberculosis is caused by a bacteria that gets into the air when a person with the disease coughs or sneezes.

Signs/Symptoms

TB has three stages:

- In the early stage, you may have no symptoms at all, even though you are infected, or you may feel as though you have the flu.
- In the second stage, you may have fever, weight loss, sweating, and tiredness.
- In the later stage, the most common sign is a cough. You may cough up yellowish-green matter (sputum) or blood. It may be painful and hard to breathe.

Care

To see whether you have TB, you will have a lung x-ray and, possibly, skin and sputum tests. The people you live or work with may also need to be tested.

Your doctor will prescribe one of several medicines that kill TB germs. You will need to stay away from other people until you have taken the medicine for a few days. You have to continue taking the medicine for up to 1 year. If the disease is not completely cured, the germs will remain in the body, eventually damaging the lungs or other organs.

Risks

Without treatment, you are more likely to have long-lasting problems with your lungs. The infection can spread to your brain, bones, spine and kidneys. In the end, it can be fatal.

WHAT YOU SHOULD DO

- Your doctor must report all cases of tuberculosis to the health department. This helps protect others from getting the disease. It also helps you get the care you need to cure your TB. **You must stick with your treatment until you are cured, even if you don't feel sick.** Otherwise, the health department can step in and make sure you get the treatment you need.
- It is very important that you take your tuberculosis medicine exactly as your doctor tells you. If you skip or stop your pills, some of the TB germs will not be killed. Remember, the germs can hide in your

body without causing symptoms unless they are completely eliminated with the right medicine. Here are some hints for remembering
your pills:

—Ask someone else, such as a family member or a friend, to help
  you keep track of your doses.
—Take your pills at the same time every day.
—Mark on a calendar every time you take the pills.
—Each night, put out the pills for the next day.
—Keep the pills in a place where you can't miss them, such as the
  bathroom or kitchen. Be sure they are out of reach of children.
—Use 7 little pill bottles and label them for each day of the week, or
  buy a pill container marked with the days of the week at a drug
  store.

• You will need to have regular checkups to make sure the pills are
  working. **It is very important that you keep all your appointments.** At the checkup, be sure to tell your doctor if you think something is wrong.
• At every checkup, you'll have your weight, temperature, and lungs
  checked. You may also have a picture taken of your lungs (chest
  x-ray) to see how you are healing. In addition, you may be asked for
  a sputum sample. It will be tested to see if you are coughing up any
  TB germs and whether the pills are working.
• Until your doctor says you can't spread your TB germs to others:
  —Stay at home. Avoid close contact with others, especially babies
    and elderly people.
  —You don't need to wear a mask. But, **always** cover your mouth
    and nose with a paper tissue when you cough or sneeze. Throw
    the used tissues away. If possible, flush them down a toilet.
  —Wash your hands with soap and water after you cough or sneeze.
  —Don't go back to work or school. You may be able to return to
    work once your coughs and sneezes are no longer infectious. If
    your boss is worried, your doctor may be able to help.
• It's important to eat a well balanced diet, but you don't have to stuff
  yourself or eat special foods. And be sure to get plenty of rest.
• Other family members, close friends, and co-workers should have a
  TB skin test. They could have caught the germs without getting sick.
  They may need to take medicine to keep TB from developing.
  People you saw only once in a while probably don't need to be
  tested.
• You can't pass TB germs to others from clothes, drinking glasses,
  dishes, handshaking, or using the same toilet.
• After you are finished with treatment, you will need to have regular

checkups for at least 2 years to make sure the TB doesn't flare up again.

Call Your Doctor If . . .

• You have any problems that may be caused by the medicine you are taking. Side effects you should tell your doctor about include nausea and vomiting, rash, urine the color of dark tea or coffee, or yellow eyes or skin.

• Your tuberculosis symptoms don't go away or get worse, even though you are taking your TB pills.

• Anyone who spent time near you develops symptoms of tuberculosis such as fever, loss of appetite, weight loss, night sweats, or cough. They will need to get tested for TB.

• You have a cough that doesn't clear up after 3 or 4 weeks following a cold.

• You have a high temperature.

Seek Care Immediately If . . .

• You have chest pain or bring up blood when you cough.

• You have trouble breathing.

• You have fever, headache, vomiting, and neck stiffness.

IF YOU'RE HEADING FOR THE HOSPITAL . . .

What to Expect While You're There

You may encounter the following procedures and equipment during your stay.

• **Chest X-ray:** This picture of your lungs and heart will show the doctor any signs of the illness. The heart is checked for its size, and the lungs for liquid.

• **Sputum Sample:** If you are coughing up sputum, your doctor may need to send a sample to the lab. This sample will be tested for TB and other kinds of germs.

• **Bronchoscopy** (bron-kos-ko-pee): For a close look at your lungs, the doctor can pass a flexible tube through your nose or mouth and down into your airways. The tube can also be used to take a sample of mucus or a small piece of lung for testing.

• **Lumbar Puncture:** In this test, fluid is taken out of an area near your spine. It is then sent to a lab and tested for blood and signs of infection.

• **Medicines:** Tuberculosis drugs will be prescribed to fight the infection. They may be given by IV, in a shot, or by mouth.

• **Taking Vital Signs:** These include your temperature, blood pressure, pulse (counting your heartbeats), and respirations (counting

your breaths). A stethoscope is used to listen to your heart and lungs. Your blood pressure is taken by wrapping a cuff around your arm.

- **Pulse Oximeter:** While you are getting oxygen, you may be hooked up to a pulse oximeter (ox-IM-uh-ter). It is placed on your ear, finger, or toe and is connected to a machine. It measures the oxygen in your blood.
- **IV:** A tube placed in your vein for giving medicine or liquids. It will be capped or have tubing connected to it.
- **Blood:** Usually taken from a vein in your hand or from the bend in your elbow. Tests will be done on the blood.
- **Blood Gases:** Blood is taken from an artery in your wrist, elbow, or groin, and tested for the amount of oxygen in your blood.
- **Oxygen:** Your body may need extra oxygen at this time. It is given either by a mask or nasal prongs. Tell a doctor if the oxygen is drying out your nose or if the nasal prongs bother you.

Tympanoplasty

See Pressure-Equalizing Ear Tubes

Ulcers

WHAT YOU SHOULD KNOW

An ulcer is an open sore in the digestive tract. Most ulcers are found in the stomach and top of the small intestine. When stomach acid comes in contact with an ulcer, it can become quite painful.

With treatment, most ulcers heal in 1 to 2 months. The most serious problems occur when there is bleeding from the stomach and when the ulcer breaks through (perforates) the stomach or intestinal wall.

Causes

Most ulcers are caused by a bacterium called *H. pylori*. Excess stomach acid makes the situation worse. Certain medicines, such as the nonsteroidal anti-inflammatory drugs prescribed for arthritis, also can cause ulcers. Smoking, drinking, consuming too much caffeine (from coffee, tea, or cola drinks) and stress play an important role in the development of an ulcer.

Signs/Symptoms

The most common symptom is pain in the upper abdomen (the area around the stomach), especially when the stomach is empty. You may also have pain after eating, especially if you eat something that upsets your stomach. Other possible symptoms include nausea, vomiting, and burping.

Care
Most ulcers can be treated at home. If your ulcer starts to bleed, however, you will probably have to go to the hospital.

Risks
With treatment, your ulcer will usually heal without any problems. Without proper care, however, you may develop a bleeding ulcer or other problems that require surgery.

WHAT YOU SHOULD DO

- Your doctor may prescribe antibiotics, drugs that block acid production, and regular antacids. You will probably have to take several drugs at different times each day. Be sure to follow directions exactly. Don't stop taking the medicines on your own, even if you're feeling better.
- You can use over-the-counter antacids, but take them only as directed by your doctor.
- Try to keep something in your stomach. Eat several small meals at regular times during the day. Missing meals and eating irregularly can make your symptoms worse.
- Avoid foods and beverages that upset your stomach. These may include acidic foods, carbonated beverages, beer and other alcoholic drinks, tea, and coffee.
- Don't take aspirin or ibuprofen. They may cause bleeding. You may use acetaminophen.
- Don't smoke. Smokers are more likely to develop ulcers, and their ulcers take longer to heal and are more likely to recur.
- Try to reduce the stress in your life. Seek professional counseling if necessary.
- Rest as much as possible. You may resume your normal activities when you feel better.

Call Your Doctor If . . .
- Your stools are black, bloody, or tarry-looking.
- You have diarrhea or constipation that may be caused by antacids.
- Your symptoms do not improve in a few weeks.

Seek Care Immediately If . . .
- You vomit blood or material that looks like coffee grounds.
- You have severe abdominal pain.

• You have cold skin, are sweating, and feel weak or faint.

IF YOU'RE HEADING FOR THE HOSPITAL . . .

What to Expect While You're There

You may encounter the following procedures and equipment during your stay.

- **Upper GI:** An x-ray of your stomach and intestines. You will need to drink a chalky liquid before the x-rays. The pictures help your doctor locate the problem.
- **Endoscopy** (end-AH-scuh-pee): Your doctor may need to examine the inside of your stomach. A tube will be passed through your mouth and into your stomach, and the doctor will use a camera to look at the ulcer.
- **Taking Vital Signs:** These include your temperature, blood pressure, pulse (counting your heartbeats), and respirations (counting your breaths). A stethoscope is used to listen to your heart and lungs. Your blood pressure is taken by wrapping a cuff around your arm.
- **Pulse Oximeter:** If you are getting oxygen, you may be hooked up to a pulse oximeter (ox-IM-uh-ter). It is placed on your ear, finger, or toe and is connected to a machine that measures the oxygen in your blood.
- **IV:** A tube placed in your vein for giving medicine or liquids. It will be capped or have tubing connected to it.
- **Blood:** Your nurse will usually take blood from a vein in your hand or from the bend in your elbow. Tests will be done on the blood.
- **Chest X-ray:** This picture of your lungs and heart shows your doctor how well they are handling the illness.
- **Blood Transfusion:** If you are losing too much blood, a transfusion may be needed.
- **Surgery:** A perforated or bleeding ulcer may require surgery. Your doctor will discuss the operation with you in advance.

After You Leave

Follow the directions listed under "What You Should Do."

Ulcers, Corneal

See Corneal Ulcer

Umbilical Cord Care

See Cord Care

Upper GI Endoscopy

See Gastrointestinal Endoscopy

Upper Respiratory Infection

See Common Colds

Urethritis, Gonococcal

See Gonorrhea

Urethritis, Nonspecific

See Nonspecific Urethritis in Men

Urinary Calculi

See Kidney Stones

Urinary Retention in Men

WHAT YOU SHOULD KNOW

When you can't empty your bladder completely during urination, the condition is known medically as urinary retention. Men with this problem may be able to pass only small amounts of urine or none at all.

Causes

Urinary retention develops when the duct that drains the bladder (the urethra) becomes blocked—often by an enlarged prostate gland. The condition may also be caused by certain medicines, an infection, an injury, or bladder stones.

Signs/Symptoms

The condition is characterized by frequent, strong urges to urinate accompanied by an inability to actually pass very much urine. There may be dribbling or leakage during the day and while you are asleep. You may need to push in order to start urination.

Treatment

The doctor will have your urine tested, and may examine your bladder through a tube threaded up the urethra. To keep the bladder drained, the doctor may insert a soft tube called a catheter. There are also various medicines that can reduce the blockage and encourage urination.

Risks

Left untreated, this condition can lead to urinary tract infections and serious kidney problems.

WHAT YOU SHOULD DO

- Do not let your bladder get too full. Urinate as much as you can whenever you feel the urge.
- If your doctor has installed a catheter, do NOT pull on it or try to remove it yourself. Keep the urine bag attached to the catheter below the level of your bladder.
- Drink enough water to keep your urine clear or pale yellow. This helps keep the catheter from clogging.

Call Your Doctor If . . .
- Your symptoms return or get worse.
- Your urine becomes cloudy and foul smelling, or you experience pain or burning when you pass urine. These are signs of infection.
- You have a high temperature.
- Your catheter comes out, or you have redness, pain, blood, or drainage where the catheter enters the penis. These are signs of infection or irritation.

Seek Care Immediately If . . .
- You cannot pass any urine or, if you have a catheter, no urine is filling the bag.
- You have fresh blood or clots in your urine.
- You develop an extremely high temperature

Urinary Tract Endoscopy

See Cystoscopy

Urinary Tract Infection

WHAT YOU SHOULD KNOW

A urinary tract infection (also called a UTI) is an infection of the bladder or kidneys. UTIs are more common among women, especially those who are sexually active. They also occur in men, however, particularly those over the age of 50. It's possible to have repeated infections.

Causes
Urinary tract infections are caused by bacteria that travel up the urinary duct (urethra) into the bladder. Among men, UTIs are more likely to develop when an enlarged prostate gland cuts off the flow of urine, causing it to stagnate and giving bacteria a chance to multiply. Among women, sexual intercourse, pregnancy, diabetes, or a past

UTI all increase the chances of this kind of infection. Women also increase their risk by wiping from back to front after a bowel movement. Holding your urine rather than urinating when you feel the need will also raise the odds of a UTI.

Signs/Symptoms
Typical symptoms include a frequent need to urinate with inability to pass more than a small amount, pain and burning during urination, and dribbling or leaking during the day and while asleep. After urinating, you may still feel the urge; and you may need to urinate often during the night. The urine may develop a foul odor or become blood-specked. If the problem is in your kidneys, you may have a pain in your abdomen or side accompanied by a fever and nausea.

Treatment
Your doctor will have your urine tested for bacteria. Antibiotics are prescribed to fight the infection. Acetaminophen can be taken for fever.

WHAT YOU SHOULD DO

- Take antibiotics exactly as directed. Be sure to take all the medication, even if your symptoms disappear. If you stop treatment too soon, some bacteria may survive and re-infect you.
- Get plenty of rest. If you have a fever, stay in bed until your temperature is normal (98.6 degrees F or 37 degrees C) and you feel better.
- Drink 6 to 8 soda-can size glasses of fluids—especially water—every day to help flush out your kidneys and wash out germs from your urinary tract. Drinking cranberry juice or taking vitamin C will help make your urine more acid and keep the infection under control.
- Urinate often—as soon as you feel the urge—and try to empty your bladder completely each time. It is a good idea to urinate before and after sex. Make sure that a child with a UTI urinates at least 3 or 4 times a day.
- Avoid caffeine and alcohol during treatment; they irritate the bladder.
- Take showers rather than baths. Each day, wash the genital area well with soap and water (use only water to wash this area in children). Do not use bubble bath or bath oils.
- Women should remember to wipe from front to back after urinating or having a bowel movement. This reduces the chance of germs get-

ting into the bladder. It's also wise to wear underwear and pantyhose with a cotton crotch.

• If you have a kidney infection—also called pyelonephritis (PIE-lo-nef-RY-ITS)—it is important to keep your follow-up visit to make sure the infection is cured. Otherwise, lingering infection could damage the kidneys.

Call Your Doctor If . . .
• You have a high temperature.
• You have blood in your urine.
• Your symptoms don't improve in a few days.
• You have nausea, vomiting, diarrhea, or a rash.
• You develop any new or unexplained symptoms. They may be related to the medication you are taking.
• Your symptoms (especially fever) return after you finish treatment.

Seek Care Immediately If . . .
• You start vomiting and can't keep down any fluids or medicine.
• You are unable to urinate.

Urticaria
See Hives

Using Crutches
See Crutches

Uterine Bleeding, Abnormal
See Dysfunctional Uterine Bleeding

Vaginitis, Candida
See Candidiasis

Vaginitis, Nonspecific
See Bacterial Vaginosis

Vaginosis, Bacterial
See Bacterial Vaginosis

Varicella
See Chickenpox

Varicose Veins

WHAT YOU SHOULD KNOW

Varicose veins are swollen, snakelike, bluish veins that you can see under the skin. These veins are most often found in the legs, but they can occur in other parts of your body as well.

Causes
Leg veins have valves that help blood return to the heart. If the valves become weak and allow blood to leak backwards, pressure can build up in the veins, making them swollen and stretched. Standing for long periods can trigger the problem. Pressure on veins from pregnancy, fluid in the belly, or tumors can also lead to varicose veins. The problem tends to run in families.

Signs/Symptoms
In addition to the veins themselves, there may be a little discomfort and aching in the legs, especially after standing; and feeling tired.

Care
Do not wear tight clothing. You may, however, wear elastic support hose (put them on before you get out of bed). Take breaks often and rest your legs by propping them up above the level of your heart. The veins can be removed surgically or eliminated with chemical shots.

Do's and Dont's
To keep from getting varicose veins, exercise regularly. If you are very overweight, you may need to lose weight.

WHAT YOU SHOULD DO

- Stay off your feet as much as possible.
- Don't stand or sit in one position for long periods of time. Don't sit with your legs crossed.
- Rest with your legs raised during the day.
- Wear elastic stockings or support hose. Don't wear a girdle, garters, or pantyhose with tight elastic tops.
- Walk as much as possible to increase blood flow.
- Raise the foot of your bed at night with 2-inch blocks.
- If you get a cut in the skin over the vein and the vein bleeds, lie down with your leg raised and press on it with a clean cloth until the bleeding stops. Then have a doctor take care of the wound.

Call Your Doctor If . . .

- The skin around your ankle itches, looks brownish, and starts to break down.
- You have pain, redness, tenderness, itching, and a hard swelling in your leg.
- You are very uncomfortable because of the leg pain.

Venereal Warts

See Genital Warts

Venous Access Ports

See Implanted Venous Access Ports

Ventricular Septal Defect

WHAT YOU SHOULD KNOW

About 40,000 babies are born in the United States each year with an abnormal heart. Nearly 9,000 of these babies have a problem called a ventricular (ven-TRICK-u-ler) septal (SEP-tul) defect or VSD. It is one of the most common defects of the heart.

In VSD, there is a hole in the wall that divides the lower right and left parts of the heart. The hole can be small or large. Because of it, arteries and veins going to your child's lungs must work harder to pump more blood.

Causes

It is not known what causes a VSD. It may be inherited. It can also be caused by an infection or use of drugs or alcohol early in the pregnancy. The heart forms during the first 14 to 60 days of pregnancy.

Signs/Symptoms

Are different for every child. Some children have no symptoms because their VSD is small. Other children may grow slowly, not gain enough weight, have little energy, get frequent colds, and have problems breathing.

Care

Treatment depends on how large the hole is, and the age and health of your child. No care may be needed if the defect is small. The hole may close on its own. However, children with a large defect may need surgery right away. Your child may be put in the hospital to have more heart tests.

Risks
Ventral septal defect can be fatal. The risks of serious illness or death are smaller if you follow your doctor's suggestions.

WHAT YOU SHOULD DO

- Ask your doctor when you should return for a checkup. Always give your child the medicines exactly as prescribed.
- Talk to your doctor about your child's activity at home, in day care, or in school.
- If your child is older, he or she will need to take antibiotics before and after dental work is done. They are needed to prevent development of an infection inside the heart.

Call Your Doctor If . . .
- Your child has a high temperature.
- Your child is not eating or drinking as usual, or is fussy.

Seek Care Immediately If . . .
- The child has trouble breathing, the skin between the ribs is being sucked in with each breath, or the lips or nailbeds are turning blue or white. **Call 911 or 0 (operator)** for help.

IF YOU'RE HEADING FOR THE HOSPITAL . . .

What to Expect While You're There
You may encounter the following procedures and equipment during your stay.
- **Taking Vital Signs:** These include the child's temperature, blood pressure, pulse (counting heartbeats), and respirations (counting breaths). A stethoscope is used to listen to the child's heart and lungs. Blood pressure is taken by wrapping a cuff around the arm.
- **Pulse Oximeter:** Your child may be hooked up to a pulse oximeter (ox-IM-uh-ter). It is placed on the ear, finger, or toe and is connected to a machine that measures the oxygen in your child's blood.
- **Oxygen:** May be given using nasal prongs or a face mask.
- **IV:** A tube placed in your child's vein for giving medicines or liquids. It will be capped or have tubing connected to it.
- **Blood:** Usually taken from a vein in your child's hand or from the bend in his or her elbow. Tests will be done on the blood.
- **Blood Gases:** Blood is taken from an artery in your child's wrist, elbow, or groin. It is tested to see how much oxygen it contains.

- **Chest X-ray:** This is a picture of your child's heart and lungs. The caregivers use it to see how your child's heart and lungs are handling the illness.
- **ECG:** Also called a heart monitor, an electrocardiograph (e-LEK-tro-CAR-dee-o-graf), or EKG. The patches on your child's chest are hooked up to a TV-type screen. This screen shows a tracing of each heartbeat.
- **12 Lead ECG:** This test makes tracings from different parts of your child's heart. It can help your doctor gage the seriousness of the problem.
- **ECHO:** Also called an echocardiogram (ek-oh-CAR-dee-o-gram). This uses sound waves to view your child's heart as it beats. It can help the doctor assess the problem.
- **Cardiac Catheterization (cath-uh-ter-i-ZAY-shun):** A test used to study the arteries sending blood to your child's heart.
- **Diuretic Medicine (di-your-ET-ic):** This medicine increases the child's urine output. It will get rid of extra fluid in the body or lungs.
- **Surgery:** An operation may be needed if your child's heart problems are serious.
- **Emotional Comfort and Support:**
  —You may stay with your child to give comfort and support. Children feel safer in the hospital if parents are close by.
  —As a parent, you may feel scared, confused, and anxious about your child's heart problem. You may blame yourself and think you have done something wrong. To work out these feelings, talk about them with your doctor or someone close to you.
  —Ask your doctor about support groups for parents who have children with heart problems.

Vertebral Compression Fracture

WHAT YOU SHOULD KNOW

A vertebral compression fracture, also called a vertebral crush fracture, is a collapse or breakdown of one or more of the bones in your spine (the vertebrae).

Causes

This type of fracture typically results when osteoporosis, the "brittle bone" disease, weakens the bones in the spine. Lack of calcium and sustained use of some medicines can also lead to weaker bones. A fall or jump may cause the fracture; but the bones sometimes collapse from the body's own weight.

Signs/Symptoms

If the injury occurs suddenly, you may have severe pain or weakness in your back, arms, or legs. If the collapse happens more slowly, the pain may be much milder. You might also experience problems with urination and bowel movements.

Care

You may need an x-ray of the spine to determine the location of the injury. Casts and splints aren't used for this type of fracture, but you may need to wear a back support. Your doctor also will probably prescribe medication for the pain and drugs that will gradually strengthen the bones.

WHAT YOU SHOULD DO

- Avoid heavy lifting and strenuous exercise until your doctor says you may resume your normal activities.
- If you are using a back support, wear it until your doctor says you no longer need to.
- You may take nonprescription medications, such as aspirin, acetaminophen, and ibuprofen, to relieve the pain.

Call Your Doctor If . . .

- The pain gets worse.
- You have problems taking your medicine.
- The pain prevents you from sleeping or resting comfortably.

Seek Care Immediately If . . .

- You have numbness or tingling in your arms or legs.
- The pain becomes so severe that you cannot care for yourself.
- You begin to have problems controlling your bladder or bowels.

Vertigo

See Dizziness

Viral Croup

See Croup

Viral Hepatitis A

See Hepatitis A

Viral Hepatitis B and C

See Hepatitis B and C

Viral Infections in Children

WHAT YOU SHOULD KNOW

There are many kinds of viruses. Colds, flu, measles, and many other diseases are all viral infections. Some infections can become serious. Others just make a child not feel well.

Signs/Symptoms

Symptoms differ from virus to virus. Often, however, the child may have a fever, headache, sore muscles, vomiting, or a runny nose. Other signs may be cough, sore throat, belly ache, or a tired feeling.

WHAT YOU SHOULD DO

- Encourage as much rest as possible while the child has a fever.
- For children younger than 4 years who cannot blow their noses:
  —Use a rubber suction bulb to suck drainage from both sides of the nose. This is especially important for infants (up to 6 months old) since they breathe mostly through their nose.
  —To loosen dried nasal drainage: Put 2 to 3 drops of warm water in each nostril using a moist cotton ball. Wait about 1 minute and gently suction out each nostril.
- Use a cold mist humidifier to keep the air moist and the nasal drainage loose.
- Have the child drink extra fluids such as fruit juices and water or eat chicken noodle soup. Do **not** give milk products since they may thicken drainage in some children.
- For coughing and sore throats:
  —Children older than 4 years of age may suck on throat lozenges or hard candy.
  —Corn syrup may be soothing for younger children. Do not give honey to infants.
- Antibiotics do not work for viral infections. To ease fever and discomfort, you may give the child over-the-counter medicines as directed by your doctor:
  —For pain or fever: acetaminophen or ibuprofen.
  —For runny nose or cough: a decongestant/antihistamine combination.

Call Your Doctor If . . .

- The child develops a high temperature.
- Nasal drainage becomes thick and yellow.
- An infant will not breastfeed or take fluids.

- The child complains of a severe headache.
- The child coughs up yellow or green mucus.

Seek Care Immediately If . . .
- The child has trouble breathing even after the nostrils are cleared.
- The child becomes more sleepy or irritable than usual.
- The child's hands, toes, or lips turn light blue.

Viral Meningitis

WHAT YOU SHOULD KNOW

Viral meningitis (men-in-JIE-tis), also called "aseptic (a-SEP-tik) meningitis," is an infection that causes irritation and swelling of the tissue around the brain and spinal cord. The symptoms are uncomfortable, but usually clear up in a week or two.

Causes
The disease can be caused by a wide variety of viruses. It sometimes takes hold after a viral infection elsewhere in the body, such as mumps, measles, or chicken pox.

Signs/Symptoms
Symptoms typically include fever, headache, stiff neck, irritability, tiredness, confusion, and vomiting. Additionally, the eyes may be sensitive to light.

Care
Rest and recuperation is the best treatment. Antibiotics will not relieve this illness because they don't work on viruses. You should rest in a dark room for 2 to 7 days.

Risks
In severe cases, viral meningitis can cause brain damage, muscle problems, or (rarely) paralysis.

WHAT YOU SHOULD DO

- Take any medication your doctor prescribes exactly as directed. You may take acetaminophen for pain.
- Stay away from others until your doctor says you can no longer spread the infection.
- Although no special diet is needed, drink about 6 to 8 glasses (soda-can size) of water a day, even if you don't feel like it.
- If you have headaches, rest in a dark, quiet room.

• To keep from spreading germs, wash your hands after each trip to the bathroom and before eating.

• As soon as you feel better, you can return to your normal activities.

Call Your Doctor If . . .

• You have new symptoms (such as a rash, itching, swelling, or trouble breathing) that started when you began taking medicine. You may be allergic to the drug.

Seek Care Immediately If . . .

• Anyone else in the family develops the symptoms of meningitis.

• Anyone in the family becomes confused or difficult to wake up, or has a high temperature.

IF YOU'RE HEADING FOR THE HOSPITAL . . .

What to Expect While You're There

You may encounter the following procedures and equipment during your stay.

• **Room:** Your room will be kept dark and quiet to make you comfortable and ease your pain. You may not want too many visitors until you feel better.

• **Isolation:** To keep from spreading the infection, you will be kept away from others. Nurses and others around you will wear face masks and gowns to keep from getting the disease.

• **CT Scan:** This computerized x-ray machine can be used to take pictures of the brain. Doctors will check the x-rays for signs of danger to the brain.

• **Lumbar Puncture:** Also called a spinal tap. In this test, fluid is taken from your spine and tested for evidence of the virus.

• **Neuro Signs:** The doctor will examine your eyes, check your memory, and see how easily you awaken. These signs show how well your brain is handling the infection.

• **Taking Vital Signs:** These include your temperature, blood pressure, pulse (counting your heartbeats), and respirations (counting your breaths). A stethoscope is used to listen to your heart and lungs. Your blood pressure is taken by wrapping a cuff around your arm.

• **Pulse Oximeter:** You may be hooked up to a pulse oximeter (ox-IM-uh-ter). It is placed on your ear, finger, or toe and is connected to a machine. It measures the oxygen in your blood.

• **Blood:** Usually taken from a vein in your hand or from the bend in your elbow. Tests will be done on the blood.

- **IV:** A tube placed in your vein for giving medicine or liquids. It will be capped or have tubing connected to it.
- **Medicines:**
  —**Pain medicine** may be given in your IV, as a shot, or by mouth. If the pain does not go away or comes back, tell a doctor right away.
  —**Fever medicine** such as acetaminophen will be given for your fever. It may be given by mouth or in your rectum.
  —**Anti-nausea medicine** may be given to get rid of nausea and control vomiting so that you do not lose too much body fluid (become dehydrated).

After You Leave
- Follow the guidelines listed under "What You Should Do."

Viral Pneumonia

WHAT YOU SHOULD KNOW

Viral pneumonia is an infection that causes irritation, swelling, and congestion in the lungs. It is also called pneumonitis (nu-mo-NI-tis). Viral pneumonia occurs most often in the winter.

Causes
The infection begins when a virus is inhaled and settles in the lungs. The illness usually starts as a cold.

Signs/Symptoms
The most common symptoms are a headache, fever and chills, muscle aches, and a cough that brings up sputum. Breathing may be difficult or painful. You may lose your appetite and feel tired.

Care
If you have no other illnesses or problems, you can be treated at home. You need a humidifier to loosen your sputum (making it easier to cough up), and rest. Antibiotics do not work against viruses. However, if you see your doctor within 48 hours of the start of your symptoms, you may be given another type of drug called Amantadine (uh-MAN-tuh-deen) which helps treat certain viruses.

Hospital Care
If your illness gets worse, or if you have other problems (such as diabetes or heart failure), you may need a stay in the hospital. There your care will be similar, but you can be carefully monitored.

Risks

Viral pneumonia lowers your body's immunity, so that other infections can take hold. Without the right care, you could develop a bacterial infection.

WHAT YOU SHOULD DO

- Always take your medicine as directed. If you feel it is not helping, call your doctor. Do not quit taking it on your own.
- If you are taking medicine that makes you drowsy, do not drive or use heavy equipment.
- If you are coughing up sputum and milk seems to make the sputum thicker, do not eat or drink dairy products.
- If you do not have to limit the amount of liquids you drink, drink 8 to 10 (soda-can size) glasses of water each day. This helps thin the sputum so it can be coughed up more easily.
- To help free your lungs of infection, take 2 or 3 deep breaths and then cough. Do this often during the day.
- Use a humidifier to help keep the air moist and your sputum thin. This makes it easier to cough up the sputum. You must keep the humidifier free of fungus. Clean it every day.
- Stay inside during very cold or hot weather, or on days when the air pollution is high. This will make it easier to breathe and will help control your cough.
- Rest at home until you feel better. You may return to work or school when your temperature is around 98.6 degrees F (37 degrees C). Slowly increase your activity. You may feel weak and tired for up to 6 weeks after your illness.
- If you have chest pain, apply a heating pad (set on low) or warm cloths to the sore area for 10 to 20 minutes, 2 to 3 times a day. This may ease the pain, making it easier to breathe.
- Because you have had pneumonia, it may be easier for you to get other lung infections. Try to stay away from people who have colds or the flu. Get shots against flu and pneumonia.
- To help free your lungs of infection, take 2 or 3 deep breaths and then cough. Do this often during the day.
- Quit smoking. It harms the lungs. If you are having trouble quitting, ask your doctor for help.
- Make an appointment for another chest x-ray, if your doctor thinks one is necessary.

Call Your Doctor If . . .

- You have a high temperature
- Your chest pain does not get better in a few days.

- You get nauseated, have vomiting, or develop diarrhea.
- You are coughing up bloody or pink, frothy sputum.
- You have problems, such as a rash, itching, swelling, or stomach pain, that may be caused by any medicine you are taking.
- Another family member shows signs of pneumonia.
- You continue to have fever and chills, and feel worse.

IF YOU'RE HEADING FOR THE HOSPITAL . . .

What to Expect While You're There
You may encounter the following procedures and equipment during your stay.

- **Activity:** At first you will need to rest in bed, with a few pillows to keep you sitting up a little. This will help your breathing. Do not lie flat. Once you are breathing more easily, you will be allowed to increase your exercise.
- **Taking Vital Signs:** These include your temperature, blood pressure, pulse (counting your heartbeats), and respirations (counting your breaths). A stethoscope is used to listen to your heart and lungs. Your blood pressure is taken by wrapping a cuff around your arm.
- **Oxygen:** Your body may need extra oxygen at this time. It is given either by a mask or nasal prongs. Tell your doctor if the oxygen is drying out your nose or if the nasal prongs bother you.
- **Pulse Oximeter:** While you are getting oxygen, you may be hooked up to a pulse oximeter (ox-IM-uh-ter). It is placed on your ear, finger, or toe and is connected to a machine that measures the oxygen in your blood.
- **ECG:** Also called a heart monitor, an electrocardiograph (e-lec-tro-CAR-dee-o-graf), or EKG. The patches on your chest are hooked up to a TV-type screen or a small portable box (telemetry unit). This screen shows a tracing of each heartbeat. Your heart will be watched for signs of injury or damage that could be related to your illness.
- **12 Lead ECG:** This test makes tracings from different parts of your heart. It can help your doctor decide whether there is a heart problem.
- **Chest X-ray:** This picture of your lungs and heart shows how well they are handling your illness.
- **Blood:** Usually taken from a vein in your hand or from the bend in your elbow. Tests will be done on the blood.
- **Blood Gases:** Blood is taken from an artery in your wrist, elbow, or groin. It is tested for the amount of oxygen it contains.
- **IV:** Is a tube placed in your vein for giving medicine or liquids. It will be capped or have tubing connected to it.

After You Leave
Follow the directions listed under "What You Should Do."

Viral Syndrome in Adults

WHAT YOU SHOULD KNOW

When a virus makes you ill, doctors often say you have viral syndrome. There are hundreds of different kinds of viruses. They can cause illnesses such as colds, the flu, shingles, and measles, or just produce a general feeling of not being well.

Causes
Viruses are the smallest of all germs. Many spread easily from person to person.

Signs/Symptoms
Each virus has its own unique symptoms. However, many viruses produce fever, headache, sore muscles, extreme tiredness, and vomiting.

Care
Antibiotics won't cure viral infections. For certain types of viruses, however, your doctor can prescribe medicine that may make the infection less severe.

WHAT YOU SHOULD DO

- You may use aspirin, acetaminophen, or ibuprofen for fever and body aches.
- Rest until your temperature is normal (98.6 degrees F or 37 degrees C). Get plenty of sleep. Your doctor will tell you if you should stay home from work.
- Drink plenty of liquids. Water, clear fruit juices, ginger ale, other sodas, and sports drinks are good choices.
- Warm baths or showers may help relieve body aches.
- Stay away from older people and young children. They can get very sick if they catch your infection.

Call Your Doctor If . . .
- You have a high temperature.
- You have vomiting for more than 24 hours and can't keep liquids down.
- You start having really bad headaches, a stiff neck, trouble breathing, or problems with seeing.

Seek Care Immediately If . . .
• Your temperature is very high.
• You blackout or faint.

Vomiting and Diarrhea in Children

See Stomach Flu in Children

Vomiting in Children

WHAT YOU SHOULD KNOW

Vomiting or "throwing up" is very common in children. There is no immediate cause for concern.

Causes
Often, the child has simply eaten something that does not agree with him or her. The vomiting could also be a sign of infection.

Signs/Symptoms
If your child has an infection such as the flu, the vomiting may be accompanied by fever, stomach or muscle pain, and diarrhea. It should stop in 6 to 24 hours. If the vomiting continues, the child may lose too much water and become dehydrated. This can be a serious problem.

WHAT YOU SHOULD DO

• The child should rest in bed until he or she feels better or there has been no vomiting for 24 hours.
• Let the child's stomach rest for 1 hour after vomiting, then give sips of liquids every 10 to 15 minutes. Gradually increase the amount of liquid you offer.
• Encourage but do not force your child to drink. If vomiting starts again, give the liquids a teaspoonful at a time.
• Give only clear liquids for the first 24 hours. The following liquids are usually well tolerated:
  —Crushed ice.
  —Gelatin water: Add 1 package of instant gelatin to a quart of water. Remember that red gelatin may stain stools and be mistaken for blood.
  —Flat carbonated liquids such as ginger ale or cola. Let the beverage stand at room temperature with the cap off or put a teaspoon of sugar or warm water into the drink to make it flat. Gas in your child's stomach can cause more vomiting.
  —Frozen juices.

—Clear beef broth, chicken broth, or bouillon cubes. If the cubes are spicy, dilute with twice as much water as you would usually use.
—Sports beverages.
• If the child wants food, start with saltine crackers. Do not give milk or solid foods for at least 24 hours.
• After 24 hours, try diluted skim milk, refined rice or cereal, bananas, or applesauce, then work toward a normal diet.
• Do not give your child fresh fruit with peels, raw vegetables, or coarse cereals until recovery is complete.
• Medicines are usually not needed to stop the vomiting, although your doctor may prescribe an antibiotic if the child has a bacterial infection. Do not give your child any medicine without first asking your doctor.

Call Your Doctor If . . .
• Vomiting is not better in 24 hours.

Seek Care Immediately If . . .
• Your child is overly drowsy or confused.
• Your child has sharp or constant abdominal pain, painful or frequent urination, labored breathing, fever that doesn't go away, a high temperature, or a severe cough.

VSD

See Ventricular Septal Defect

Wart Removal

WHAT YOU SHOULD KNOW

A wart is a small, hard, rough lump on your skin. Although you may get a wart anywhere on your body, they are most common on fingers and hands. You may or may not need treatment. Warts can be a long-term problem.

Causes
Warts are caused by a virus called Human Papillomavirus (PAP-ih-LOW-muh-VI-russ), or HPV.

Signs/Symptoms
The wart may be reddish-brown, black, gray, or the same color as your skin. Warts can grow and spread. You may develop a number of them or find only one.

Care
Warts sometimes go away without treatment. You can remove some with over-the-counter medicine. Others may need to be removed by your doctor. The two most common procedures are electrocautery (burning the wart away) and cryotherapy (killing the wart with frost).

Risks
Surgical removal of a wart poses a small risk of infection. Follow your doctor's instructions to prevent this problem.

IF YOU'RE HEADING FOR THE DOCTOR . . .

What to Expect While You're There
- **If electrocautery is planned, be sure to tell the doctor if you wear a pacemaker for your heart**.
- During Your Wart Removal:
  —The wart and the area around it will be cleaned. The doctor may give you numbing medicine so you will feel little pain.
  —In electrocautery, a tool with a thin, needle-like, hot tip will be touched to the wart. The area around the wart may look as though it is "bubbling."
  —In cryotherapy, an extremely cold fluid such as liquid nitrogen will be applied to the wart. You may feel a mild sting and the area may turn white.
  —After the tissue has been killed, your doctor may remove the dead skin and may send a sample to the lab for tests.
  —The doctor may cover the area with a bandage and give you instructions for taking care of the area. You may need another treatment if the wart reappears.
  —The treatment will take from 15 to 30 minutes.

After You Leave . . .
- If there is bleeding during the first 24 hours, press a clean tissue or cloth to the area for 10 minutes.
- Keep the treated area clean with soap and water. You may cover it with a small adhesive bandage to protect it for a few days. If the bandage gets wet, change it promptly.
- After cryotherapy, do not apply any medicine, creams, or lotions to the treated area.
- A scab will form over an area treated with electrocautery. It will drop off by itself, leaving a small scar. Healing time is 2 to 3 weeks. If you receive cryotherapy, a blister will form at the site. Do not pick at the blister or try to break it open. It will break by itself in 10 to 14 days, leaving a scab.

Call Your Doctor If . . .

- You have increasing pain, swelling, redness, or drainage in the treated area.
- The warts don't disappear completely, or more warts appear.
- The blister that forms after cryotherapy becomes large or painful.

Seek Care Immediately If . . .

- You develop a high temperature.

Warts, Genital

See Genital Warts

Warts, Plantar

See Plantar Warts

Whiplash

WHAT YOU SHOULD KNOW

Whiplash is a sprain in the upper part of the spine. It occurs when the neck is whipped forward and back, stretching the muscles and connecting tissue. The problem is known medically as cervical spine strain.

Causes

Neck sprains are usually the result of a car accident or contact sports.

Signs/Symptoms

Possible symptoms include neck pain and stiffness, dizziness, headache, problems swallowing, nausea, and vomiting. The pain may not start right away.

Care

Your doctor is likely to have you wear a cervical (neck) collar for a while to allow the strained muscles to heal.

WHAT YOU SHOULD DO

- Wear your cervical collar until the doctor says you can do without it.
- Your doctor will tell you how active you can be. If your neck hurts a great deal, you may have to take it very easy until the pain lessens, or even rest in bed.
- Apply ice or heat (whichever feels better) to the sore muscles for 15 to 20 minutes each hour for the first 1 to 2 days. You can put ice in a plastic bag and place a towel between the bag of ice and your skin.

For heat, you may use a warm heating pad, whirlpool bath, or warm, moist towels.

• Gentle massage may help your neck.

• You may use over-the-counter medicines such as acetaminophen or ibuprofen to ease the pain. Take them exactly as directed by your doctor.

• Sleeping without a pillow may help relieve the pain. You may also sleep with a cervical pillow (a special pillow you can buy at a medical supply store). You can also try tightly rolling up a small towel (so that the roll is 2 inches thick) and placing it under your neck.

Call Your Doctor If . . .
• Your neck pain is getting worse.

Seek Care Immediately If . . .
• You have pain, numbness, tingling, or weakness of your arms, face, or scalp.
• You have shortness of breath, a hoarse voice, or problems swallowing.
• Your headaches get worse or you have problems seeing.

Whooping Cough

WHAT YOU SHOULD KNOW

Whooping cough, also known as pertussis, is an infection of the air passages and lungs. Thick sputum plugs the air passages, causing severe coughing spells. There is no cure for whooping cough, but antibiotics can help early in the disease.

Causes
Whooping cough is spread in the air from an infected person. It is most serious in infants.

Signs/Symptoms
Whooping cough begins like a cold. Your child could have a runny nose, slight fever, and a cough. These signs do not get better after a few days. The cough gets worse after 10 to 14 days.

During a coughing spell, your child's face or nailbeds may turn red, blue, or white from not getting enough oxygen. When the coughing spell ends and the child takes a breath, it may make a "whooping" noise.

Coughing spells lasting up to a minute may go on for 2 to 10 weeks. Some children vomit after a coughing spell.

Ear infections are common with this illness. Signs of an ear infection are ear tugging, ear pain, and fever. Call your doctor if your child has these signs.

Risks
The risks of serious illness or death from this illness are very small if you follow your doctor's suggestions.

WHAT YOU SHOULD DO

- Try to stay calm and have your child rest as much as possible. Breathing problems and coughing will become worse if the child is crying and afraid.
- Do not let anyone smoke near the child. Smoke can make the breathing problems and coughing worse.
- Your child may need to go into the hospital, where the cough can be treated and breathing can be monitored.
- Whooping cough is no longer common because most children get shots to prevent it. If your child has not had a pertussis (per-TUSS-is) shot and has a cough for more than a few days that is getting worse, you should check with your doctor.

Call Your Doctor If . . .
- Your child has a high temperature.
- The child is tugging his or her ears or has ear pain.
- Vomiting lasts more than a few hours.
- The child is not drinking liquids.
- The cough is getting worse.
- The cough is interfering with the child's sleep and rest.

Seek Care Immediately If . . .
- Call 911 or 0 (operator) for help if your child has any of the following signs: trouble breathing, the skin between the ribs is being sucked-in with each breath, or lips or fingernails are turning blue or white.

IF YOU'RE HEADING FOR THE HOSPITAL . . .

What to Expect While You're There
You may encounter the following procedures and equipment during the child's stay.
- **Visiting:** You may stay with the child to give comfort and support. Your child will feel safer in the hospital with you nearby.

- **Room:** Your child will be kept away from others to avoid spreading the disease. Nurses and others will wear a face mask and gown. This may scare the child.
- **Hand Washing:** Wash your hands after visiting to keep from spreading the infection.
- **Taking Vital Signs:** These include the child's temperature, blood pressure, pulse (counting heartbeats), and respirations (counting breaths). A stethoscope is used to listen to the heart and lungs. Blood pressure is taken by wrapping a cuff around the child's arm.
- **Oxygen:** Your child will probably be put in either a clear plastic mist tent or a high humidity room. This helps make breathing easier. Oxygen may be given using nasal prongs or a face mask.
- **Pulse Oximeter:** Your child may be hooked up to a pulse oximeter (ox-IM-uh-ter). It is placed on the ear, finger, or toe and is connected to a machine that measures the oxygen in the child's blood. There is no pain.
- **Chest X-ray:** This picture of the heart and lungs shows how your child's heart and lungs are handling the illness.
- **IV:** A tube placed in your child's veins for giving medicine or liquids. It will be capped or have tubing connected to it.
- **Blood:** Usually taken from a vein in your child's hand or from the bend in his or her elbow. Tests will be done on the blood.
- **Blood Gases:** Blood is taken from an artery in your child's wrist, elbow, or groin. It is tested for the amount of oxygen in it.
- **ECG:** Also called a heart monitor, an electrocardiograph (e-lec-tro-CAR-dee-o-graf), or EKG. The patches on your child's chest are hooked up to a TV-type screen. This screen shows a tracing of each heartbeat. Your child's heart will be watched for signs of injury or damage that could be related to his or her illness.
- **Medicines:**
  —Your child will get antibiotics in the early part of the disease.
  —Antibiotics may also be used if your child has another infection, such as an ear or lung infection.
  —Cough medicines are not given for whooping cough. They provide no help.
- **Postural Drainage:**
  —Your child may have postural (POS-ture-ul) drainage (PD) to loosen sputum in the lungs every few hours.
  —Keeping the child's head lower than the feet, a nurse will gently tap your child's back. This will not hurt the child.
  —Your child may cough more after this is done.

After You Leave
- Be sure to give the child any medicine prescribed by your doctor.
- Your child could continue to cough for 10 weeks. Do not give cough medicine unless it's suggested by your doctor. Coughing helps keep sputum from clogging the lungs.
- If your child is having a coughing spell:
  —Put the child on his or her tummy in the crib or bed with head to one side. This is a safe position because it will prevent choking if the child vomits. Raise the foot of the crib or bed. This will help drain the lungs. You can also hold the child in a sitting position.
  —Help older children sit up and lean forward during a coughing spell. This makes it easier to cough and bring up sputum from the lungs.
- Use a cool mist humidifier in the child's room. Place it out of reach by the bed. Fill it with cool water. Direct the mist stream towards the child's face. Using the humidifier will help loosen the sputum in the child's throat.
- Your child needs rest and plenty of liquids. Feed him or her about six small meals daily. Small meals may help prevent vomiting after a coughing spell. Wait a short while before giving the child food after a coughing spell.
- Your doctor will tell you when to send your child back to school.

Wife Beating

See Domestic Violence

Withdrawal, Alcohol

See Alcohol Abuse

Withdrawal, Barbiturates

See Barbiturate Abuse

Withdrawal, Cocaine

See Cocaine Abuse

Withdrawal, Narcotics

See Narcotic Abuse

Withdrawal, Tranquilizers

See Benzodiazepine Abuse

Wound, Puncture

See Puncture Wound

Wound Care

WHAT YOU SHOULD KNOW

Any tear, scrape, or cut in the skin is considered a wound. There are many types. Abrasions are wounds in which the outer layer of the skin has been rubbed or scraped off. Lacerations are cuts through the skin. Puncture wounds are cuts made by round, sharp objects such as needles or nails. Most wounds take 2 to 6 weeks to heal.

Signs/Symptoms
Pain, bleeding, bruising, and swelling are all to be expected.

Care
If the wound is large, deep, or won't stop bleeding, you may need to have it closed with stitches (sutures) to speed healing and to keep it from getting infected. Using stitches also reduces the amount of scarring. You may need a tetanus shot if you have not had one in the past 5 to 10 years.

WHAT YOU SHOULD DO

- Keep the wound and bandage clean and dry. If the bandage gets wet and you need to change it, unwrap it slowly and carefully. If it sticks and starts to hurt, use water to loosen it gently. Pat the area dry with a clean towel before putting on another bandage.
- If possible, keep the wound lifted above the level of your heart for 24 to 48 hours. This will help ease pain and swelling and help healing.
- Leave the dressing on for several days.
- Clean the wound gently 3 to 4 times a day:
  - Flush the wound thoroughly with clean water. Wash the area around the wound with soap and water or a cotton tipped swab dipped in a mixture of half water and half hydrogen peroxide.
  - If you have a mouth or lip wound, rinse your mouth after meals and at bedtime. Ask your doctor what mixture to use. Do NOT swallow the mixture.
  - If you have a puncture wound, soak it briefly 3 to 4 times a day.
- If you have a scalp wound, you may wash your hair gently after you get home. Then keep your hair dry until the day you are to have your stitches removed, when you may wash it gently again.

- Do not go swimming or soak the wound for long periods.
- If the wound has stitches, your doctor will tell you when to return to have them taken out.
- If you have been given a tetanus shot, your arm may get swollen, red, and warm to the touch at the shot site. This is a normal reaction to the medicine in the shot.

Call Your Doctor If . . .
- Bleeding in the wound area is getting worse.
- You develop a high temperature.
- You have any signs of infection (increasing pain or soreness, swelling, redness, pus, a bad smell, or red streaks coming from the injured site).
- You have numbness or swelling below the wound.
- You cannot move the joint below the wound.

Wrist Injury

WHAT YOU SHOULD KNOW

A wrist injury can involve either a sprain or a strain. Sprains result from suddenly stretching or tearing the ligaments that hold the bones together. A strain is an injury to the muscles or the tendons that connect the muscles to the bones. In most cases, either type of injury will take about 6 to 8 weeks to heal.

Causes
Sprains are usually caused by an accident. Strains usually result from over-use.

Signs/Symptoms
Typically, there will be pain, tenderness, swelling, or bruising of the injured wrist. If the injury is serious, you may have trouble moving the wrist.

Care
You'll probably need to wear a splint or ace bandage to keep the wrist from moving. The doctor may take an x-ray of the wrist; and if you also injured the skin, you may need a tetanus shot.

WHAT YOU SHOULD DO

- Put ice on the injury for 15 to 20 minutes each hour for the first 1 to 2 days. Place the ice in a plastic bag and place a towel between the bag of ice and your skin.

- After the first 1 to 2 days, you may put heat on the injury to help ease the pain. You may use a heating pad (set on low), a whirlpool bath, or warm, moist towels for 15 to 20 minutes every hour. Do this for 48 hours.
- For 48 hours, keep your arm lifted above the level of your heart whenever possible to reduce the pain and swelling.
- Wear your splint until you see a doctor for a follow-up visit. If your fingers get numb or tingly, you may need to loosen your splint. If you do not know how to do this, call your doctor immediately for instructions.
- You may take over-the-counter medications to relieve the pain. If the doctor prescribes any medicine, take it exactly as directed. If it makes you drowsy, don't drive.
- If you have been given a tetanus shot, your arm may get swollen, red, and warm to the touch at the shot site. This is a normal reaction to the medicine.

Call Your Doctor If . . .
- If the pain or swelling grows worse.
- The fingers below the injury are colder than those on your other hand.

Seek Care Immediately If . . .
- The fingers below the injured wrist are swollen and very red.
- The fingers are swollen, turn white or blue, and feel cool.
- The fingers are numb or tingling.

Wrist Sprain or Strain

See Wrist Injury

Wryneck

See Torticollis

Yeast Infection

See Candidiasis

Zygomatic Fracture

See Facial Fracture

Signs and Symptoms Index

Index

The PDR® Family Guide to Over-the-Counter Drugs™

For the first time, the most trusted name in medical publishing, Physicians' Desk Reference®, has produced a comprehensive, authoritative, and reliable consumer guide to over-the-counter drugs. Its features include

- The uses, active ingredients, proper dosages, and side effects of each medication

- Handy comparison tables to help you select the best product for each ailment

- Symptoms of vitamin deficiency—and the signs of overdose

- Special cautions for seniors, expectant mothers, and infants

- And much more!

Published by Ballantine Books.
Available wherever books are sold.